Implausible Professions

arguments for pluralism and autonomy in psychotherapy and counselling

extended second edition

edited by
Richard House
and
Nick Totton

PCCS BOOKS

First edition published 1997
This edition published in 2011 by PCCS Books, Ross-on-Wye HR9 5LA

Reprinted 2015
PCCS Books Ltd, Wyastone Business Park, Wyastone Leys, Monmouth NP25 3SR

Tel +44 (0)1600 891 509
contact@pccs-books.co.uk
www.pccs-books.co.uk

Implausible Professions: Arguments for pluralism and autonomy in psychotherapy and counselling (extended 2nd edition)

ISBN 978 1 906254 33 9

Cover designed by Denis Postle – Printed by Lightning Source

Acknowledgements
The following chapters have appeared previously; we are grateful to editors and publishers for permission to reproduce them.
Colin Feltham, 'Challenging the core theoretical model', in *Counselling*, 8 (2), 1997.
John Heron, 'The politics of transference', in *Self and Society*, 20 (1), 1992.
Richard House, 'The dynamics of counselling research' (as 'The dynamics of professionalisation: a personal view of counselling research') in *Counselling*, 8 (3), 1997.
Richard House, '"Audit-mindedness" in counselling: some underlying dynamics', in *British Journal of Guidance and Counselling*, 24 (2), 1996.
Richard House, 'Training: a guarantee of competence?' is an abridged version of 'The professionalisation of counselling: a coherent "case against"?', *Counselling Psychology Quarterly*, 9 (4), 1996.
Peter Lomas, 'The teaching of psychotherapy', in *Personal Disorder and the Family*, Transaction Press, 1997.
Katharine Mair, 'The myth of therapist expertise' is an abridged version of her chapter of the same name in *Psychotherapy and its Discontents*, W Dryden and C Feltham (eds), published by Open University Press, Milton Keynes, 1992.
Richard Mowbray, 'Too vulnerable to choose?' is a modified version of Chapter 17 from his *The Case Against Psychotherapy Registration: A Conservation Issue for the Human Potential Movement*, published by Trans Marginal Press, London, 1995.
David Smail, 'Psychotherapy and tragedy', was first presented at a memorial conference for Richard Marshall in 1996; an earlier version appeared in the Newsletter of the British Psychological Society Psychotherapy Section.
Brian Thorne, 'The accountable psychotherapist' was first presented to the Annual Meeting of the Ashby Trust, 1991; an earlier version appeared in *Self and Society*, 23 (4), 1995.
David Wasdell, 'In the shadow of accreditation', in *Self and Society*, 18 (1), 1990.

Contents

Dedication

We wish to dedicate this book to one of the contributors to the first edition, the late psychotherapist, trainer and celebrated writer, **Peter Lomas**, 1923–2010 – highly esteemed and much-missed advocate of independent thinking, pluralism and autonomy in the fields of psychotherapy and counselling.

Introduction to the Second Edition

Nick Totton

After publication day, authors and editors frequently experience a sense of anti-climax. Instead of the intended splash, the waters seem to have closed silently over one's book, and nothing more is heard except for perhaps a couple of polite reviews. It is easy to wonder whether it was worth it – whether the book made a blind bit of difference.

This was emphatically not the case with *Implausible Professions*! Not only was the book repeatedly and positively reviewed; much more importantly, it was noticed by and had an effect on many, many people. It is fair to say that its publication in 1997 changed the terms of the debate on psychotherapy and counselling (mainly referred to hereafter as 'therapy'): by giving a voice to what had previously been relatively unarticulated arguments against the direction in which we were being taken, *Implausible Professions* created a permanent shift in the centre of gravity for therapy in the UK. Without this book, of course (in conjunction with Richard Mowbray's *The Case Against Psychotherapy Regulation* [1995]), something else would no doubt have happened to create that shift: the time was right, and we happened to be able to seize, or be seized by, the moment. What is important is that the shift *did* happen, and certainly contributed to holding back the drive towards state regulation for a good deal longer than many people expected at the time, as well as validating the ways in which many practitioners had long been working, but which were starting to be thrown into question by the tabulators and regulators.

It can only be an enormous pleasure to write an introduction to this second edition. The need for one confirms the value of the original book, and confirms that the passage of time has not made it irrelevant, that the case it makes for pluralism and autonomy in psychotherapy and counselling is still of importance. What slightly tarnishes this pleasure, of course, is exactly the same thing: that the case is not yet accepted across the field, that there are still those who argue for yet more standardisation and control – the measure of this being that state regulation of psychotherapy and counselling has continued to be proposed, and now seems likely to become a reality.

A great deal has changed in the last 14 years in relation to therapy regulation. This book was originally conceived as a counterbalance to the positions taken by the UK Council for Psychotherapy (UKCP), the British Association for Counselling and Psychotherapy (BACP) and the British Council for Psychotherapy (BCP), who were at that point the main or only proponents of state or statutory regulation. Now, in 2011, it is the government, and its designated agency the Health Professions Council (HPC), who propose regulation, and while BCP are still its enthusiastic supporters, UKCP at least – since the election to its chair of Andrew Samuels, a contributor to this volume – has shifted its position to one of wary scepticism about statutory regulation, together with a commitment to the continuing accreditation of those who choose not to register with HPC.

State regulation has come a great deal closer, but it has not yet arrived. I still believe that in the end it may not arrive, and if it does, in any onerous form, there are likely to be large numbers if practitioners who refuse to engage with it, which will mean that they have to relinquish their existing titles of 'counsellor' and 'psychotherapist' and choose new ones. This will lead to a massive reordering of the field, and, I hope, a reaffirmation of what I see as its true values, those laid out in the pages of this book. It may be time for a parting of the ways between practitioners invested in the speedy alleviation of symptoms and the return of their clients to the workforce, and practitioners committed to a long-term and open-ended exploration of their clients' processes. There is plenty of room for both, and indeed for other approaches to therapy as well – that is what pluralism means, but pluralism also means acknowledging real differences.

Perhaps the most useful thing to do in this new introduction is to explore what seem to be the biggest current issues around pluralism and autonomy. A great deal of thinking and debate about these themes has gone on in the 14 years since the first edition appeared; and while the content of the book is still sound, some aspects have emerged during that time which are either new, or more important than they seemed then. Among these are:

- the negative role of the NHS
- the pernicious state of much of the voluntary sector

- the widespread inadequacy of existing self-regulation
- the identification of two different activities operating under the same label of 'therapy'

I shall briefly explore each of these in turn.

Therapy and the NHS

It has become much clearer in the intervening years that the NHS is a reactionary force in relation to psychotherapy and counselling. In retrospect, in fact, we made a very bad decision when we chose to bring therapy within the NHS. Of course, this decision was not on the whole conducted consciously and strategically, and to the extent that it was, the motives were by and large positive – to increase the availability of psychotherapy or counselling which was free at the point of use, and also culturally accessible, in GPs' premises, in a way that it would not be in ordinary consulting rooms.

The motives were positive (though not entirely altruistic: they were also bound up with a search for more jobs for practitioners), but the negative results have outweighed the benefits by a fair proportion. Negative for the *clients*, in that most of the work offered on the NHS has been pared down to a time-limited, outcome-focused, defensively structured version of therapy, where the client generally has no choice of either practitioner or modality; we can confidently expect this situation to become progressively worse with the spread of the misnamed Improving Access to Psychological Therapies Programme (IAPT). Negative for the *practitioner*, because even the most skilled and well-intentioned are being steadily straitjacketed into this impoverished way of working; because pay and conditions are generally very unsatisfactory; and, above all, because the identification of therapy and counselling as medical practices, together with the need and desire of the NHS to regulate its employees, has provided the seedbed for state regulation.

In hindsight, therapy has been considerably damaged by its involvement with the NHS. The cause of offering therapy free at the point of use could have been far better served in one of two ways: either by creating practical support and cultural encouragement for therapists to offer and advertise one or two free sessions as part of their caseload, or by campaigning for the creation of a National Psychological Service, parallel to but separate from the NHS, run by practitioners with a far deeper understanding of what therapy can and cannot do.

Therapy and the voluntary sector

The biggest gap in the first edition was probably the lack of attention paid to the voluntary sector, which at that point was only beginning to grow into the monster it has since become. The provision of therapy in the UK is the complete reverse of what common sense would expect: the most complex and challenging clients are frequently seen by the least skilled and experienced practitioners, some of them not even having completed their training, while the most skilled and experienced often work largely with 'normal neurotics'.

This grotesque situation has come about through the lack of both public and private funding for community-based therapy and counselling. What funding there is is largely restricted to start-up money: bizarrely, you can (sometimes) get funds to start a service, but not to run it, and certainly not to pay practitioners. This has dovetailed neatly with the large numbers of trainees and newly graduated therapists desperate for 'hours' to complete their qualification. This generally very keen but not necessarily highly competent group is forced to work without payment with often very difficult material, and usually without the sort of supervision they need (quite often with no more than line management). Can this exploitative forced labour be the best way to meet the needs of distressed people?

Self-regulation

At the same time it has also become much clearer that some traditional aspects of how therapy is organised are not satisfactory. Specifically, procedures for handling conflicts between practitioner and client are generally inadequate. Conventionally there has often been an element of the gentlemen's club about the hearing of complaints: practitioners have been 'investigated' by peers who often know them well, or at any rate are members of the same organisation, and not unlikely to bring to the situation a presumption of competence and ethical behaviour. Even more culpably, there has sometimes been a sense that even when misconduct is glaringly apparent, it should be hushed up for the sake of the organisation or the profession.

None of this will do' and it must be admitted that the push for professionalisation and regulation has brought a lot of these problems out into the open – as part of a wider social trend towards transparency about abusive behaviour. The trouble is that the alternative models proposed for dealing with complaints – for example the Health Professions Council's fitness to practice hearings – are quite unsuited for the job of exploring conflicts between client and therapist. Their exclusive focus on identifying malpractice and protecting the public forgets the primary goal of existing complaints procedures: meeting hurt and angry clients' need for acknowledgement and reparation. As well as the public in *general*, complaints procedures need to look after *particular* members of the public who feel mistreated, and, of course, to look after the practitioners who may have made a mistake.

What hurt clients very often want is an apology. The 'fitness to practice' type of structure more or less guarantees that they won't get it – because in an adversarial system, such an 'admission of guilt' would be highly unwise. Contrariwise, practitioners will be handicapped in explaining themselves by their ethical unwillingness to dissect a client's emotional problems in a court-like environment.

The biggest difficulty, though, is that approaches to complaints based on 'common sense' are unlikely to meet the needs of therapy, which is generally not so based. It is not wholly through incompetence or self-interest that we have been struggling with issues of accountability for so long: there are several aspects of what we do – its profound confidentiality, its emotional intensity, the role of transference and counter-transference – which make it extremely hard to shine a light on what has gone wrong in any particular situation. One could conclude from this that therapy, as traditionally practised, is a bad thing; but if we believe it to be helpful, then we need to be clear that making therapists conform to everyday common-sense rules effectively means proscribing therapy.

Two sorts of therapy

The tension between the requirements of the public and voluntary sectors (and of insurance companies) and the historical nature of psychotherapy and counselling has created stresses which seem likely to result in the sheering away from each other of two quite different ways of working. Subpopulations of therapists who inhabit different work environments are adapting to those environments, and developing two quite distinct activities, both valid and valuable in their own context, and both unfortunately going by the same name of 'therapy'. By identifying these two different groups we might be able to avoid a lot of the bickering and name-calling which plague the field, and ultimately to agree on peaceful coexistence, each in our own ecological niche.

I have argued elsewhere (e.g. Totton, 2004) that these two approaches can best be seen as the 'expert systems' approach and the 'local knowledge' approach. The more recent arrival on the scene, expert systems therapy, has evolved in an environment that demands expertise, demonstrated partly through qualifications and partly through quantified research into outcomes and effectiveness; an environment where both clients and purchasers are demanding maximum amelioration of distress in minimum time. Hence the appropriate users are people who don't prioritise self-knowledge and psychological exploration – individuals with other, equally valid focuses to their lives, who simply want to be able to get on with things. Expert systems therapy, therefore, is a lean, mean evolutionary machine, which avoids detours and distractions, and privileges symptom removal over the uncovering of meaning. Its practitioners are often enormously skilful at what they do, by virtue of their tight and creative focus on effective technique.

Local knowledge therapy has evolved in a very different world, one in which clients – usually self-financing – have chosen to seek, alongside and even sometimes in preference to symptom removal, *understanding* of their symptoms and experiences, placing them within the wider context of their life as a whole, their family and social networks, the entire social and cultural framework, and indeed human existence in general. The name 'local knowledge', borrowed from sociology and anthropology, refers to a reliance on intuition and wisdom in preference to technique and research: an emphasis on *self*-knowledge for both practitioner and client.

Expert systems therapy operates at a point of convergence between clients who often want to avoid dependence on their therapist and return as fast as possible to a state of ordinary functioning, and service providers who need quick and cost-effective ways of restoring their users as fast as possible to a state of ordinary functioning. No one in this context is in a position to question what exactly 'ordinary functioning' implies. Local knowledge therapy, however, by virtue of its privileged situation, can ask these sorts of questions; for example, it can use the values and understandings of therapy as a measure against which ideas of 'ordinary functioning', and other social norms and standards, can be critiqued.

This way of working is authentic and important, but very different from the function of expert systems therapy, which is explicitly to *help* people deal with the *effects* of the way in which we live – or of their brain chemistries, or poor strategic choices, depending on which paradigm one uses. It employs a considerable array of techniques to help clients manage their distress, ideally to such an extent that they no longer experience it and are able to operate successfully according to their own conscious preferences.

This is clearly an important, respectable and comprehensible goal. The goal of local knowledge therapy is much harder to articulate, which is perhaps one reason why the situation has become so confused. This way of working is not actually about helping at all; or rather, paradoxically, it knows that in order to be *helpful* it has to avoid as far as possible actually *helping*. This is linked to the widely acknowledged paradoxical theory of change (Beisser, 1970): that a person is able to change once they have accepted themselves as they are.

Such paradoxes are central to the sorts of therapy celebrated in this volume, and many of them are explored in the chapters that follow. We are proud to have facilitated the publication of a book which stands up clearly for the strangeness, variousness and valuableness of therapy, and proud of its effect on the debates in which it intervened. Our thanks again to all the authors, and to Pete and Maggie of PCCS Books.

References

Beisser, A. (1970) 'The paradoxical theory of change', in J Fagan and I Shepherd (eds) *Gestalt Therapy Now: Theory, Techniques, and Applications* (pp. 77–80). Palo Alto, CA: Science and Behavior Books.

Mowbray, R. (1995) *The Case Against Psychotherapy Regulation: A Conservation Issue for the Human Potential Movement*. London: Trans Marginal Press.

Totton, N. (2004) 'Two ways of being helpful', *CPJ,* 15 (10): 5–8.

Introduction to the First Edition

> This profession, which is not one, cannot even be named.
> (Andrew Samuels)

The project of this book originated as one of **opposition**; but it has developed first into one of **refoundation**, and then into one of **innovation**.

Opposition

What we initially wished to oppose can be summarised as the 'professionalisation' of psychotherapy and counselling in Britain: a process which has often been presented as a natural and evolutionary one, but which – like so many supposedly 'natural' human events – is in fact a thoroughly deliberate strategy, operating on two levels, institutional and cultural. The institutional strategy is expressed in the creation of three organisations, the UK Council for Psychotherapy (UKCP), the British Association for Counselling (BAC), and the British Confederation of Psychotherapists (BCP). In their different ways, and with various degrees of co-operation and rivalry, these organisations all promulgate the idea that psychotherapy is a profession; that this profession needs regulation; and that they are the people to do it – preferably with the help of government.

In our view, and that of many other practitioners and supporters, this would be a disaster. The reasons for this view are laid out at length in several of the chapters which follow. By now, it seems fairly clear that these organisations will not succeed in their goal of regulation and control, at least not fully. The government is not interested in backing them: at a BCP-promoted conference on 'Regulation of Psychotherapy in Europe', held in London on 7th June 1997, Anne Richardson, a Senior Policy Advisor for the Department of Health, made it clear that psychotherapy and counselling will not come under statutory regulation. She pointed out that 'there is no agreement here in the UK, or it would appear in Europe, about what exactly does or should constitute the activity of psychotherapists.' Ms Richardson went on:

> There are no plans to regulate what, after all, we have to call an activity, rather than a *title*. I mean psychotherapy is something that people do. It's something doctors, psychologists, nurses, social workers, lay psychotherapists, do. Lots of different people practise this activity. Many – most – some with training, some without training, with different kinds of training. Psychotherapy is an activity, not a job title. It's important to say it would be extremely difficult to regulate by statute something which is an activity like that. Could you imagine trying to write a law? It would be impossible. Another thing that militates against [statutory regulation] is the increasing evidence of the effectiveness of a variety of approaches which some people wouldn't call psychotherapy. Some sorts of stress management – you might not call it psychotherapy – some forms of psycho-educational approaches you might not call psychotherapy but others would and do. And there is good evidence for the effectiveness of some of these approaches with mental illness groups. So if you were to regulate or legislate, you might stop that, prevent that diversity and that would be unwelcome.
>
> (Richardson, 1997)

The institutional strategy for professionalisation is left in tatters. However, this institutional strategy has always depended upon a cultural strategy which is, if anything, more dangerous still. If a strong enough climate of opinion can be created to the effect that psychotherapy and counselling *are* professions like law or medicine – which is what the Department of Health has, it seems, rightly decided not to be the case – and that practitioners require the sort of accreditation, standardised training and presence on a register which organisations like UKCP are promoting, then practitioners who do not agree and do not conform will steadily be forced out of business. Even more importantly, valuable and effective styles of work will no longer be available to clients who might otherwise choose them – in the same way that the monopoly of allopathic medicine forced practices like homeopathy and herbalism into the shadows.

Richard Mowbray's crucial book *The Case Against Psychotherapy Registration: A Conservation Issue for the Human Potential Movement* (Mowbray, 1995) in our view comprehensively demolishes the arguments put forward for statutory registration. We commend it to any interested reader of this book. We believe that it strips all intellectual credibility from the institutional strategy of registration. What we initially wanted to do in this book was to extend the demolition programme to the whole issue of professionalisation: to present work which argues equally strongly that the 'professionalisation' model in no way suits the undertaking of psychotherapy and counselling (however much it may suit the training organisations who would benefit from their collective monopoly).

If it is true, as many people argue in different ways, that psychotherapy is ineligible as a profession because there is no general agreement about what psychotherapists do, then there are many possible ways to understand this situation. One can describe it, like Edward Erwin, as 'a state of disarray' (Erwin, 1997: 2); and, like Emmy van Deurzen, argue that 'we have to transform what used to be a craft or an art based on moral or religious principles into a scientifically based accountable professional expertise' (Deurzen, 1996: 17). One can even pretend that this has already been achieved, like the European Association for Psychotherapy, who make the wild claim that 'psychotherapy is an independent scientific discipline ... training in psychotherapy takes place at an advanced, qualified and scientific level' (EAP, 1997).

A third and, we believe, rather more productive response to the situation is a *pluralistic* one, which recognises and embraces the reality that psychotherapy and counselling are not, and in principle never can be, scientific disciplines with a reliable, replicable, predictable and generally agreed body of expert knowledge (though, of course, *some forms* of psychotherapy conceivably might be; but this would not privilege them over other forms). There is ample evidence and argument to support this both in what follows and elsewhere (e.g. Christensen and Jacobson, 1994; Shepherd and Sartorius, 1989).

Refoundation

Several chapters of this book do in fact make those arguments. Very quickly, though, it became apparent that we wanted and needed to do something more: to re-establish some values which have always been at the centre of our craft, ever since Freud wrote:

> Let us allow patients themselves to discover that it is damaging for

> them to look for mental assistance to people who have not learnt how to give it. If we explain this to them and warn them against it, we have spared ourselves the need to forbid it. On the main roads of Italy, the pylons that carry high-tension cables bear the brief and impressive inscription: *Chi tocca, muore* [Who touches, will die]. This is perfectly calculated to regulate the behaviour of passers-by to any wires that may be hanging down.
>
> (Freud, 1926: 154)

This way of understanding – that therapy is a matter for self-regulation, not compulsion – operates right across the field of psychotherapy and counselling. We see it just as clearly, for example, in Carl Rogers, a towering figure in humanistic psychotherapy and inventor of the term 'counselling' (because of his own ineligibility to be a psychotherapist – Spinelli, 1996: 55), who wrote in 1973 that:

> I have slowly come to the conclusion that if we did away with 'the expert', 'the certified professional', 'the licensed psychologist', we might open our profession to a breeze of fresh air, a surge of creativity, such as has not been known for years. In every area – medicine, nursing, teaching, bricklaying, or carpentry – certification has tended to freeze and narrow the profession, has tied it to the past, has discouraged innovation. ... The question I am humbly raising, in the face of what I am sure will be great shock and antagonism, is simply this: Can psychology find a new and better way?
>
> (Rogers, 1973)[1]

And shortly before his death, Carl Jung, another of the great founding figures, wrote in a letter:

> In medicine every conceivable method can be employed without one's being affected by it in any way. This is not possible in psychology, where everything depends on the dialectical process between two personalities. Holding lectures, giving instruction, pumping in knowledge, all these current university procedures are no use at all here. ... Under these circumstances any organisation that proposes collective methods seems to me unsuitable, because it would be sawing off the branch on which the psychotherapist sits.
>
> (Adler, 1976: 534)

Wilhelm Reich, another great pioneer, wrote of the 'professionalisation' process in psychoanalysis:

> Slowly but surely [it] was cleansed of all Freud's achievements. Bringing psychoanalysis into line with the world, which shortly before had threatened to annihilate it, took place inconspicuously at first. … *Form eclipsed content; the organisation became more important than its task.*
>
> (Reich, 1942/1973: 125, emphasis added)

It is also worth quoting a less well-known figure, Robert Knight, in his 1952 Presidential Address to the American Psychoanalytic Association:

> In the 1920s and early 1930s … many analysts were trained who might today be rejected. Many training analyses were relatively short, and many gifted individuals with definite neuroses or character disorders were trained. … In contrast, perhaps the majority of students of the past decade or so have been 'normal' characters, or perhaps one should say had 'normal character disorders'. They are not introspective, are inclined to read only the literature that is assigned in institute courses, and wish to get through with the training requirements as rapidly as possible.
>
> (Knight, 1953)

This can certainly be applied to the present day, and to other forms of psychotherapy besides psychoanalysis. It is the 'normalisation' of psychotherapy and counselling which we aim to throw into question, returning to the clear perception of many of its founders that what they had created was 'wild', extraordinary, and unsuitable for domestication.

Innovation

The third stage in the development of our project was to see that this *re*-foundation of psychotherapy and counselling also implies a *new* foundation. There are implications still to be fully developed in what we do as practitioners, and what we have discovered in doing it; and perhaps in many ways the most important chapters here are those which take up these implications and present them as new contributions to both theory and practice.

These are the ways of thinking and organising which we have called in our subtitle 'pluralism and autonomy'. Many other terms are relevant here – 'self-regulation', 'horizontal organisation', 'networking', even 'mutual aid'. From some points of view these are 'new paradigm' concepts; from other points of view they have a long and healthy tradition of their own. What *is* new, we feel, is the argument that there is an *inherent relationship* between psychotherapy and counselling on the one hand, and pluralism and autonomy on the other.

For a working definition of 'pluralism', we can look to Andrew Samuels' important chapter (IV.1: 223), where he writes:

> Pluralism is an attitude to conflict which tries to reconcile differences without imposing a false resolution on them or losing sight of the unique value of each position. Hence, pluralism is not the same as 'multiplicity' or 'diversity'. Rather, pluralism is an attempt to hold unity and diversity in balance... [T]he trademark of pluralism is competition and its way of life is bargaining.

'Autonomy', we could say, is the other side of pluralism: it follows from Samuels' definition that pluralism is incompatible with any kind of compulsion or coercion. We can look at this from the right or from the left, so to speak – free market or civil liberty, competition or co-operation: it is not a political position in the narrow sense, but it is a position in relation to *power* (see Chapter II.5). Another important term here is Wilhelm Reich's 'self-regulation', which carries with it something from child rearing, something from ecology: the sense that balance and health, if things are left alone, *will happen of their own accord.*

A number of the contributions which follow argue and demonstrate, from many different points of view, why this sort of position can be seen to flow naturally from our craft as psychotherapists and counsellors, and why the top-down, conformist, coercive model used by UKCP in particular is incompatible with the best values of our craft. This includes material which lays out the *personal* damage caused by coercive accreditation models. Other pieces – or sometimes the same ones – try to spell out what an alternative might be: how *else* practitioners could organise, in a way which meets the need for accountability while also honouring the nature and meaning of what it is we do.

The great positive contribution of the professionalisation debate is that it has brought into awareness, in however obfuscated a form, the real need for greater accountability on the part of what Denis Postle calls 'psycho-practitioners'. There is very little argument about this (though see Richard Mowbray's two chapters, this volume). What many of our contributors *do* argue with is the model of accountability being offered by UKCP, BAC and BCP: an essentially legalistic, after-the-horse-has-bolted model which focuses on establishing 'guilt' or 'innocence' in relation to a rigid code laid down in advance. We have seen over many years how limited the effectiveness of such a model is in relation to lawyers, say, or doctors; how little real satisfaction it produces for any of the parties involved. We want and need something better – an ongoing, flexible, personal, problem-solving model for monitoring and conflict-resolution. Several of the chapters in our final section make suggestions towards such a model.

Contents

The sections into which we have organised the book are, as so often, somewhat arbitrary. Several pieces really 'belong' in more than one section. What we have tried to do is to offer some sort of progression, not so much historical as logical – starting out with work (some of it several years old) which outlines the destructive and distorting effects of 'professionalisation' and coercive accreditation; going on to work which challenges the arguments on which these approaches are founded; and then to material which tries in various ways to move from one model to another, 'from professionalisation to pluralism'. Our fourth section includes three substantial pieces, by three very well-known figures, and another piece about the now half-forgotten work of an important pioneer, which lay down conceptual bases for a new and radical approach; while the final section shows some of the ways in which these concepts can be, and are being, put into practice.

Although there is some very important material here from the psychodynamic tradition, the great majority of the chapters that follow come from the humanistic psychotherapy and counselling world. We don't feel that this particularly reflects a balance of opinion; it is probably more that psychodynamic and analytic practitioners are less willing to take a public stand. It is worth mentioning, though, that we had been going to include an excellent and hard-hitting article by Chris Oakley entitled 'Psychoanalysis: a rendezvous with disappointment' (Oakley and Oakley,

1994) which the author withdrew because he has become convinced that '*no* regulation, not even self regulation' is appropriate for psychotherapy (personal communication). Which goes to show that however radical this book may be, there is always someone more radical …

Getting published

Richard Mowbray's crucial book *The Case Against Psychotherapy Registration*, which we mentioned earlier, is self-published. We decided that it would be easier, and make this book more accessible, to approach a commercial publisher. Nearly two years later we began to think that Mowbray had been right! We offered the book to every major publisher we could find with a serious psychotherapy and counselling list. Many were encouraging; none were prepared to publish. Most of them said, as publishers do, that it 'didn't fit their list'. Maybe they were all sincere; but we did start to wonder what 'fitting their list' really meant, when an editor for one of the leading firms in the field wrote:

> I am sure your book will be an interesting and thought-provoking collection. I'm afraid, though, that _____ would not be able to pursue the idea to publication. We … have close links with the UKCP, the BAC and other regulatory bodies who are co-publishing or planning to co-publish with us and it would not therefore be appropriate for us to take on this title.

So much for pluralism. Another large publisher was very enthusiastic, but rejected the book after a negative response from readers – one of whom, we could tell from internal evidence in their report, is a leading light in UKCP! A third publisher was initially keen but finally told us that they had been 'advised not to publish'.

Thanks

We have all the more reason, then, to thank Maggie and Pete of PCCS Books for their enthusiasm and integrity in publishing *Implausible Professions* – as well as for the supportive, co-operative and empowering way in which they have done so. We also want to thank the many people who have encouraged and helped us at every stage of the process; and our contributors for their patience, open-mindedness, and hard work; and to thank, and honour, the series of initiatives which laid the ground for this book: articles in the humanistic journal *Self and Society* (Brown and Mowbray, 1990; Kalisch, 1990, 1992; Heron, I.1, this volume; Postle and Anderson, 1990; House and Hall, 1991; Totton, 1992; Wasdell, I.2, this volume); the two Cambridge 'Dynamics of Accreditation' conferences in the early 1990s (Cannon and Hatfield, 1992; House, 1992; Cannon and Hatfield, III.5, this volume); the Norwich Group Process Group led by Robin Shohet (House and Hall, 1991); the founding of the Independent Practitioners Network in 1994 (Totton, V.3, this volume); and the publication of Richard Mowbray's *The Case Against Psychotherapy Registration* in 1995.

Above all, we would like to thank each other. We are two strong-willed individuals with often very different views about both style and content. The fact that we have successfully produced this book is in itself a strong argument for pluralism as a creative process!

We have been involved in the fight against professionalisation for several years now. Recently, we have had a strong sense that the tide has changed. There are still many problems; but now, rather than fighting *against* – always a dispiriting activity – we feel we are fighting *for* something: for the values and organisational styles outlined in this book. We hope that they will also be of value to you.

References

Adler, G. (ed.) (1976) *C. G. Jung Letters, Vol. 2, 1951–61*, London: Routledge & Kegan Paul.

Brown, J. and Mowbray, R. (1990) 'Whither the human potential movement?', *Self and Society*, 18 (4): 32–5.

Cannon, C. and Hatfield, S. (1992) 'Some thoughts after the 2nd National Conference on the Dynamics of Accreditation, Cambridge, June 1992', *Self and Society*, 20 (4): 28–34.

Christensen, A. and Jacobson, N. (1994) 'Who (or what) can do psychotherapy; the status and challenge of non-professional therapies', *Psychological Science,* 5: 8–14.

Erwin, E. (1997) *Philosophy and Psychotherapy: Razing the Troubles of the Brain,* London: Sage.

European Association for Psychotherapy (1997) 'Strasbourg Declaration', *International Journal of Psychotherapy*, 2 (1).

Deurzen-Smith, E., van (1996) 'The future of psychotherapy in Europe', *International Journal of Psychotherapy*, 1 (1): 15–21.
Freud, S. (1926) 'The question of lay analysis', in *Two Short Accounts of Psycho-Analysis*, Harmondsworth: Penguin, 1962.
Heron, J. (1990) 'The politics of transference', *Self and Society*, 18 (1): 17–23, reprinted as Chapter I.1, this volume.
House, R. (1992) 'A tale of two conferences: organisational form and accreditation ethos', *Self and Society*, 20 (4): 35–7.
House, R. and Hall, J. (1991) 'Peer accreditati on … – within a humanistic framework?', *Self and Society*, 19 (2): 33–6.
Kalisch, D. (1990) 'Professionalisation: a rebel view', *Self and Society*, 18 (1): 24–9.
Kalisch, D. (1992) 'The living tradition and the division of the spoils: professionalisation again', *Self and Society*, 20 (4): 36–7.
Knight, R. (1953) 'The present status of organized psychoanalysis in the United States', *Journal of the American Psychoanalytic Association*, 2.
Mowbray, R. (1995) *The Case Against Psychotherapy Registration: A Conservation Issue for the Human Potential Movement*, London: Trans Marginal Press.
Oakley, C. and Oakley, H. (1994) 'Psychoanalysis: a rendezvous with disappointment', *Journal of the Irish Forum for Psychoanalytic Psychotherapy*, 4 (2): 31–48.
Postle, D. and Anderson, J. (1990) 'Stealing the flame', *Self and Society*, 18 (1): 13–15.
Reich, W. (1973) *The Function of the Orgasm*, London: Souvenir Press. (Original work published 1942)
Richardson, A. (1997) 'The significance for the United Kingdom – a view from the Department of Health', address to Conference on 'Regulation of Psychotherapy in Europe' organised by the British Confederation of Psychotherapists, 7 June (transcript).
Rogers, C. R. (1973) 'Some new challenges to the helping professions', *American Psychologist*, 28 (5): 379–87; reprinted in H. Kirschenbaum and V. L. Henderson (eds) (1990) *The Carl Rogers Reader*, London: Constable, pp. 357–75.
Shepherd, M. and Sartorius, N. (eds) (1989) *Non-Specific Aspects of Treatment*, Toronto: Hans Huber.
Spinelli, E. (1996) 'Do psychotherapists know what they're doing?', in I. James and S. Palmer (eds), *Professional Therapeutic Titles: Myths and Realities*, British Psychological Society Occasional Papers Vol. 2, Leicester: BPS, pp. 55–61.
Totton, N. (1992) 'Therapists on the couch', *i to i*, July–Sept.

Endnote

1. Thanks to Rosie Atkins for this quotation.

Part I
The Dynamics of Professionalisation

The Politics of Transference I.1

John Heron

In 1971 the government published a report on the scientologists, who were at that time causing much public disquiet. It was written by a well-known QC, J. G. Foster, who knew very little about psychotherapy, and therefore took advice from the psychoanalytic lobby. Following this advice, he condemned the scientologists on the grounds that they were exploiting emotionally vulnerable people and *abusing the dynamics of the transference.* And he recommended the statutory registration of psychotherapists in private practice in order to protect the public from this kind of abuse (Foster, 1971).

This led to the formation of a working party on the statutory registration of psychotherapists in private practice, attended by all the primary established bodies in the field. Their report hit my desk at the British Postgraduate Medical Federation, where I was Assistant Director, some time after 1977. The majority of organisations involved supported nominal registration – that is, the names 'psychotherapist' and 'psychoanalyst' would be registered, with a list of associations providing approved training and accreditation. The report argued that this was all necessary in order to protect the public, quoting with approval the 1971 recommendation.

The behaviour therapists disagreed in a minority report. They wrote that since there was substantial research evidence that psychotherapy did not do anyone any good, there could be no case for giving it statutory recognition. Privately, they put it to me in much stronger terms. They said that statutory recognition, far from protecting the public, would lead to widespread exploitation, because it would legitimate psychotherapists taking money under the pretence of offering a service that did some good – when studies showed that it did no better than having no therapy at all.

They also said, in more radical tone, that psychoanalysts in particular were hypocritical in wanting to protect the public from transference abuse,

This paper was first published in *Self and Society*, 18 (1), 1990: 17–23.

when their own therapy was riddled with this very phenomenon. They let their clients slip into emotionally regressed attitudes, sustained them there over long periods by manipulative interpretations, and exploited this state of disempowerment to make money by recommending an increase in the number of sessions per week. What the psychoanalysts really wanted, said my behaviour therapy sources, was to manoeuvre the government into protecting their lucrative monopoly on transference abuse. Strong stuff indeed, but with an important grain of truth, in my judgment and my experience.

The report of that working party came to nothing. A private member's bill, the Bright Bill, based on it was put forward, but the government, having been advised that there was too much dissension in the field to warrant statutory intervention, made sure that there was no time available for the bill to be taken up by Parliament. The Royal College of Psychiatry was secretly opposed to a bill, for fear that it would expose many of their members, consultant psychiatrists, who were, alongside their NHS appointments, in lucrative private practice as psychotherapists without any proper training whatsoever.

However, in several European countries, authoritarian and restrictive legislation was already afoot, and in some cases in place. This has led to the fear that as the UK participates more fully in the European Community, it may have to take on board after 1992 a pan-European model of accreditation or statutory registration. Thus the Association of Humanistic Psychology Practitioners, getting itself ready for 1992 and beyond – or for any separate UK registration – through affiliation with the Standing Conference for Psychotherapy, says that applicants must show they have had a long training and supervision in the understanding and handling of transference and counter-transference, if they want to be accepted as a member. The concept of transference again becomes central to the political argument.

There is, however, a disturbing paradox here. For it is fear that has, in my experience, characterised the response of psychotherapists to the whole political process of professionalisation. They fear loss of livelihood, loss of status and recognition, loss of legitimacy. And in this fear I detect a strong element of transference itself: the acting out of infantile survival patterns in the face of all powerful authority figures. So the political argument for professionalisation, based on legally accredited competence in handling transference, is itself a rationalisation of a more deep-seated transference phenomenon. This is the paradox. One can scarcely have much confidence in psychotherapists whose need to have their management of transference government approved is itself a sign of unresolved transference material.

The case against statutory registration of psychotherapists, especially the case built on the exclusive professionalisation of transference competence, is as strong as ever it was. The phenomenon of transference is very widespread throughout our emotionally repressive society, whose rigidity is sustained by distorted and unprocessed psychosocial dynamics. People carry around a great deal of buried infantile distress which drives them to act out in adult life submissive and dependent behaviours in the presence of those on whom they unawarely project oppressive parental status. Most professions – medicine, law and the judiciary, education, social services, politics, to name but a few – exploit this. The professionals, caught up in the same widespread patterns of repression, deal with their own infantile insecurity by identifying with their internalised authoritarian parent, and exercise too much power and control over their clients – upon whom they unawarely project the repressed, hurt child within.

If the insecure child within psychotherapists drives them to use this whole distorted system to legalise a new, exclusive, highly trained and protected profession to handle transference, they too will fall foul of their own introjected authoritarian parent – which will subtly contaminate the way they theorise about, and work on, their clients' transference material. In the guise of protecting their clients from the unqualified, they will oppress them. They will use the transference dynamic improperly to sustain it. This is the half-a-head-out, half-a-head-in phenomenon: the therapists both have insight into a distorted dynamic process and at the same time fall foul of it within themselves when working on it in others. Put in other terms, it means that a lot of their counter-transference is not spotted for what it is and is displaced unawarely into a warped form of therapy. This is a peculiarly unfortunate kind of helping treason.

Competence in handling transference by its very nature cannot, without serious distortion, be professionalised and legalised in an emotionally repressive society. The professionalisation of it takes it away from the public domain into mystification and expert knowledge accessible only to thc few. And this exacerbates and reinforces the very processes which it is supposed to be dealing with. There is no better way to sustain compulsive infantilism in society (and thus an endless supply of clients) than by setting up a highly specialised, government-protected profession that alone is qualified to deal with it. This is the ancient corruption of priestcraft: to organise your hierarchy in such a way that you generate the sins you are appointed to redeem. It is significant that the pressure for statutory registration in this field always comes *in the first instance* from those who are already caught up in some kind of transference abuse and want to preserve and protect the improper exercise of professional power.

The concepts of psychotherapy and therapy are historically close to the concepts of psychopathology, treatment and the patient. The tendency of such association is to relegate the notion of transference to the domain of those who are in a state of psychological deficit, with emotional problems, and who have fallen out of the mainstream of social life. This obscures, and distracts awareness from, the fact that transference is a psychosocial dynamic that affects every aspect of life in our society. And the relegation reinforces the bad old distinction between education and training on the one hand, and emotional therapy and treatment on the other. Once this distinction is made, then education – which is of universal application – excludes the acquisition of emotional competence, which is purveyed only by an esoteric profession for a disturbed minority of citizens. This creates the absurd anomaly that the majority remain emotionally incompetent, and only patients with problems qualify for affective growth.

There is another profound anomaly in the argument that seeks to protect the public from transference abuse in psychotherapy. It overlooks the fact that one area where transference abuse readily occurs is in the sphere of religion and the spiritual life. Gurus, perfected masters, evangelical preachers, traditional priests of all persuasions, mediums entranced by spirit guides, the hierarchs in psychic and occult groups, charismatic teachers with a spiritual message – all these abound in our society today. They generate and often exploit, wittingly or unwittingly, a great deal of transference material. The exploitation is for purposes of power, control and dominance; and often for money as well. This indeed is where the story began in the UK in 1971, with a concern about the scientologists – who were operating as a church.

There was, however, no talk in 1971 or thereafter about the statutory registration of practitioners of the spiritual and religious life, about protecting the public from the transference abuse perpetrated by many of them. The reason is not far to seek, for such talk would offend one of our deepest and most cherished traditions – that of religious liberty and toleration, the right of every person to affirm and practise whatever creed they choose. To define a religious practitioner, and specify the training required, for statutory purposes would inevitably protect some limited dogmatism by law, and cause an outcry that the state was busy with religious oppression and persecution. A deeper reason is perhaps our tacit awareness that everyone has a right at some time to be a spiritual practitioner for others – praying, blessing, invoking, exhorting, healing – and that this universal right transcends matters of legislation.

So in this field the claims of religious tolerance and liberty are so strong that they override any concern about protecting the public from transference abuse. We leave people to find their own way, through trial and error, and to exercise the right of the pilgrim to undergo – for however long a period – whatever travails and snares are to be found upon the path. Why, then, such protective paternalism in the field of psychotherapy?

The answer is uncompromising and rigorous. To define transference for purposes of training and accreditation, in order to underwrite statutory registration of psychotherapists, will enshrine a limited dogmatism in law. This is logically inescapable: for any definition is bound to exclude the transference dynamic – for both putative practitioners and the public – involved in the very pursuit and application of such legislation. In other words, the widespread social and political dimension of transference will be absent from the definition. Hence psychotherapists, in possession of a half-truth, repress their anxiety involved in handling the whole truth, through the social defence mechanism of statutory restriction. In claiming legal protection for themselves as personal change agents, they abdicate their responsibility as social and organisational change agents. The legislative claim is in reality nothing to do with protecting the public, but everything to do with protecting the unresolved transference material – in its social and political dimensions – of the psychotherapists themselves.

What, then, is the way forward? There seem to me to be some simple and quite fundamental principles to guide us. The first is that, both theoretically and practically, the intrapsychic and interpersonal dimensions of transference are to be seen always in relation to the society-wide and political dimensions. This leads on to the second principle, which is that the right to be emotionally competent – which includes the ability to understand and master the dynamics of transference – is the birthright of every person in society. Until this claim is acknowledged, the whole social, organisational and political process will be distorted by people unawarely acting out compulsive victim, compulsive oppressor, compulsive rebel and compulsive rescuer roles.

This in turn leads to the third principle, that the right to emotional competence is an inalienable and central part of the right of everyone to a proper education. What we need, therefore, is an educational system for all in which emotional and transference competence is the hub around which intellectual, technological, interpersonal, organisational and political competence revolves.

These three principles entail certain consequences for current practice. We need to interrupt every tendency to hive off the handling of transference into restrictive psychotherapy. We need progressively to introduce it into general education. One obvious place to start is in adult education through the provision of personal development workshops for the general public. This, of course, has been going on now for several decades in the UK, both in independent and in institutionally based centres. What is perhaps needed more and more on these courses is that in-depth work on emotional competence should relate the intrapsychic and interpersonal aspects of transference to the social and political aspects.

The other obvious place to start is in continuing education, especially in-service further training for the teaching, helping, management, political and other service professions. What is needed here are more and more experiential courses in which professional and personal development are seen as inseparably combined, in which skill on the job has transference competence as a central component.

The psychotherapists can aid all this educational development by ceasing to call themselves psychotherapists and by abandoning the term 'therapy' and the lugubrious and out-moded language of 'psycho-pathology', 'cases' and 'case-work', 'referrals' and 'supervision'. They could serve the purposes of social transformation much better if they were to call themselves affective educators, facilitators of personal growth, practitioners of emotional competence, and thus stake out a claim to be central to much-needed educational reform. They could quite overtly – as a matter of policy and public nomenclature – supplement and augment, through intensive one-to-one tutoring and facilitation, the development of emotional competence through group-based programmes in adult education and professional in-service education. And they could still reach out, using an educational model and working over long periods, to those with special emotional difficulties.

For it is clear that good psychotherapy does not and should not involve a treatment-and-cure model. This model derives from physical medicine, where the physically diseased and passive patient is treated by the expert doctor who thus procures a cure. Even in medicine today this model is now outmoded, with a new emphasis on education for patient power and active self-direction in promoting the healing process. Where psychotherapy has been contaminated by the treatment model, it has made the patient too passive – lying back and free associating, and the therapist too active and controlling – with a series of unilateral, theory-laden interpretations imposed upon the client's mental process.

To treat the psyche like a *body* with the fluid of association flowing through it – a fluid into which interpretations are injected – is to adopt the method of indoctrination and subtle dominance. It induces *passive* regression and may prolong it with a degree of disempowerment that can turn into sustained depression and, in some instances, depressive suicide. Some psychotherapists today still use this method.

By contrast, to relate to the psyche as a *person* is to enable, educe and cultivate the client's emerging awareness, insight and skill in dealing with deep-seated emotional processes. The client is being facilitated, through *active* regression, in self-directed emotional learning and growth. This educational model – of the client acquiring understanding and skill – is the one which *in practice* a large number of humanistic psychotherapists today, to a greater or lesser degree, espouse. It is surely time they made this explicit, dissociated themselves from indoctrination-psychotherapy, and abandoned the narrow and ultimately self-defeating pursuit of statutory legitimacy.

Of course, on the wider canvas of emotional education, there are still very important issues about the competence, training and accreditation of the affective educators, whether working with groups or one-to-one. But these matters should be entirely outside the jurisdiction of government and of state legislation, as they are in relation to the competence, training and accreditation of spiritual teachers.

Our society has already grasped the point that general education and religion relate to such fundamental human rights that anyone can, and should be allowed to, set themselves up as an independent educator or an independent religious teacher. For this is the only way to honour the right of people to acquire knowledge and spiritual practice from any source they choose. It also honours the responsibility of people to sort out the consequences of whatever choices they make. The extension of education from intellectual to emotional competence only serves to take this right even deeper – into the domain of self-knowledge and personal mastery.

The right to emotional growth is too profoundly related to the exercise of human autonomy for the state to have any say in who is or is not fitted to facilitate it – just as the right to spiritual growth is too deeply engaged with the inner freedom of the soul for the state to prescribe who is allowed to foster it. These two rights are closely related, for emotional growth rooted in human autonomy sooner or later leads over into spiritual growth expressing the freedom of the soul. It is the business of the state *only* to affirm and protect the unfettered exercise of these twin rights. It is the business of the facilitators of these kinds of growth to develop forms of training and accreditation that are both responsible and at the same time capable, in terms of their content and method, of unlimited progression and unfoldment.

The 1989 guidelines for membership of the Association of Humanistic Psychology Practitioners, in the section which gives details for applying for full membership, represent a sorry mess. This section falls between the stool of self-assessment and self-selection of practitioner categories, and the stool of imposed criteria for the category of psychotherapist imported from the UK Standing Conference for Psychotherapy. These criteria are not only imposed, they also appear to be restrictive and outmoded, implying a total separation – within a closed, hierarchical professional enclave – of psychodynamics from socio-political dynamics. It is all very unhealthy, and looks as though humanistic practitioners are incongruently choosing a form of professionalisation quite at odds with the interrelated values of self-realisation and social transformation which have so far distinguished humanistic psychology.

Reference

Foster, J. G. (1971) *Enquiry into the Practice and Effects of Scientology*, House of Commons Report 52, London: HMSO.

In the Shadow of Accreditation | 2

David Wasdell

The field of accreditation in psychotherapy is fraught with fears, threats and anxieties, some acknowledged, some unconscious. Two distinct trends or patterns of behaviour seem to be emerging. The first is a commitment to the highest possible standards within the profession, the improvement of quality, the upholding of ethics, continued learning and the sustained provision of a high-quality service to the whole population. Accurate and widely disseminated information is also needed so that potential clients can make appropriate choices in the continued search for health, wholeness and the realisation of human potential. Opinions may differ sharply as to how best to achieve these ends but the professional integrity behind the commitment to common goals cannot be called in question.

There is, however, a second and more shadowy side to the accreditation scene. Here the dynamics and motivation are largely unconscious, dominated by the processes of transference, projection and collusion. This paper is an attempt to probe a little further into the dark side of the force that is driving the complex set of dynamics in play. The analysis is based on a series of conversations and interviews, backed by literature review, a study of the history and emergence of the institutions of professionalism and accreditation within the field, and observation of those group and institutional processes which arise in conferences debating the critical issues involved.

Grounds of accreditation?

The assessment of competence in the area of counselling, psychoanalysis and psychotherapy is extraordinarily difficult. There is a confusing plethora of schools, beliefs, practices and doctrines – a glittering galaxy of psychoclass fragments gathered collusionally around the memory of

---

This paper was first published in *Self and Society*, 20 (1), 1992: 3–14.

charismatic leaders whether dead or alive. Each grouping is more or less convinced that their own way of going about the therapeutic task is correct, while the approaches of all others are wrong and ineffective. In this sense the group norms of the particular fragment to which a therapist belongs carry in their construct the common coding of anxiety defences of that particular group. Denied negativities are duly projected into the environment and focused into the set of out-groups, the corporate carriers of the shadow. Attitudes to accreditation inevitably reflect the splitting, projection, displacement and paranoia already inherent in the complex inter-group and inter-institutional dynamics of the field. Under these conditions, no in-group is likely to take kindly to accreditation procedures based on the criteria of other groupings or institutional sectors, let alone staffed, administered or imposed by outsiders, whose competence is called in question by the very fact that they are outsiders. Incestuous processes of in-group mutual-accreditation proliferate, reinforced by self-assessment, peer-assessment, client-feedback and institutional authorisation. Recognition of such sub-group accreditation by other sub-groups and institutions in the field is, however, just as fraught as external accreditation itself.

The same arguments and objections apply, raised now to the inter-group and inter-institutional level of dynamic, rather than held at the individual level. If accreditation by the outsider is bedevilled by projection, accreditation by the insider is fraught with collusion. If we turn to client-feedback and outcomes research, we find little help. Few clients have the experience to make effective comparisons between a number of therapists, which might be used for the basis of evaluation of one against another. Client assessment is also coloured to a profound extent by the inter-personal relationship established between client and therapist. Client feedback is therefore as much a statement of the current processes of transference and counter-transference, as it is an objective evaluation of the skills, practice and competence of the therapist concerned. A client may terminate a therapeutic engagement in angry protest at what is perceived to be therapeutic incompetence, only to realise years later that the therapist concerned had put their finger on issues of counter-dependency in an intervention which, with hindsight, had been the creative turning point of the client's life.

Outcome research in the therapeutic world is a minefield of methodological problems. It involves long-term monitoring of the client's condition before, during and after the therapeutic process, followed by some kind of comparison of those 'results' with a control group which does not in fact exist. It is virtually impossible to answer the question, 'What would have happened to those particular clients if they had not been working with this particular therapist, had not been engaged in therapy at all, or had been working with someone from a different school, training or approach?' It is impossible to identify a group of people within the population as a whole who have identical problems proceeding to different outcomes in the absence of therapy. In any case the numbers of clients involved with a potential therapist are small and the time base of longitudinal studies quite out of the question in any procedure of accreditation, particularly in view of the fact that accreditation would normally take place at the start of the person's professional career before they had engaged significantly with many clients in the first place.

So, accreditation procedures tend to be forced back on to the most easily measured parameters, which in this situation are the least significant. Books read, courses attended, training analysis, or number of hours spent under supervision, intellectual understanding of the issues involved – none of these are necessary, let alone sufficient, criteria of competence in the therapeutic engagement. One thing that does emerge from outcomes studies is that it is not so much the paradigm, the ideological framework, or the particular skill-set involved that makes a difference, but the quality of the interpersonal relationship established between therapist and client. Seen in this light, truly the therapist has no clothes and accreditation is an attempt to generate a veritable Emperor's wardrobe of nonsense.

Client choice

Against this background the task facing a potential client is indeed daunting. There is a bewildering array of therapies and approaches from which to choose, with almost no available criteria of comparison or effectiveness. Even if such criteria did exist, the level of self-awareness in the prospective client would have to be very high indeed if the comparative information were then to be related to the particular needs which motivated the client to seek to employ a therapist. Once a particular approach has been selected, there may be a large number of individual practitioners associated with the particular method chosen. Comparative information which might enable the choice between therapists within a particular school is also unavailable. So the degrees of freedom involved in the choice are extremely high, information is minimal, uncertainty is massive and all at a point in the person's life where anxiety is already great. The capacity for making judgements about the appropriateness or otherwise of any particular therapist from any particular school is likely to be clouded by the very condition which motivated the client to seek a therapist in the first place. A national register of accredited psychotherapists would hopefully solve all such problems, reducing the anomie and anxiety and ensuring that any client who wished to engage a therapist could pick a name from a list in full confidence that the service rendered would be competent, uniform and effective. Tragically, any such confidence is misplaced. A register of accreditation would provide a token or symbolic form of arixyolite, while in fact hiding the realities of confusion, uncertainty and unpredictability that underlie the choice-making procedure. In this sense, the drive towards accreditation that stems from client anxiety is a defensive manoeuvre, colluding with the public desire for a simplified and irresponsible decision making process.

The bottom line

There is a very powerful feedback loop involved once the idea of accreditation is raised. Therapists who depend for their livelihood upon the fees paid to them by clients (or the wages given to them by their employers, it all depends on your point of view) become distinctly 'twitchy' once one group parades itself as 'accredited' and clients begin to stipulate accreditation as part of their choice-making process. What begins as a trickle ends in a paranoid stampede to get the appropriate letters after one's name and the papers of accreditation and affiliation firmly established and publicly noted. The risk is a rapid diminution in the client base and eventual starvation. In that sense the drive towards accreditation may stem from the very lowest levels of Maslow's hierarchy of need. It is a bandwagon, to fail to board which is to put at risk the very means of earning a living. Once the movement towards accreditation has passed a certain critical point, therefore, it is the bottom line of economics that drives it towards universal adoption, rather than anything inherently appropriate or professionally significant in the actual process of accreditation itself. The result is one group of therapists who are accredited, who get business and survive, and another group of therapists, who may be equally competent but are not accredited and therefore do not get business and do not survive. The boundary between the two is a false, or pseudo, dichotomy, designating a distinction between the in-group and the out-group that is lacking in meaning, since the quality and lack of uniformity of therapy inside and outside the boundary is unlikely to differ significantly.

Of rejection and discreditation

From the therapist's point of view, however, a different range of motives and anxieties presents itself. Leaving aside for the moment the professional adult search for excellence and the open and confident submission of one's practice to examination by one's peers, other more shadowy motives emerge. There is the hysterical desire to belong to a group and the fear of rejection. From these roots springs the complaint that therapists offer to the accrediting procedures precisely those facets of their practice which are deemed to match the criteria of acceptance, whether or not they reflect the practice of the therapist concerned. There is a presentation of a 'false self' and a suppression of potentially damaging information, in an attempt to press through the needle's eye of accreditation. In that coveted space beyond, guarded by the generalised boundaries of the in-group, the newly accredited therapist feels freer to practise in ways which may or may not be coherent with the principles of accreditation employed.

Underlying and driving this position is the fear of being found to be discreditable, of being cast out of the profession. 'It is better not to seek accreditation, than seeking it, to fail.' Resistance to accreditation by any procedure may arise from the sense of professional maturity and integrity which sees the whole procedure as a redundant irrelevancy. It may also stem from anxiety about being discovered to be incompetent. 'If people really knew the mistakes I make, the mess I get into, the difficulties I have engaging with clients, they could not possibly accredit me.' Some of the most robust rebellion against accreditation may well be a displacement of some such fear lurking in the shadows. So much of the emotion associated with examination inherent in the very notion of accreditation reaches back to those most primitive levels of being acceptable or not acceptable in the first experienced environment. Those who know themselves to have been profoundly and deeply acceptable and affirmed will therefore be quite confident in approaching any procedure of accreditation. The therapist whose imprinted experience is of profound rejection may be stimulated into primal terror at the very thought of exposing him/herself to an assessing environment. The infantilising transactions and the processes of projection and transference stimulated within the accreditation procedures run profoundly counter to the mature interdependence of adult/adult engagement which the profession seeks to engender as a norm of social relationships. It is this kind of distortion in the professional dynamics, in which the procedures adopted are completely out of gear with the underlying value system, that provides a pointer and a clue to the origin of the shadow of accreditation.

The European connection

There are different patterns of legal control operating under the different legislative systems within the European Community. In England and Wales, the individual is free to advertise services and to receive payment for them unless legislation is enacted specifically forbidding the particular activity. Just as a person is presumed innocent until proven guilty, so the assumption about any remunerative activity is that it is legal unless declared unlawful. The situation is quite different in the majority of Common Market countries. Here legislation concerning remunerative activity is proactive. The question about the legality of any particular mode of employment is therefore, 'Has this been legally endorsed as a remunerable activity within the public sphere?' If not, it is illegal. Procedures of accreditation, control and legalisation are quite distinct within the two legislative situations. Within the realm of English Common Law anyone may offer their services in a therapeutic capacity unless already forbidden so to do by existing law. Within other Common Market countries no one may exercise a profession as a therapist unless legally entitled so to do.

Against this background the whole debate about accreditation can be seen as one facet of the struggle at the boundary between English customs, constitution and Common Law, and the practices, customs and legal statutes of other European partners. Attempts to negotiate around the whole area of accreditation within psychotherapy which do not take this meta-level, or contextual, dynamic into account may in fact not be dealing with the right level of engagement. Equal outrage is experienced by the makers of potato crisps, whose flavours have been rendered illegal within the Community's pedantic forest of laws.

Accreditation and the dynamics of social systems

Some of the most powerful dynamic forces within the shadow of accreditation stem from the corporate processes of the profession as a whole. The greatest strengths of counsellors, analysts and therapists lie in the area of one-to-one engagements, working with great sensitivity and awareness in creative relationships with individual clients. Groups are sometimes used, but usually for 'therapeutic' or personal development purposes in which the group setting is a context in which the individuals are supported to work on their own process. The focus is not on the dynamic of the group as a whole. Very few therapists have developed the skills of group analysis, together with intervention strategies based on a deep awareness and understanding of inter-group, organisational, institutional and social dynamic processes. This blind spot renders the profession peculiarly vulnerable to dynamic collusion in its social behaviour. If you bring a group of therapists together there is extremely sharp awareness of the individual processes going on, but comparative unconsciousness of the group dynamics in play. The weakness shows itself with great intensity in the difficulties experienced in the politics of therapeutic organisations and in conferences, large workshops, annual gatherings and congresses, held by different sectors of the profession. It is particularly noticed in those events which span, and therefore incorporate the dynamics from, a wide cross-section of the different groups and institutions within the profession as a whole. It is therefore likely that the UK Standing Conference and the issue of accreditation, which have gathered the broadest spectrum of professional interests into a single focal point, might constitute an arena for the acting out of the corporate unconscious of the profession.

It is, of course, the areas of the common unconscious which dominate these group and institutional processes, whereas the whole training and intent of individual therapists sharpen their awareness of the individual and deviant patterns of the client. There seem to be three strands of this common unconscious dynamic which weave and interrelate in the psychodrama of accreditation. They are generated firstly by dynamics originating from within the profession, secondly by those emanating from the client base, and thirdly by the processes of the wider society as a whole. In practice the three areas are overlaid on each other with complex patterns of introjection, projection, transference and counter-transference. The boundaries between the three strands are not absolute, and each area affects and is in turn affected by dynamics from the other two. However artificial the separation of the strands may be, it is a useful way of beginning our analysis, provided we remember that it is indeed an artificial device.

Boundaries and dynamics of the profession

The as-yet-unresolved and unconscious areas of an individual, repressed and denied at the intrapersonal level, are displaced and projected into the life of the group and acted out in the psychodrama of the interpersonal dynamic.

Where these unconscious patterns resonate most deeply between the highest numbers of individuals, they set up powerful group norms and processes which energise and drive the dynamics of the group as a whole. These are the areas of common collusional repression and denial, followed by group displacement and projection across its boundary into the outside world. In the field of such groups and organisations, institutions and systems, the commonly repressed unconscious content of the intra-group levels is deposited and pooled into the inter-group and institutional process and acted out in the psychodrama of the inter-group. The higher the aggregation of the system, the more the dynamics enacted stem from the most profoundly common collusional processes of the individuals concerned. It is hardly surprising, therefore, that the societal dynamics of the profession are least open to insight from within the profession. Individuals professionally involved in one-to-one relationships find themselves at the mercy of unconscious, irrational and often destructive forces being acted out at the corporate dynamic level of those organisations which bring psychotherapists, counsellors and analysts into organisational relationships. These dynamics are not unique to the profession of psychotherapy. The area represents the most common processes of human unconscious dynamic which can be observed throughout the whole range of group, organisation, institutional and social life, and which at a higher level of aggregation dominate international relationships and the inter-cultural and inter-ideological processes of our global village. For those with eyes to see, therefore, the inter-institutional psychodrama within the world of psychotherapy holds a kind of holograph or mirror of the common unconscious of society as a whole. Insofar as these dynamics remain unconscious within the profession, they represent the ground of corporate collusion between the profession, its client base and its social environment. Insofar as the profession becomes aware of these processes, withdraws and owns the displaced and projected material which gives them power and deconstructs the associated defences, is the profession as a whole able to engage across its boundary with integrity, insight and authenticity, instead of the present position of mirroring, collusion and counter-transference.

The words 'profession' in general and 'accreditation' in particular have to do with boundaries. They differentiate between the inside and the outside. Within the profession there are many sub-boundaries which distinguish one sub-set or in-group from another. Until quite recently, these sub-professional boundaries had been the dominant carriers of the dynamic. The emergence of an external or extra-professional threat typically generates a meta-boundary and suppresses the splitting at the sub-group boundary. It is just such a process that now appears to be in place with the engagement between the UK and its partners within the European Community creating the meta-system dynamics which we are now experiencing. As a result the profession as a whole is beginning to distinguish itself from the social environment. Motivation is in part paranoid, driven by the (quite realistic) anxieties concerning the prohibition of conducting unauthorised or unaccredited therapy for payment. At another level, anxieties have been expressed about 'the maintenance of our craft'. It is a phrase which became highly significant within the debates at the Association of Humanistic Psychology Practitioners a couple of years ago. Initially it seemed a very genuine and straightforward concern, but as it was examined, all kinds of difficulties emerged. Who were the 'we' who exercised ownership? Was it the group of humanistic practitioners gathered in the particular conference, not all of whom in any case would identify or want to be identified with each other as exercising the same 'craft'. What about the people who were within the field of humanistic psychology but were not able to attend that particular conference; were they also part of 'we'? Or did this first-person-plural pronoun stand in for a much wider gathering? In which case how was the boundary actually to be managed?

Then there was the issue of the 'craft'. We began to become aware of all the nuances of the old trade guilds, ideally separating the skilled from the unskilled, in practice protecting the interests of an elite by disempowering non-members. 'Craft' could stand for a set of skills. It could also stand for 'guile'. We began to recognise the devious dynamics involved in craft-maintenance and professional boundary preservation, with all the shadowy Machiavellian jockeying for power, resources, status and exclusiveness that professionalism at its worst can represent. Then again the word 'craft' began to be identified with the little boat, the fragile craft tossed on a stormy sea – the lifeboat with limited resources, dedicated to survival under paranoid conditions. If skills were disseminated too widely, the livelihood of professional members would be in jeopardy. If too many differences were allowed among the crew, then piloting the craft through the stormy waters ahead would be impossible.

So the dynamics which emerge at the professional boundary are inconsistent with the value system overtly espoused within that boundary.

At another level the dynamics which emerge in the group, inter-group, institutional and professional behaviours enact the corporately bonded defence constructs of the common unconscious. The more insightful the group becomes, the more primitive its common defence construct, since the corporate dynamic reflects the most common, as-yet-unresolved, core of the unconscious. Professionals who are acutely alert to and have worked through the unconscious processes stemming from post-natal traumata will act out in their common behaviours patterns of corporate defence stemming from pre-and perinatal material. Groupings who share in common a process of integration of the perinatal impingement will reflect much more primitive patterns of regression and idealisation in their corporate behaviour. So it is that the corporate professional dynamics encode structures of anxiety defence, to disturb which is to expose the people involved to restimulation of as yet intolerable and unresolved level of terror, rage and grief, and to be precipitated as a body into common patterns of psychodrama and abreaction of common imprinting.

These levels of group psychodynamics are shared across the professional boundary with the client group and the wider society. Issues arise of power and powerlessness, omnipotence. There are fears about survival or destruction, blaming, scapegoating, inappropriate struggle for resources and irrational anxieties about implosion, chaos, fragmentation and annihilation. Patterns of splitting from this primitive level of defence are absolutised. Issues tend to be polarised into black and white, good and bad, us and them, inside and outside. As the dynamics build up in intensity, so inter-group negotiation becomes more and more fraught. As the profession as a whole increases the strength of its overall boundary and represses internal splitting, so the us/them, inside/outside projections are focused into relationships between the profession and its client system.

Phrases emerge like 'accreditation gives permission to go into the outside world', as if the profession is bounded by some kind of mega-womb within which the professionals unconsciously regress into idealised dependency, with more and more time and energy vested in intra-professional engagement and less and less resources available to cross the boundary into the working interface with the client group.

Client group transference

In the one-to-one therapeutic engagement the distinction between the therapist and the client is clear. The limits of therapeutic competence are determined by the therapist's own awareness of unconscious process. In so far as both therapist and client are unconscious of what is going on, there will be collusion, transference and counter-transference and a mutual reinforcement of the defensive procedures in play. Growth and development in the skill of the therapist depends on the working through of their own internal defensive materials, which in turn leads to the withdrawal of collusion and the deconstruction of the counter-transference within the relationship. It is of course a life-long process, never completed and calling for sustained commitment to personal and professional development on behalf of the therapist.

That being said, however, it is inevitable that any therapist at any point in their personal development carries introjected transference, unresolved and acted out in counter-transference from the set of clients with which they are engaged. In this sense the therapist acts as a carrier of the unconscious processes of the client set. When therapists meet in a group they therefore carry into the group process the unconscious projections of their combined client field, mirrored by, colluding with and stimulating the as-yet-unresolved unconscious residue of the therapists' own internal worlds. The group, inter-group, institutional and professional dynamics of therapists may be seen therefore not only as generated by the intrapersonal unresolved unconscious of the therapists, but also reinforced by, and collusionally empowered by, the internalised transference from the client group as a whole.

It is this powerful collusional bonding between the unconscious of the intraprofessional dynamic and the unconscious of the client environment that makes the intra-professional processes so occluded and so resistant to intervention and resolution. If therapists gained access to this level of material, they would not only have to deal with the reintegration in their own personae of repressed traumatic imprints, but also and in the same period of development, would have to interface their client set with the same areas of the unconscious. Recognising that these dynamics are indeed the common areas of unconscious material, it is not simply the client set but also the familial, collegiate and social context of the therapists themselves that reinforce and empower the occluded common dynamic. So the unresolved infantile needs of the client base are transferred into the therapeutic community. At the client–therapist interface there is a child–adult distortion of the transactional analysis.

However, because of the common restimulation of the repressed as-yet-unacceptable parts of the child within the therapeutic set, the profession as a whole is dominated by regressive dynamics and acts out the unaccepted parts of its child in common psychodrama. In that sense the unconscious corporate dynamics of the profession mirror the behaviour of the regressed client, so reinforcing and maintaining the common defences against anxiety. There is, therefore, a very real sense in which however effective the therapist is in individual dealings with the client, the profession as a whole reinforces the common defences and acts as a powerful preservative node within the neurotic and psychotic levels of social behaviour. Not only are the unresolved infantile projections of the client base reflected in the corporate dynamics of the profession, the client community also projects its anxieties about dealing with the unconscious, its fear of the unknown, its terror of re-engaging the terrifying. The profession acts as a corporate receptor of such projected anxiety and therefore acts out in its institutional dynamic a pattern of paranoid response reflecting the intense anxiety focused into it from its environmental boundary. The defences against anxiety evidenced in the dynamics of the profession are therefore not simply generated by the intra-professional processes but are also an encoding of extremely powerful defences against the projected and transferred levels of anxiety from its client environment.

Systems of social collusion

An individual therapist, working with a presenting adolescent as client, will recognise that the child has been offered for therapy by the family system within its wider social setting. In that sense the client is a carrier of messages from a wider environment into the therapeutic context. In other situations those deemed 'mad' by their social environment carry by projection the parts denied and displaced from that environment. Excreted and exorcised, they are placed in some kind of institutional container and subjected to the same defensive repression and alienation as the disowned areas of irrationality within the population as a whole. These dynamics are clear and well known in the boundary transactions between the mental hospital and its surrounding community. A similar pattern of displacement, projection, disowning and dumping occurs within the less clearly institutionalised processes of therapy. In this sense the client group carries by displacement the feared unconscious processes of society. These elements of the disowned corporate unconscious are offered for treatment, resolution and containment by the therapeutic profession. The profession therefore shoulders the displaced responsibility of the community as a whole for owning and integrating its unacceptable parts.

Any given client is a carrier not only of their own intrapersonal material but also bears by displacement their familial and social context. There is often a sense of shame at having to have therapy in the first place and a whole host of subtle signals are mounted at the boundary of the client, so preserving the family and the society from any conscious awareness of unconscious material lying behind its own defences. In this sense therefore the whole process of professionalism, accreditation and the engagement with clients serves the unconscious societal task of defence maintenance. When these processes are aggregated and summed across the whole field of psychotherapy it is possible to recognise that the aggregate dynamics of the profession as a whole mirror most profoundly the most common societal defence maintenance processes. It is therefore possible to interpret the psychodynamics of the profession as collusional counter-transference, maintaining the pathology of the social system, reinforcing norm patterns of neurotic and psychotic behaviour and reinforcing the stasis-maintenance dynamics of the community. Caught in this collusional dance, it is hardly surprising that the profession of therapy has so little impact on the behaviour of social systems. So the processes of professionalism and accreditation come to represent the internalisation of the shadow of the social environment.

If the social system as a whole is seen as a corporate client of the profession as a whole, then it is clear that client and therapist are locked in a collusional pattern of transference and counter-transference, mirroring each other's neurosis, preserving each other's defences and effectively blocking any possibility of progress towards maturation, health, wholeness and the releasing of human potential. Breaking out of the present deadlock requires dedication to excellence and competence, not only in the field of individual dynamics but also in the understanding and management of the psychodynamics of social systems. It is essential to gain access to, and resolution of, the most profoundly occluded areas of our common unconscious if we are to cast any light on the shadow of accreditation.

Too Vulnerable to Choose? | 3

Richard Mowbray

> Recently, when I mentioned to a friend who is basically sympathetic to my view that people should feel as free to 'shop around' for psychotherapists as for those providing any other service, she said that she thought this conclusion was questionable because 'how can you expect someone who is seriously distressed to make a good choice?'. My answer is, why shouldn't they? There is absolutely no evidence that emotional distress necessarily implies incompetence or an inability to judge what is helping or hurting in an attempt to alleviate that distress ...
>
> (Robyn M. Dawes, 1994: 125)

Practitioner selection for the 'decisionally challenged'

Protagonists of statutory control of psychotherapy, counselling or psychology frequently present the image of the potential purchaser of these services as being in such a state that they are incapable of making a sensible choice of practitioner. They are presented as vulnerable, distressed, traumatised, disturbed, lacking in autonomy or 'rationally impaired'. Holmes and Lindley, for example, hold that:

> The patient is usually not in the position of a free purchaser. She is in distress, and is prone to grasp uncritically at any offer of help. The market does not protect old ladies whose pipes burst in winter from exorbitant and incompetent plumbers, and *a fortiori,* the desperation of someone in need of therapy may frequently lead to bad therapy choices being made by patients.
>
> (Holmes and Lindley, 1989: 118)

This chapter is a modification and extension of 'Practitioner Selection and the Perils of Transference', Chapter 17 of *The Case Against Psychotherapy Registration: A Conservation Issue for the Human Potential Movement*, London: Trans Marginal Press, 1995.

The Foster Report, which started the registration ball rolling in the UK, holds that:

> ... it will not have escaped attention that those who feel they need psychotherapy tend to be the very people who are most easily exploited: the weak, the insecure, the nervous, the lonely, the inadequate, and the depressed, whose desperation is often such that they are willing to do and pay anything for some improvement of their condition.'
>
> (Foster, 1971: 178)

There is a certain circularity about all this. If someone is seeking psychotherapy or counselling, they are *ipso facto* insufficiently 'together' to be fully responsible for choosing their practitioner!

Granted that some seekers are in such a state of distress that their adult functioning falls below a minimum level needed to retain adult responsibility for their choices and for whom the social role of being 'sick' (Parsons, 1953) is appropriate – they are indeed 'patients' in relation to the potential practitioner (see the discussion of SAFAA, below). However, it is disingenuous to presume that *all* or most seekers are so impaired in their decision-making that they are sitting ducks for exploiters and that therefore special legislative arrangements should be made. This is all the more so if, as is the current tendency, the term 'psychotherapy' is being stretched to cover self-actualising approaches such as in the humanistic area as well as remedial treatments for 'psychological disorders' or 'mental illnesses'.

In addition, the potential customer for psychotherapy or counselling is presented as being faced with a dauntingly difficult task of selection in a disorganised and complex field, crowded with a plethora of different types of work to choose from. Hence the need for systems of accreditation to sort the wheat from the chaff and ease the burden on this less than adequately functioning individual:

> [A psychotherapy profession] would also help to overcome a real difficulty which exists for the consumer faced with the variety of psychotherapies ... The person in search of help is faced with an array of different treatments, and is often not in a position or state to evaluate the distinctions between them, and so make an informed choice of therapy...
>
> (Holmes and Lindley, 1989: 217).

However, as David Wasdell points out (Wasdell, 1992: 5; see Chapter I.2, this volume), the notion that the registration of psychotherapy would really help the potential client to choose is illusory and misleading. There are no easily applied external qualifications that you can trust. Having selected a type of work that suits your intentions and values, the basis for deciding on a practitioner must essentially be personal. Moreover, since the available evidence does not strongly favour any particular approach as being generally more effective than any other, the choice of what type of work to undertake is less critical than it might at first appear, and can be approached on the basis of what sort of work attracts you or by experimenting and trying out several types. In addition, rather than assuming that the consumer cannot become sufficiently well informed to become 'aware' enough to 'beware', and must instead leave fundamental parts of the selection process to a statutory board, the potential consumer can be 'informationally enriched', as discussed below.

The perils of transference

'Transference' is a term derived from psychoanalysis that refers to the unconscious assignment to the practitioner (or other person) of feelings about important and usually powerful figures in one's past (such as parents). Although this term is usually used in relation to a therapeutic setting, the phenomenon to which it refers is not confined to that context but is widespread, though seldom acknowledged elsewhere for what it is. Transference is also a phenomenon which varies in its manifestation, depending upon the expectations associated with the setting. The more it is 'the done thing', the more it will be done.

Much of the discussion about the statutory control of psychotherapy has been heavily influenced by the psychoanalytic model in which transference is actively encouraged, since the analysis of the transference is the primary *modus operandi* of that approach: '... "Deep" transference is an extension and exaggeration of everyday transference which occurs mainly, but not exclusively, in analytic therapies whose arrangements, for cxample the passivity and reticence of the analyst, are especially designed to evoke it' (Holmes and Lindley, 1989: 117). Frequent, regular sessions also tend in this direction. The Foster Report was heavily influenced by the psychoanalytic lobby and the Sieghart Report (Sieghart, 1978), cited by UKCP as justification for the pursuit of registration, was the outcome of a working party dominated by analytic bodies. Holmes and Lindley (one of them a psychoanalytically trained consultant psychiatrist/psychotherapist, the other a philosopher) favour a statutory profession, and likewise seem to view these matters through a lens coloured by that model. However, from perspectives other than that of psychoanalysis, such as 'holotropic therapy' for example, transference would not be regarded as something to be encouraged but rather as a complication of the therapeutic process, a form of resistance rather than as necessary to successful treatment (Grof, 1988: 225). In humanistic and transpersonal approaches such as gestalt, psychodrama or psychosynthesis, the relationship between the client and practitioner would be regarded as important, for example as a 'container', but transference would not be regarded as the main instrument of the work as in analytic approaches. Though awareness of the phenomenon would be included, actual encouragement of a transference would not necessarily be involved or considered appropriate.

Early in his career, Freud himself regarded transference as a form of resistance that impeded progress. The fact that he later abandoned this viewpoint should not be automatically taken as a sign of its redundancy. After all, Freud also abandoned the 'seduction hypothesis' of hysteria (that emphasised the importance of memories of actual childhood sexual abuse) in favour of a 'phantasy' interpretation, and he felt that this marked the beginning of psychoanalysis as a therapy and a profession (Masson, 1984).

There is no conclusive evidence that psychoanalysis or related psychodynamic psychotherapies are more effective than other forms of therapy (not to mention cost-effective!).[1] Indeed there are signs of a decline in confidence in such approaches as a form of psychological treatment. For example, the use of psychodynamic approaches for treating depression now provides cause for a legal suit in the US courts (Griffin, 1996). Therefore, although such approaches constitute the largest grouping in UKCP, and BCP is entirely composed of them, it hardly seems appropriate that these forms of psychotherapy should be used as the touchstone for legislative decisions. The more so if the 'psychotherapy profession' is supposed to include a gamut of other approaches, such as the humanistic ones mentioned above, as intended by UKCP.

Encouraging transference involves encouraging regression and dependency. Holmes and Lindley refer to therapy creating a temporary dependency *en route* to a state of increased 'autonomy', the promotion of autonomy being the essential goal or outcome of psychotherapy. In a section describing 'some common elements in various types of psychotherapy', they say that: 'Psychoanalytic therapy attempts, through the concept of *transference*, to make the issue of dependency-in-the-service-of-autonomy a central vehicle for therapeutic change …', and that: '… it remains true that some of the ethical dilemmas of psychotherapy do arise out of the *cultivation of dependency* in the service of increased autonomy' (Holmes and Lindley, 1989: 5–7). Despite Sir John Foster's claim that 'More than ever today, psychotherapists regard the ultimate dissolution of the transference at the end of treatment as the most difficult, and yet most crucial, part of their task' (Foster, 1971: 177), the concept of 'counter-transference', and the usual inhibition of post-therapeutic contact between therapist and client, carry an implication that the 'resolution of the transference' is actually a theoretical possibility rather than necessarily the norm.

Autonomy, here, is a variable state of being. With regard to the safe selection of a therapist, discouraging transference and concomitant regression, and encouraging what adult functioning and autonomy the person *already* has, is the more appropriate stance. This means not colluding with any urges in the prospective client to forsake what adult status and responsibility they do have and the responsibility for choices that only they can make – including the choice of a practitioner.

Institutionalising the transference

The accreditation route fostered by UKCP, UKRC et al. promotes the myth that the public can be protected from the difficulties of choice in this area.

The promotion of this myth is indicative of a process that I refer to as *institutionalising the transference*. This represents a further effect of registration/licensing in this area that, if anything, actually *increases* the potential risk of harm to the public over and above the negative side-effects of registration/licensing that generally occur (see Mowbray, 1995: 86–8).

Many institutions, individuals and professions appeal to and exploit transference – for good or ill. As we have seen, some types of psychotherapy and related fields address transference itself and work with it directly, and indeed an awareness and understanding of transference can be regarded as a basic competence in this field – and should be a basic social competence. As John Heron explains (Heron, 1990: 19; see also his Chapter I.1, this volume), promoting the handling of transference as the rightful province of a special professional enclave mystifies it and removes it from the public domain – where an awareness of it as a pervasive phenomenon rightly belongs. Demonstrating this awareness collectively as practitioners (and individually) would mean refusing to collude with a 'fear of freedom' that makes people yearn for someone else to relieve them of the burden of decision and take charge of their lives.[2] It would also involve practitioners refusing to act out their own urges towards aggrandisement.

Instead, we have the very occupations which should know better pursuing the myth of accreditation in this area and seeking 'official recognition', statutory privilege and monopoly. By so doing, transference would become institutionalised in the sense that the practitioner's status as 'expert' would become endorsed by the state and his or her authority commensurately enhanced. Transference, and regression, are encouraged by anything that encourages you to 'look up' – from the couch onwards! Potential clients can become lulled into a false sense of security and suspension of judgement by such a system. It encourages them to defer to the authority of the practitioner and the institutions backed by the state that give him credibility – to 'leave their brain at the door' – in a way that fosters dependency and a letting down of appropriate self-protective guards.

As with transference, so with hypnosis, suggestion and subliminal influence. These are not techniques or phenomena confined to the 'therapy' room. Nor are they phenomena so discrete that they can be readily defined for the purposes of law without infringing on civil liberties. Can hypnosis and meditation, for example, be legally differentiated? Our culture is awash with appeals deliberately aimed to bypass conscious awareness. Our media are full of subliminal cues and emotive inducements, and our politics full of 'feel-good factors'. Perhaps politicians and advertising agencies should be licensed.

The golden rule is to let personal judgement or recommendation be your guide. The personal qualities of the practitioner are crucial. Remain circumspect and do not allow status to cloud your personal assessment of the practitioner and what they do and say. As sociologist Eileen Barker of INFORM – Information Network Focus on Religious Movements – has said of the so-called 'mind-control' techniques used in some cults: 'the point is, the techniques they use are not irresistible' (*Focus*, 1995: 36).

The latest 'hazard' of psychotherapy and counselling to cause concern is the notion of the 'false memory syndrome'. Alongside the encouragement of transference, interpretation is a favoured psychoanalytic technique. In the past, Freudian dogma has led psychoanalysts to erroneously interpret the emerging memories of sexual abuse of some of their patients as 'phantasy'. The 'false memory syndrome' can be seen as a consequence of the further misapplication of that technique, whether by psychoanalysts or others, but in this case the error is in the reverse direction. A medical model notion of the practitioner as diagnostician of the underlying cause of symptoms is also implicit here, and it is the attribution of a status of 'expert' to the practitioner that is likely to raise the client's suggestibility and make them more vulnerable to such errors.

Worse still, with respect to any particular client/patient, the attribution of a status of 'expert' to registered professionals in the mental health area (whether psychologists, psychiatrists, counsellors or psychotherapists) is largely erroneous. A professional expert should be able to make predictions about an individual case that are superior to the predictions of people without that status. On the assumption that they have acquired such superior abilities through their training, qualifications and experience, such professionals are called upon to make judgements about individuals in courts of law and by third party funders as well as in the 'consulting' room. However, these 'experts' do not know best. As Robyn Dawes shows, the notion that professional training yields understanding, not just about people in general but about a particular individual, is contrary to the scientific evidence:

> ... in predicting what people will do, clinicians are worse than statistical formulas ...
>
> (Dawes, 1994: 102)

> ... no one has yet devised a method for determining who will change, or how or when. Professional psychologists cannot predict that. (If any have been able to do so, it has been kept secret from the research literature.)
>
> (Ibid.: 105)

> While licensing has given professionals permission to proffer an opinion [on the status of recovered memories] as if it were fact, it has apparently

> taken away from many of them the ability to say three little words: 'I don't know.'
>
> (Ibid.: 175)

Basic SAFAA

In *The Case Against Psychotherapy Registration* (Mowbray, 1995), I put forward a proposal for distinguishing between those who can be regarded as competent to choose and capable of entering into a contractual basis for working on themselves with a practitioner, and those who are unwilling or unable to do so. This SAFAA criterion, *Sufficient Available Functioning Adult Autonomy*, refers to a requirement for a 'sufficiently available functioning adult' in the sense of both sufficient ability to be in contact with the 'here-and-now' and 'consensus' reality, and to be self-responsible and self-directing.

Such a requirement does not preclude the exploration of deep feelings, states of regression, projections or transference issues. The trick is that such feelings are explored on a 'twin-track' basis – that is, whilst also retaining the ability to be 'in touch' with the present both perceptually and emotionally. It is not the *presence* of intensely experienced feelings or distress that is the limiting criterion but rather the *absence* of access to a functioning 'adult' self.

SAFAA is not a pejorative diagnostic label but rather a functional criterion to allow for 'safer' working through appropriate discrimination. The requirement is minimal and not fixed. Someone's availability of sufficient autonomous adult functioning may vary with time and circumstances, and what constitutes 'sufficient' may vary depending upon the nature of the work being contemplated by the recipient. So, sufficient for *what* is the pertinent question.

From the practitioner's point of view, indications of sufficient available functioning adult autonomy on the part of the potential client would include: an ability to function 'in the world' such as to be self-supporting, cope with a job and generally 'have a life', of some sort, 'out there' including relationships and other means of personal support; the ability to sustain strong feelings without acting them out against self or others in violent or other destructive ways; and the ability to make a commitment and to adhere to agreements, including those contracts and safety rules involved in undertaking the form of work in question. An interview of some sort may be necessary to be sure, as best one can, that the SAFAA criterion is met.

In conjunction with clarity as to the aims of a particular form of work and the essential underlying model (a human potential/personal growth model, a social adjustment, 'normalising' model or a medical model focused on the alleviation of psychological disorders such as specified in the *DSM*, the American Psychiatric Association's Diagnostic and Statistical Manual), SAFAA also provides a means for distinguishing human potential work from psychotherapy regarded as psychotherapeutic treatment (Mowbray, 1995: 172–84).

Non-credentialed registration

There are undoubtedly those whose autonomy really is already well below a necessary minimum for adequate adult functioning and self-protection. The functional distinction between recipients provided by the 'SAFAA' criterion of 'good-enough adult' forms a basis for distinguishing those activities and situations where diminished responsibility on the part of the 'patients' is accepted. What can be called a 'non-credentialed registration' system might usefully be applied in these situations, and provides a form of practitioner regulation that may be appropriate to state (or other third party) funded settings (Hogan, 1979: 361–2, 371–2; Mowbray, 1995: 209–12).

Non-credentialed registration emphasises an absence of entry requirements, and is a system whereby a right to practise or use a title is easy to acquire but can be withdrawn in the event of evidence of harm. Such a system avoids the drawbacks of restricting entry to the occupation on the basis of qualifications that may not be related to competence or performance, whilst allowing a means of halting those who do prove, for whatever reason, to be harmful.

A non-credentialed system would avoid restricting eligibility for working with 'patients' to practitioners with high training and qualification 'overheads' which have not been shown to be particularly relevant to basic competence in this area – such as clinical psychologists and doctors or members of such organisations as UKCP or BAC/UKRC. Such a system could provide an economical basis for meeting the increasing demands for 'counselling' or 'psychotherapy' rather than drug-based approaches in the NHS (Pedder, 1994).

Relevant information and full disclosure

In addition to their appeal to the authority of status, with its manifold drawbacks as discussed above, the criteria for selection promoted by registering bodies, whether voluntary or statutory, are generally so divergent from what are known to be the relevant factors to look for in a practitioner that these bodies are essentially functioning as major sources of misinformation rather than promoting a better-informed consumer choice.

This situation could be improved through measures to enhance public knowledge of which criteria are actually most pertinent to consider when looking for a practitioner to work with.

In addition to the dissemination of such information through books such as this volume and *The Case Against Psychotherapy Registration*, 'full disclosure' provisions enacted as part of general legislative improvements in the area of consumer law would also be helpful. The same issue of access to pertinent information about the relevant criteria for selection applies to many different purchase decisions, and would be beneficial in most if not all markets, not just this one.

The need for truthful product or service 'labelling' is an essential element in such 'full disclosure' provisions, and the epistemological status of any statements or claims about the product, service or practitioner, in the sense of the evidence or arguments for the claims being made, can be specified as a necessary part of such provisions. Claims to scientific validity should be backed up by empirical or experimental evidence and references should be cited, along with any contrary opinions. If the statements made are a question of belief, this should be acknowledged. Perhaps they are based on clinical experience? If so this could be specified. Such provisions would be a way of ensuring appropriate classification and substantiation of the numerous claims that emanate from practitioners and their organisations.

'Full disclosure' principles can provide an alternative model for practitioner organisations generally. All too often, such organisations present themselves as quasi-licensing bodies offering assurance of competence in the traditional professional mode. Instead of the usual list of 'approved' practitioners, such organisations could provide a list of practitioners which explicitly disclaims any recommendations as to competence but which provides full disclosure information for each practitioner. The role of the organisation would be to specify which information was pertinent to competence in their view (and their evidential basis for claiming so), to verify the information provided by each member and to exclude practitioners in the event of falsehood – or to add the record of it to their disclosure statement.

Responsible choice

The need to protect 'the vulnerable' is the mantra most favoured by registration advocates. However, vulnerability in this context is not an isolated condition of personal make-up. It is proportional to the power that the prospective client gives away to the practitioner. Official recognition based on unconfirmed criteria *begets* vulnerability.

Safety here lies in retaining an appropriate degree of circumspection – appropriate to the degree to which competence *can* be assured. Supporting the potential client's existing autonomy, whatever degree of 'adult' they already have, by empowering them with relevant information to help them make the judgements that *only they* can make, is more appropriate than enhancing the official status of the practitioner with the accompanying assumption that competence has been assured. Greater safety in this area lies in an encouragement to evaluate rather than the encouragement to take on trust that is fostered by conventional registration schemes.

As Schutz says:

> In the present situation [USA 1979], I rely on the state to tell me who is competent. I passively submit myself to a professional, and if I do not like what he does, I sue him for malpractice. My role is very inert and childlike. If I, as a consumer, know that I am responsible for selecting a counselor, I am likely to assume a more responsible stance. In many cases, the very act of being responsible will have a therapeutic effect.
> (Schutz, 1979: 157)

References

Dawes, R. M. (1994) *House of Cards: Psychology and Psychotherapy Built on Myth*, New York: Free Press.

Feltham, C. and Dryden, W. (1993) *Dictionary of Counselling*, London: Whurr.

Focus: The Magazine of Discovery (1995) 'The Far-out World of Cults', February.

Foster, J. G. (1971) *Enquiry into the Practice and Effects of Scientology*, House of Commons Report 52, London: HMSO.

Fromm, E. (1942) *The Fear of Freedom*, London: Kegan Paul.

Griffin, J. (1996) *Treating Depression without Drugs*, West Sussex: European Therapy Studies Institute.
Grof, S. (1988) *The Adventure of Self Discovery*, New York: State University of New York Press.
Heron, J. (1990) 'The politics of transference', *Self and Society,* 18 (1): 17–23; reprinted as Chapter I.1, this volume.
Hogan, D. B. (1979) *The Regulation of Psychotherapists*, Cambridge, MA: Ballinger.
Holmes, J. and Lindley, R. (1989) *The Values of Psychotherapy*, Oxford: Oxford University Press.
Masson, J. (1984) *The Assault on Truth: Freud and Child Sexual Abuse*, New York: Farrar, Straus and Giroux.
Mowbray, R. (1995) *The Case Against Psychotherapy Registration: A Conservation Issue for the Human Potential Movement*, London: Trans Marginal Press.
Parsons, T. (1953) 'Illness and the role of the physician', in C. Kluckhorn and H. Murray (eds), *Personality in Nature, Society and Culture*, New York: Knopf.
Pedder, J. (1994) quoted in Sinason, V., 'A standard practice', *The Guardian*, 12 March.
Reich, W. (1950) *Character Analysis*, London: Vision Press. (Original work published 1933)
Reich, W. (1972) *The Mass Psychology of Fascism*, London: Souvenir Press. (1st edn, 1933).
Roth, A. and Fonagy, P. (1996) *What Works for Whom? A Critical Review of Psychotherapy Research,* New York: Guilford Press (2nd edn, 2006).
Russell, R. (1981) *Report on Effective Psychotherapy: Legislative Testimony*, Lake Placid, NY: Hilgarth Press (with 1993 update).
Schutz, W. (1979) *Profound Simplicity*, Big Sur, CA: Joy Press.
Sieghart, P. (1978) *Statutory Registration of Psychotherapists: The Report of a Profession's Joint Working Party*, London: Copyright Paul Sieghart in trust for the professional bodies that composed the working party.
Smith, D. (1993) 'Does therapy work?', *Sydney Morning Herald*, 1 June, p. 12.
Wasdell, D. (1992) 'In the shadow of accreditation', *Self and Society*, 20 (1): 3–14; reprinted as Chapter I.2, this volume.

Endnotes

1. See for example, Hogan, 1979; Holmes and Lindley, 1989; Roth and Fonagy, 1996; Russell, 1981/1993; Smith, 1993; Feltham and Dryden, 1993: 150.

2. The notion of a 'fear of freedom' was explored by Wilhelm Reich in the 1930s during the rise of Fascism in Europe (Reich, 1950, 1972) and borrowed, in part, by Erich Fromm for his book of the same name (1942). Reich stated that: 'in those with neurotic character structures [i.e. most people] there is at the same time *fear of freedom* and *fear of responsibility (pleasure anxiety)*' (Reich, 1950: 255; original emphasis).

Reflections on Fear and Love in Accreditation | 4

Robin Shohet

This is a very short piece. What I have to say is quite simple. It is based on an assumption that any action or thought that springs from fear is ultimately unproductive. If this is so, and I cannot prove it, but suggest that it is an interesting and useful hypothesis, then the whole debate around accreditation is not whether to be for it or against it, but how we can have the views we do have and not polarise (a manifestation of fear).

A while ago I wrote an article entitled 'How green is your mind?' (Shohet, 1995). In it I argued that the source of pollution is not external, but in our minds. I asked people to imagine they were a car and their brain/thoughts/mind were the exhaust pipe. Every time they had any negative thought, criticism or judgement, their exhaust pipe would give off fumes. Most of us would, I imagined, be polluting the planet. I argued that we create a duality (say green people and polluters) and make the other wrong to make us right. Because we are projecting (greens projecting their own polluter, for example), we become frightened of the other because they are carrying disowned parts of ourselves, and we therefore wish to attack or control them. I asked people to imagine that it is this negative thought form of making others bad or wrong, based on fear, which leads to the external pollution. By making the other other, so to speak, we can disregard them. As the Upanishads say, 'Where there is another, there is fear'. And so what I want to ask is, are you in any way part of making otherness – either by making your assessors other, people who do not agree with you other, the system other, other schools of psychotherapy other? In what subtle ways might you be threatened by this otherness and retaliate by making yourselves 'right'? And in case there should be any doubt, I do it frequently, but have become interested in this question of otherness, rather than whether accreditation is right or not. Again quite simply a stance for or against is no longer so relevant to me as one which says, 'Am I afraid, and therefore defending by making others defensive by judging or attacking them in some way?'

I think the accreditation debate has raised a lot of fears. This in itself is not a bad thing. It is when they are unrecognised, rationalised, justified or buried that the distortions begin to happen. A while ago I helped to organise a conference on the dynamics of accreditation. We set up an exercise where people talked about their love of their work. It was a privilege to be there. I have always found people to be very honest when trusted, and my fear (!) is that accreditation can have built in a lack of trust, so that people will hide their shortcomings and therefore their potential growing points. Just as an exercise, could you now imagine three times when you have worked extremely badly with a client, maybe abused your power. Would these go on an application form? If not, then there is fear.

I have come to a pause in my writing. I wonder now if there is some fear as the above came out effortlessly. I ask myself, am I beginning to make you other (i.e. start censoring, which means being fearful of your responses). I wonder is this because it is easy for me to talk about fear, but not so easy to talk about love, which I believe is fear's opposite. Being a psychotherapist has taught me much about love for which I am extremely grateful. I hope that amidst the trainings and the techniques and the schools and the procedures that love does not get lost.

• • •

This was the piece I originally submitted. I thought it said all I wanted to say, namely fear comes from making the other person 'other'. At the end I implied that the way through this was love, fear's opposite. I felt no need to develop any arguments, as this was a personal point of view, and even if people did not agree with what I wrote about love, then I imagined few would disagree that there was fear around, even if they disagreed with the reasons I gave. I submitted the piece. It was rejected by the editors of this book because of its brevity. I commented that I thought we were in a parallel process. I had failed 'my assessment' because the guidelines on length had become more important than the quality of what was being written. The editors quite rightly pointed out that they had set out their structure very clearly (minimum 2,500 words), and my short piece would look out of place. I said this was a fear response, a concern with appearances. I also realised later that the deadline had been brought forward without consultation – a form of moving goalposts that happens in accreditation. We were stuck, as I said I would not write more.

As we polarised it occurred to me that I must be frightened (it was much easier to spot their fear). I consciously remembered that I had a good relationship with one of the editors. I liked him and his work, and that his asking me to write a piece sprang from our connection. The less I made him 'other', the more possibilities opened up, including writing about our process together, and his suggestion I write more about love. In our subsequent exchange of faxes he wrote, 'I'm realising what a fine line there is between setting clear and "healthy" boundaries and guidelines, and over-controlling a process to the extent that all life is taken out of it.' Thank you for your honesty and flexibility. From my point of view I see how I respond to threat (moving deadlines) with a 'take me or leave me' attitude that sets up the other person (I did not even consider negotiating a shorter piece).

I describe this to show how each of us could (and did for a time) have got into a process that did not look like fear, but both of us realised was. And we got through through relationship.

I would like to give an example of how accreditation has affected what I do most for a living – namely teach supervision courses. Through our centre, three of us have been teaching for over 20 years, and in the last two or three years we have been getting requests for some form of certification. Up until then we had deliberately not been involved in any accreditation process, but we see that participants had a real need. Together the three of us agreed certain criteria. One of the results is that people have been rushing to do their minimum requirements so as to get their certificate. Attendance on courses has shot up, but sometimes people have not been ready to do the advanced course in particular. I can see the pleasure in learning that has been a feature of our work for so long, being replaced by a fear of getting it right, filling requirements. A side effect which we had not realised was that it was also very good for business. By consciously addressing the fear around this issue, I hope to dissipate some of it. Perhaps some of it is inevitable, I don't know. What is interesting is that because people are coming on our courses to get the certificate, we cannot easily withdraw from the process, even though we are having misgivings. The process is beginning to have a life of its own. And even as I write this, I wonder if there isn't a fear – if I stop the process, numbers will go down.

For a while I have been giving talks on the subject of the Addictive Organisation. I talk about how organisations take on a life of their own behaving like addicts, creating splitting, division, denial, etc. I think inevitably with accreditation we are creating more institutions/

organisations. A while ago I came across a quotation from a book entitled *Conversations with God*. I had a little bit of an edge about putting God as the source, but I think it is relevant as to how we create otherness as a survival technique.

> *Author:* No doctor wants to deny a cure. No politician wants to see his people die.
> *God:* No individual doctor, that's true. No particular politician, that's right. But doctoring and politicking have become institutionalised, and it's the institutions that fight these things, sometimes very subtly, sometimes even unwittingly, but inevitably ... because to those institutions it's a matter of survival.
>
> And so, to give you just one very simple and obvious example, doctors in the West deny the healing efficacies of doctors in the East because to accept them, to admit that certain alternative modalities might just provide some healing, would be to tear at the very fabric of the institution as it has structured itself.
>
> This is not malevolent, yet it is insidious. The profession doesn't do this because it is evil. *It does so because it is scared.*
>
> (Walsch, 1997, emphasis added)

Wilfred Bion has a wonderful quotation that we should enter the therapy room without memory, desire or understanding. I believe the more afraid we are, the harder it is to do this, because it requires a great deal of trust in self, other and the therapeutic process. Very hard, and yet without it, what messages are we giving?

Which brings me back to love. I know very little about it, yet paradoxically it is a state of being which at core I believe we know most about. Because we (I) do not have the courage to live it, we create expertise and experts, which are poor substitutes. As in the first 'piece' I wrote, I feel very unsure writing about it. So much opportunity to be seen as flakey as opposed to the solid facts and criteria of the real world. (Or am I polarising unnecessarily?)

I'll end with a story about a client whom I had been seeing for twelve years face to face. When I moved to the North of Scotland we corresponded weekly for over a year. She died three weeks ago. I had known for two days that she was in a coma and dying but could not get to see her. On the Tuesday night I got very agitated. I wanted to write but knew my letter would not arrive in time. I suddenly thought of faxing. I faxed the hospice, and ten minutes after my fax was read to her she died. Even though she was in a coma, people who were there said it was as if she had been waiting for it.

Now I know that I often made mistakes with her. I often wondered about the whole issue of dependence, the dangers of collusion, over-identification. I think I might have failed an accreditation process with her as a case history. Certainly I would be very reluctant (frightened) to really name how important she was in my life. I would be very wary of acknowledging to someone who was assessing me, and who did not know the rest of my work well, how much uncertainty I felt in our work towards the end. And most of all, I wonder whether I would have had the courage, and indeed why I felt it would need courage, to say I loved her.

• • •

After I had written this, I showed it to a friend. She brought up the issue of confidentiality. For a while I went into a complete spin. How could I not have thought about this? I had better omit the piece about my client or change details so she would not be recognisable. It was only later that I realised that fear had again intruded. There would be some people who would recognise who I was talking about. Why would that matter? Had I said anything about her that was disrespectful, or revealed anything that I shouldn't?

For many years now at the beginning of my groups, I suggest that we do not have a confidentiality contract. It could not be enforced, and was reliant on people's goodwill. So why not have a goodwill contract where we contracted not to speak about ourselves or each other with disrespect? A contract where we committed ourselves to be mindful when talking of others in the belief that anything we said about them would probably be true on another level about ourselves? I think there is great value in confidentiality, but I think we also need to examine the fear around it. I even wonder if it is the unprocessed fear that causes so many confidences to be broken.

A final word. In writing about fear and love, I am entering territory that is far from clear for me. I know that this piece is, accordingly, less polished than I would normally have liked. In demanding a lot of myself, I will have demanded much of the reader. Bits have got added as more and more fears got recognised. There is no neat ending because the issues of fear and love are lifelong ones.

References

Shohet, R. (1995) 'How green is your mind?', *One Earth Magazine*, Summer.
Walsch, N. D. (1997) *Conversations with God*, London: Hodder and Stoughton.

The Dynamics of Counselling Research: A Critical View I.5

Richard House

> It is only with the heart that one can see rightly; what is essential is invisible to the eye.
>
> (Antoine de Saint-Exupéry)

Introduction

In the past few years, the field of counselling has been moving towards a more self-confident professional status, and there are many aspects of this process which are to be welcomed – not least because it helps to enhance the credibility of counsellors working in a variety of settings. In this chapter, however, I want to express some personal reservations about this process, and about the *form* that moves towards professionalisation are taking in the counselling field.

First, there has been the hasty embracing of the principle and practice of accreditation (see, for example, Dryden, 1994: 194), with at best only lip service being paid to the unconscious dynamics driving such a process (for a notable exception see Wasdell, 1992; Chapter I.2, this volume). This neglect seems at the very least surprising in a 'profession' in which one of the central leitmotivs is reflexive self-understanding, and mature awareness of what drives our beliefs, feelings and motivations.

More recently, we are seeing another imprudent rush, this time into a concern with research, audit and evaluation – and most notably, *empirical* research or counselling evaluation; and, in my own professional field, an explosion of concern with the cost-effectiveness of general practice counselling and psychotherapy (see, for example, Fahy and Wessely, 1993).

This chapter was first published as 'The dynamics of professionalisation: a personal view of counselling research', *Counselling, 8* (3), 1997: 200–4.

Counselling approaches and market ideology

Robert May of Amherst College (quoted on a Routledge advertising leaflet) has recently written that 'we see counselling and psychotherapy more and more pushed towards a purely surface-oriented, symptom-focused and cost-driven approach'. In the medical literature, we are increasingly seeing statements like the following: 'All therapies must prove their worth ... The new rigours of the purchaser–provider split mean that all such treatments will now be subject to ... cost–benefit analyses' (Fahy and Wessely, 1993: 576). And it comes as no surprise that the logic of controlled scientific evaluation and market rationality leads inexorably to the conclusion that:

> The psychotherapy that has adopted the market approach par excellence is behaviour therapy. The practice of graded exposure to phobic stimuli incorporates the routine measurement of symptoms during treatment and the recording of hours of therapy. Cost–benefit information is thus readily available.
>
> (Ibid.)

Such a claim for the objective scientific validity of behaviour therapy ignores the fact that the theory and practice of behavioural therapy are shot through with unacknowledged and, to say the least, highly questionable epistemological and ontological assumptions, and that as a form of therapy it contains 'very serious limitations in its capacity to address some aspects of the human situation that are basic to the conduct of psychotherapy in the contemporary world' (Woolfolk and Richardson, 1984: 778; see also Spinelli, 1994: 243–54).

Nearly 30 years ago, Anthony Storr wrote that 'the idea that ... cure in psychoanalysis is analogous to the cure of physical disease ought to be finally discarded' (Storr, 1968: 60); and that:

> the exploration of ... symptoms inevitably leads on to a consideration of the whole person .... Abolition of [a] single symptom ... even if this were possible, would not relieve the patient of the bulk of her emotional problems. *The same is true of by far the majority of neurotic symptoms.*
>
> (Ibid., 51, 56, emphasis added)

Many counsellors of various orientations would surely view these arguments as being as relevant to counselling practice as they are to psychoanalysis, and to the extent that this is so, then considerable doubt is cast upon the relevance of the kinds of symptom-orientated 'objective' evaluation studies referred to above, with their extremely limited and limiting conceptions of 'cure' and the therapeutic change process.

Yet in the world of *realpolitik*, it has been argued that '[NHS purchasers] may need to resist the demand for more counselling services until better evidence of efficacy and safety is available' (Fahy and Wessely, 1993: 577). Thus, as Hicks and Wheeler (1994: 29) write:

> the reality remains that any service, *just to survive,* must be as cost effective as possible ... a scientific approach may be required if counselling is to optimise its practice and to survive in the current climate of welfare cuts. Indeed, counselling may have to justify *its very existence* ... .
> (emphases added)

The phrase '(just) to survive' is most telling, for it is revealing of the fear-driven dynamics that are in part, and quite understandably, precipitating the increasing preoccupation with evaluation and audit, just as, according to Wasdell (1992; Chapter I.2 this volume), it is deep unconscious levels of anxiety that are in part driving the often unquestioned embracing of the principles of accreditation and registration (ibid.). For if our very *survival* is at stake, then the pull to embrace what may feel like an alien set of values may be irresistible – notwithstanding the fact that those same values may well be substantially antithetical to our own deepest-held humanistic, person-centred principles and moralities. In their article, Hicks and Wheeler pay no attention to the possible dysfunctional dynamics that may well be driving the trend towards what they term 'research-mindedness' – an omission which I am attempting to rectify in this chapter.

Dilemmas and dangers for humanistic practitioners

I do not want to minimise the profound dilemmas and difficulties in all this for the person-centred or dynamically inclined practitioner working in health-service settings (I am one such myself): for do we embrace the agenda of undiluted market rationality and risk betraying in the process the foundational principles of our practice and world-view; or do we stand up for and defend humanistic and holistic principles, at the risk of being replaced in the marketplace by more mechanistic therapeutic approaches whose values and view of the person are very different from, and largely incompatible with, our own? There are, alas, no simple answers to these dilemmas, and it is for each practitioner to decide how to respond to such challenges.

I believe that there is a vital need to pause and reflect upon the dynamics of the trend towards audit and evaluation, and also critically to question the values and implicit assumptions that underlie the kinds of empirical methodological approaches which are actively being advocated and taught in increasing areas within the counselling field. In the remainder of this chapter I attempt to articulate the reasons for my concerns. I write as a professional counsellor, and, in a previous incarnation, as an academic empirical researcher with a Ph.D. in regional economics. I therefore write from a vantage point that includes both extensive experience of relatively high-powered academic empirical research and also a thorough immersion in the ethos of humanistic counselling, psychotherapy and personal development.

Recent issues of *Counselling* have contained strongly expressed arguments in favour of the growth of research, audit and evaluation in the field of counselling (Hicks and Wheeler, 1994). Dryden (1994: 194) has also argued for counsellors taking an increasing interest in evaluation and audit. He writes, 'Potential employers will want harder evidence and it is likely that counsellors will be required to provide such evidence in the not too distant future .... [C]ounsellor training courses will need to put evaluation and audit on the curricula' (ibid.).

There can be a seductive fascination and excitement with the world of seemingly 'objective' statistical techniques; and so it was of no surprise to read in Hicks and Wheeler's article that trainees who had previously been highly sceptical of, and resistant to, doing counselling research 'became more excited by the empirical methods used' (ibid.: 31).

One of the greatest dangers of predominantly or exclusively quantitative research is that we end up knowing the *price* (or numerical value) of everything, and the *value* (or essential quality) of nothing. The desire to quantify, irrespective of the appropriateness of such an approach to the subject matter under consideration, is one which has to be self-consciously and tirelessly guarded against – for the seductive power of quantification, and the appeal that it makes to the scientistic, technocratic mind at this point in the evolution of human consciousness, is such that we can so easily be seduced into entirely inappropriate research procedures without even realising it. We would also do well to bear in mind that 'Attempts to equate scientific knowledge with ... some inflexible standard of verification have proven lacking' (Woolfolk and Richardson, 1984: 777); and that 'all knowledge, *even scientific knowledge,* cannot be isolated from its psycho-social context' (Spinelli, 1994: 84).

Anyone of humanistic persuasion who is familiar with the empirical research literature in any of the social sciences (including many branches of the psychology discipline) can only surely wince at the aridity and disembodied irrelevance of a significant proportion of the conventional literature in the academic journals; and I submit that it would surely be a tragedy if our field, based as it is on person-centred, holistic values, were to go down the same road of sterile and soulless empiricism.

The neurotic psychodynamics of modernity and scientism

Modernity and modernism constitute a world-view which:

> is dominated by science and scientific technology and the modes of thought peculiar to them ... the quest for certitude, and a devaluation of the traditional past ... technique and technical considerations achieve paramount importance .... The aims of prediction and control and a style of planning and decision-making *in which emotional and aesthetic considerations are subservient to the rational* and pragmatic are essential features (of modernity) .... *Science becomes the ultimate source of knowledge.*
>
> (Woolfolk and Richardson, 1984: 778, emphases added)

The psycho-social analyst David Wasdell argues that the dynamics of the global social system are (d)riven by shared, species-wide developmental traumata which are normally repressed from awareness, and the effects of which only tend *overtly* to manifest themselves dysfunctionally under conditions of high stress and anxiety, and diminishing resources. Although Wasdell focuses exclusively on pre- and perinatal traumata, his argument can very plausibly be extended to the post-natal world of human experience (House, 1996; Chapter I.6, this volume); and without wishing to be overly reductionistic, it is logically and evidentially compelling to view our dysfunctional *ideological belief systems* as being in some sense rooted in and driven by species-wide developmental traumata, and the associated 'deformations of mind' which accompany them. To quote Wasdell:

> Where the primary trauma is shared in common, the cyclic psycho-drama is enacted in common. With the common ground [of shared developmental traumata – RH] collusively denied, the dynamic process is *corporately constructed.* It is supported by symbolism and mythology and *socially reified into an unquestionable ideology*.
> (Wasdell, 1991: 1, emphases added)

I am proposing that the objectivist epistemology of empiricist methodology, and its associated zeal for quantification, can be understood in this light, and that it is only through the experiential task of working through and integrating the repressed and unintegrated material of early developmental experience that we will be in a position individually and collectively to heal our individual and collective psychic dis-integration and move towards a wholeness from which it is far more likely that an epistemology and methodology which is truly humanistic in nature will organically emerge.

Thus, Janus (1989: 52) has written that 'research in the psycho-social field always entails the involvement of the researcher himself and is a process of consciousness transformation. The actual research process changes the researcher, and *is thus also limited by his personal resistance*' (emphasis added). As I read it, his point seems to imply that the methodologies that we choose and the research procedures we embrace are not a coincidence or some kind of random event: rather, they closely and faithfully reflect our own personal character structures, defences and the extent (or otherwise) of our own personal psychological integration.

I fear that unless we pause and take careful stock of the dynamics driving the evaluation bandwagon, and the implicit and anti-humanistic assumptions that so often underlie so-called 'objective' empirical methodologies, we could conceivably end up with a plethora of sterile research studies which are substantially antithetical to the values of person-centred and dynamic counselling – and worse, we might well be doing a kind of violence to the values on which humanistic therapeutic philosophy is based. There are some disturbing signs of the possibility of such 'violence' being done to humanistic principles in the position paper by

Hicks and Wheeler (1994). Thus, they write of what sounds suspiciously like a non-democratic imposition of 'research-mindedness' when they write of '*top-down directives* ... emphasising the role of research as a means by which ... resources (can be) used with optimal effect ....' (emphasis added). Would these authors *normally* advocate 'top-down directives' in their professional practice as counsellor trainers? We must all pay close heed to the possibility of an anxiety-driven reaction to the various 'scientific' critiques to which our field is currently being subjected (Spinelli, 1994: 66–93) if we are not to risk being drawn into potentially dysfunctional and neurotically driven acting-out which might well betray the very values which I believe to be foundational to our field.

Towards humanistic counselling research?

> There are inherent difficulties in any attempt to fashion a meaningful understanding of existence in terms of the moral and epistemological categories provided by scientific culture.
> (Woolfolk and Richardson, 1984: 783)

I agree with Dryden (1994: 195) that 'the increasing attention being given to qualitative research will ... help to introduce reluctant counsellors to the world of research as it is ... more in keeping with the spirit of counselling than quantitative research'. But what might a thoroughgoingly *humanistic* research methodology look like? Some useful pointers are contained in the paper by Gillian Thomas (1994), in which she describes a qualitative phenomenological approach to researching into counselling for irritable bowel disease. And Moustakas has recently also made a major contribution to the literature on phenomenological research methodology (Moustakas, 1994).

There is, further, a substantial literature on qualitative research philosophy and methodology; and the pioneering volume edited by John Rowan and Peter Reason (1981) on 'new paradigm research' provides an excellent base from which to develop the kinds of sensitive, person-centred research on which a humanistic evaluation practice should surely be based. In addition, there is the journal *Collaborative Inquiry* (based at Bath University's Centre for Action Research in Professional Practice), which advocates collaborative, self-reflexive research of the kind that will certainly appeal to the humanistically minded practitioner; and last but not least, it is now possible to carry out qualitative Ph.D. research in counselling and psychotherapy at Regent's College, London.

I disagree with Hicks and Wheeler (1994: 30) when they write that 'only quantitative research can lead to predictions concerning best treatment procedures'. Such a view assumes that a quantifying methodology is the appropriate approach for evaluating the efficacy of humanistic–dynamic counselling; yet the kinds of factors that a humanistic perspective holds to be decisive in facilitating therapeutic change (most notably, the healing quality of a relatively non-neurotic loving reparative therapeutic relationship) represent *human qualities* that are quite beyond the ambit of controlled and 'objective' scientific measurement and mechanistic modes of understanding. Similarly, Castoriadis (1995) has recently argued that positivist scientific practices, which place such emphasis on the principles of falsifiability, replicability, predictability and substitutability, are quite inappropriate for studying the human psyche and the therapeutic change process. And a recent paper by Bromley (1990) has set out a detailed, carefully argued case for a clinical, case-study approach to evaluation, which allows for 'the scientific study of the individual without recourse to experimental and quantitative investigation' (p. 299).

Hollway (1989) has forcefully argued that there has been an almost 'intentional blindness' within the psychology discipline to the *conditions of production* of psychological knowledge. Any counselling training/degree course which is advocating or insisting upon its trainees/students carrying out research into counselling would do well to leave considerable space for reflection upon the dynamics of the research process itself – focusing on both the researcher's own particular personality dynamics in so far as they resonate with and determine the choice of research methodology, and also the wider cultural dynamics and ideology of modernity which underlie orthodox and received research practice. At the very least, I would advocate a close and critical reading of Carl Rogers' seminal paper, written 40 years ago now (Rogers, 1955), in which he explores the tensions he experienced between his subjective therapist self and his hard-headed, scientific self: for this paper serves as an excellent introduction to the issues raised in the present chapter. Academic departments in counselling, counselling psychology and psychotherapy should surely pay close and attentive heed to the 'conditions of production' (to use Hollway's phrase) of research knowledge, if the kind of sterile and disembodied empiricism described earlier is to be avoided.

The postmodern turn

There is also a steadily growing body of literature in the psychology field which offers a potentially devastating critique from the postmodernist standpoint of empirical social-scientific research (see, for example, the papers in Kvale, 1992). Anyone who is concerned to promulgate and advocate research-mindedness in the counselling field should at the very least be fully aware of the postmodernist challenge to empiricism, and be prepared and able to offer a coherent and sustainable response to the formidable postmodernist critique.

Some commentators are rightly concerned that a full embracing of the 'anti-epistemology' of postmodernist thinking might lead to a sort of formless relativism in which we end up in a solipsistic position where it is impossible to say *anything* about the world beyond the subjective and purely private. Smith (1994), for example, has recently attempted to steer a sustainable course between the Scylla of disembodied empiricism and the Charybdis of postmodernist relativism. Thus, he refers to a truly 'human science' as somehow being able to combine 'the usual conception of science as aiming at progressive approximation of truth in regard to causal analysis of conditions and consequences' with 'intrinsic reference to human meanings and values' (Smith, 1994: 114). There certainly exist a number of dynamically inclined studies which do attempt to incorporate some kind of qualitative element into their research procedures (e.g. Ryle, 1989; Firth-Cozens, 1992), but I am not at all sure that any of these studies respond adequately to the kinds of anti-empiricism arguments outlined in this chapter.

Perhaps postmodernism is a kind of 'reaction-formation' against the excesses of the soulless scientism of modernity; and it seems to me that the fields of counselling and psychotherapy are in a unique position to develop an embodied, humanistic approach to research that transcends the ideology of objectivism, and which honours both our need for communicable intersubjective knowledge about the world and our core humanistic principles, which elevate the values of holism and human meaning above those of mechanism and quantifiability.

John Heron's recent book (Heron, 1996) provides an inspiring cutting-edge perspective on what a viable and sophisticated post-positivist research process can look like. What is distinctive about Heron's book is the ease and fluidity with which he moves between mature and profound philosophical analysis of what constitutes valid scientific knowledge, on the one hand, and eminently practical, down-to-earth elucidation of his co-operative inquiry methodology, on the other. Heron's Chapter 10, 'A post-conceptual worldview', should be compulsory reading for anyone who intends to conduct research in the counselling and psychotherapy field. For in it he sets out with admirable clarity the tenets of so-called 'New Paradigm philosophy' which is challenging, quite fundamantally, our conventional ways of seeing and experiencing the world (see also DiCarlo, 1996; Woodhouse, 1996; and my Chapter IV.3, this volume).

Even within the realms of psychoanalytic orthodoxy we are beginning to see significant stirrings. In her recent book, Joyce McDougall (McDougall, 1995) poignantly calls her Chapter 14 'Beyond psychoanalytic sects in search of a new paradigm', and in it, she writes:

> ... dedicated researchers in every field tend to find what they are seeking in order to confirm their theories .... We discover only what our theories permit us to find .... Our cherished concepts appear to be continually self-confirming .... It would be presumptuous to imagine that it is our theories that bring about psychic change and symptomatic cure!'
> (1995: 235–6)

And Ian Parker (1995) and his colleagues have recently launched a devastating 'deconstructive' critique of the notion of 'psychopathology', which throws into severe doubt many of the taken-for-granted ideological assumptions of the psychotherapeutic world-view.

In this country the Scientific and Medical Network (which organises the annual Mystics and Scientists Conferences, as well as a host of other conferences and workshops which explore the interpenetration of the scientific and the spiritual-mystical) is at the cutting edge of these exciting new-paradigm developments. And I believe that it is these kinds of perspectives that offer by far the most fruitful avenues for future research in our field, rather than the sterility and soullessness of a positivist world-view which is becoming increasingly discredited in the 'hard', as well as in the social, sciences.

Conclusion

Those who are responsible for the funding of counselling and psychotherapy, steeped as they are in the often unquestioned ideology of modernity and technocratic culture, will very likely fail to be impressed by the arguments expressed in this chapter. Elsewhere (House, 1996; Chapter I.6 this volume), I have discussed at length the preconditions for policy-makers being in a position to question the ideologies that drive their policy-making practices. If recent American experience (Eckert, 1994) is anything to go by, however, where for some years there has been a relentless drive towards ever shorter-term, focused, 'scientifically evaluated' cognitive-behavioural therapeutic approaches, the omens for the future of humanistic person-centred practice are far from encouraging.

I would conclude by saying that as soon as we unquestioningly accept the agenda of the current *Zeitgeist* of 'cost-effectiveness', audit, 'objective' evaluation, management control systems, and all the other leitmotivs of the market economy and cultural system, we immediately do a (quite possibly terminal) violence to the humanistic principles on which our practice is founded. And the supreme irony would be that we end up destroying the very foundational values of the field whose status we are actually endeavouring to elevate through our burgeoning preoccupation with research and evaluation. What a tragedy that would be for all of us.

I realise that I have expressed the 'anti-empiricist' position in stark and uncompromising terms, and at some length; but this is in part because the views I have expressed do not seem to be receiving anything like the attention in our field that I believe they warrant, and that one would expect in a field whose central concern is with open, reflexive, undefended enquiry and understanding. I would welcome a frank and open debate with the proponents of the 'research and evaluation tendency'. Dryden (1994: 194) refers to the stimulation of some 'lengthy debate for the future good of our field', and the foregoing chapter should be seen in this light.

To end with a most apt quotation from Carl Rogers (1955: 260):

> For science too, at its inception, is an 'I–Thou' relationship with the world of perceived objects, just as therapy at its deepest is an 'I–Thou' relationship with a person or persons. And only as a subjective person can I enter either of these relationships.

References

Bromley, D. B. (1990) 'Academic contributions to psychological counselling. 1. A philosophy of science for the study of individual cases', *Counselling Psychology Quarterly*, 3 (3): 299–308.

Castoriadis, C. (1995) 'The new wave of criticism of psychoanalysis', paper presented to 'The End of Psychoanalysis?' conference, University of London Union, Psychoanalytic Forum with Institute of Romance Studies, March.

DiCarlo, R.E. (ed.) (1996) *Towards a New World View*, Edinburgh: Floris Books.

Dryden, W. (1994) 'Possible future trends in counselling and counsellor training: a personal view', *Counselling*, 5 (3): 194–7.

Eckert, P. A. (1994) 'Cost control through quality improvement: the new challenge for psychology', *Professional Psychology: Research and Practice,* 25 (1): 3–8.

Fahy, T. and Wessely, S. (1993) 'Should purchasers pay for psychotherapy?', *British Medical Journal*, 307 (6904): 576–7.

Firth-Cozens, J. (1992) 'The role of early family experiences in the perception of organizational stress: fusing clinical and organizational perspectives', *Journal of Occupational Psychology*, 65 (1): 139–48.

Heron, J. (1996) *Co-operative Inquiry: Research into the Human Condition*, London: Sage.

Hicks, C. and Wheeler, S. (1994) 'Research: an empirical foundation for counselling, training and practice', *Counselling*, 5 (1): 29–31.

Hollway, W. (1989) *Subjectivity and Method in Psychology: Gender, Meaning and Science*, London: Sage.

House, R. (1996) '"Audit-mindedness" in counselling: some underlying dynamics', *British Journal of Guidance and Counselling*, 24 (2): 301–7; reprinted as Chapter I 6, this volume.

Janus, L. (1989) 'The hidden dimension of prenatal and perinatal experience in the works of Freud, Jung and Klein', *International Journal of Prenatal and Perinatal Studies*, 1: 51–65.

Kvale, S. (ed.) (1992) *Psychology and Postmodernism*, London: Sage.

McDougall, J. (1995) *The Many Faces of Eros: A Psychoanalytic Exploration of Human Sexuality*, London: Free Association Books.

Moustakas, C. (1994) *Phenomenological Research Methods*, Thousand Oaks, CA: Sage.

Parker, I., Georgaca, E., Harper, D., McLaughlin, T. and Stowell-Smith, M. (1995) *Deconstructing Psychopathology*, London: Sage.

Rogers, C. R. (1955) 'Persons or science? – a philosophical question', *American Psychologist*, 10: 267–78 (reprinted as Chapter 10 in his *On Becoming a Person*, London: Constable, 1967).

Rowan, J. and Reason, P. (eds) (1981) *Human Inquiry: A Sourcebook for New Paradigm Research*, Chichester: Wiley.

Ryle, A. (1989) *Cognitive-Analytic Therapy*, Chichester: Wiley.

Smith, M. B. (1994) '"Human science" – really! A theme for the future of psychology', *Journal of Humanistic Psychology*, 34 (3): 111–16.

Spinelli, E. (1994) *Demystifying Therapy*, London: Constable; reprinted by PCCS Books, 2005.

Storr, A. (1966/1968). 'The concept of cure', in C. Rycroft (ed.), *Psychoanalysis Observed*, Harmondsworth: Penguin, pp. 50–82.

Thomas, G. (1994) 'A counsellor first ...', *Counselling*, 5 (1): 44–6.

Wasdell, D. (1991) 'The pre- and perinatal ground of capitalism and the free market economy', London: Unit for Research into Changing Institutions (Meridian House, 115 Poplar High Street, London E14). http://www.meridian.org.uk/Resources/PsychoSocial_Analysis/Capitalism/contents.htm

Wasdell, D. (1992) 'In the shadow of accreditation', *Self and Society*, 20 (1): 3–14; reprinted as Chapter I.2, this volume.

Woodhouse, M. B. (1996) *Paradigm Wars: Worldviews for a New Age*, Berkeley, CA: Frog Ltd.

Woolfolk, R. L. and Richardson, F. C. (1984) 'Behavior therapy and the ideology of modernity', *American Psychologist*, 39 (7): 777–86; reprinted in R. House and D Loewenthal (eds) (2008), *Against and For CBT: Towards a Constructive Dialogue?*, Ross-on-Wye: PCCS Books, pp. 52–71.

'Audit-Mindedness' in Counselling: Some Underlying Dynamics 1.6

Richard House

Introduction

In this chapter I offer a polemical critique of the ideology of audit and cost-effectiveness as currently conceptualised in the 'outcomes' field. I then go on to explore the conditions which must be satisfied if the inadequate conception of efficacy that currently holds sway is to be transformed into a more human/e/istic and less unconsciously pathological approach to counselling evaluation. For reasons that will be become clear later, I invite the reader to be aware of her or his own particular emotional response to the ideas and arguments as they unfold in this chapter.

Efficacy, quantity versus quality, and positivism

> Men develop a capacity for mastering the universe and a compulsive preoccupation with what can be predicted, possessed, piled up and counted in order to deny the strength of their early physical and emotional link with the mother.
>
> (Maguire, 1995: 60)

A technocratic mentality is holding increasing sway as technological rationality runs rampant through our culture and institutions; yet comparatively little consideration has been given to the splitting of intuition and feeling from rationality, of quantity from quality, which seem to be defining features of the modern age. A few (all-too-rare) Western philosophers have attempted to heal the split between the intellect and the emotions, between head and heart, that is so endemic and entrenched in the modern Western psyche (see, for example, McGill, 1954;

This chapter was first published in the *British Journal of Guidance and Counselling*, 24 (2), 1996: 277–83.

Solomon, 1976), yet the current *Zeitgeist* is unambiguously one of schizoid splitting, ever-increasing specialisation and *dis*-integration.

Despite our heavy preoccupation with quantity rather than quality, with price rather than value, there is extensive research evidence demonstrating that despite the apparently insatiable human striving for material aggrandisement, rated levels of human subjective satisfaction or happiness by no means necessarily increase correlatively with higher material living standards (House, 1984, Chapter 3). There is now a rapidly growing 'alternative economics' movement which is questioning orthodox, conventional measures of income and wealth in a quite fundamental way, and attempting to incorporate more qualitatively meaningful, sensitive and realistic representations of people's quality of life.

In an extraordinary paper, David Wasdell (1991b) argues forcefully that the defining features of capitalism and the free-market economy can be traced back to the underlying unconscious dynamics of pre- and perinatal developmental traumata. For Wasdell, these underlying dynamics constitute what he terms the 'normal pathology' of human psychological development (Wasdell, 1990), in that they are species-wide, and provide the seedbed for much of our common beliefs, attitudes and behaviours. I do not subscribe to an over-simplistic reductionist and psychologistic view which would crudely reduce culture and ideology to underlying psychodynamic processes, for it seems much more plausible that the specific characteristics of cultures and ideologies are substantially overdetermined. Nonetheless, the argument, based on psychodynamic thinking, for *some* kind of causal link between species-wide psychopathologies of human development on the one hand, and our ideological belief systems on the other, is a logically and evidentially compelling one.

Wasdell's argument can be extended to embrace human psychological development more generally. Thus, the effects of *post-natal* object-relations distortions and deficits, 'wounded child' issues, and the 'deformations of mind' that result therefrom must surely be directly implicated in both the genesis and maintenance of dysfunctional ideological belief systems. To quote Wasdell (1991b: 1) at length,

> Unresolved trauma laid down at any stage of human development drives a subsequent cyclic pattern of repetition. Fixatedly frozen at a point in time representing the last tolerable moment before being overwhelmed

> by hyper-stress, *the person continues to act in the here and now as if facing the next moment of the there and then* .... Where the primary trauma is shared in common, the cyclic psycho-drama is enacted in common. With the common ground collusively denied, the dynamic process is *corporately constructed.* It is supported by symbolism and mythology *and socially reified into an unquestionable ideology.*
> (emphases added)

I believe that the artificial and mechanistic splitting of quantity from quality, and the mindless and disembodied empiricism which sometimes accompanies it, is but a special case of the more general formulation articulated by Wasdell. If it is the case that the splitting of quantity from quality does such violence to the world that it cannot give us anything approaching a realistic description of reality, it follows that we should subject our current 'scientific' methodologies and ontologies (meaning 'beliefs in what exists') to searching and highly critical scrutiny.

From a humanistic or existential standpoint, it can be argued that those aspects of counselling which are most important for client well-being, and which clients themselves repeatedly report as being of central import, are *inherently and in principle unquantifiable* (Spinelli, 1994) – factors like existential aliveness, the quest for personal identity, spiritual well-being, the enhanced meaningfulness of lived experience, and the experience of being loved, for example. Storr (1968: 76) has written that 'it is love which really heals the patient'. And if this is so (House, 1995b), then the technique-oriented approaches of 'scientifically based' evaluation (of which cognitive-behavioural approaches are currently the crowning glory) may well substantially miss the point in their attempts 'objectively' to measure therapeutic outcomes purely in terms of measurable variables such as symptom removal and the like. It simply makes no sense to evaluate humanistic, dynamic or existential counselling in terms of symptom modification or removal alone.

Those commentators who insist upon 'symptom removal' as the universal criterion of counselling efficacy (e.g. Fahy and Wessely, 1993) are making the quite unwarranted assumption that *their* world-view of what constitutes successful therapeutic change has some kind of universal scientifically based legitimacy, rather than being just one (highly partial and unavoidably ideological) way of apprehending the world. Storr (1968: 51) writes that:

> the exploration of … symptoms inevitably leads on to a consideration of *the whole person*, his development, temperament, and character structure …. [A]bolition of [a] single symptom … even if this were possible, would not relieve the patient of the bulk of her emotional problems. *The same is true of by far the majority of neurotic symptoms.*
> (p. 56, emphases added)

And later, 'the term "cure" is … meaningless when we come to consider the manifold problems of the human condition, and the difficulties we all have in living' (p. 82). And in similar vein, Donald Winnicott (1986: 120) writes that 'In terms of society's sickness, the care-cure may be of more importance in the world even than the remedy-cure, and all the diagnosis and prevention that goes with what is usually called a scientific approach'.

To the extent that the prevailing *Zeitgeist* and its associated methodologies are preoccupied with quantification and measurability, symptom removal and mechanistic conceptions of the person more generally, then it is arguable that those methodologies will quite possibly yield results, lead to policy prescriptions and feed ideologies whose values are totally antithetical to the development of the truly human(e) society which, I assume, we all so long for.

Lather (1992) outlines a postmodernist critique of the human sciences (and of psychology in particular): 'scientific thought is now an archaic mode of consciousness' and 'truth is viewed as at least as rhetorical as it is procedural' (p. 89). A new 'model' of science is beginning to emerge, in which:

> Binary either/or positions are being replaced by a both/and logic that deconstructs the ground of both reductionist objectivism and transcendental dialectics. Linearity and teleology are being supplanted by chaos models of non-linearity and an emphasis on historical contingency. Power is assumed to permeate all aspects of our efforts to know, and language is theorised as constitutive rather than representational, a matrix of enabling and constraining boundaries rather than a mirror.
> (Ibid.: 90)

The positivist model of science is thus coming under increasing criticism from a variety of quarters (House, 1997 [Chapter I.5, this volume]), even from within the physical sciences themselves, and has long since been discredited in the 'philosophy of social science' literature (e.g. Keat and Urry, 1975). The positivist approach to 'scientific' evaluation adopts an extremely limited stance on what a scientific research procedure might actually consist in. Recently, the psychoanalyst Cornelius Castoriadis (1995) has persuasively shown that positivist methodologies which emphasise the cannons of replicability, predictability, substitutability and falsification are *in principle* quite inappropriate for studying and understanding the human psyche and the therapeutic change process. Thus, for example, the phenomena of paradox, overdetermination, contradiction, both/and logic and dialectical reasoning describe aspects of human experience which a positivist ontology, constricted as it is within the confines of its Aristotelian-logical structure, is quite incapable of encompassing.

A more pluralistic approach to scientific investigation is open to a range of perspectives, and there is a substantial literature on qualitative methodologies which attempt to respond to at least some of the shortcomings of positivist and empiricist approaches (e.g. Rowan and Reason, 1981; Moustakas, 1994). So what are the implications of these arguments for the policy-making process? How can we even begin to integrate what is so deeply personal with the political process?

Policy-making, change and the dynamics of pain and victimhood

> Certain social and cultural developments ... have weakened our capacities for working through the processes of psychological separation, and have rendered people more prone to seek regressive solutions to the pains of life.
>
> (Richards, 1994: 16, citing Lasch, 1979)

How, then, might the attitudes of policy-makers change such that they are able to 'hear' and be influenced by these arguments? My answer to this question is, perhaps, sobering and far from optimistic. For just as, in the process of psychotherapeutic change, I believe that an experiential, deeper-level shift in 'the self' must occur *before* the ideologies and belief systems which are founded upon that deeper self can change in any sustainable way, just so, it is only when policy-makers discover a far greater capacity for an open, non-defensive self-awareness of the deep unconscious forces that underlie their beliefs, attitudes and behaviours that any meaningful changes of the kind advocated in this chapter can take place.

The cognitive level of human beingness, with its associated belief systems and ideologies, far from being independent of, or even relatively autonomous from, the person, is, I believe, founded upon, informed by and *indissolubly linked with the whole person* – by which I mean body and spirit, feelings and emotions. It follows that any approach to attitude change which focuses purely on the cognitive-intellectual level, and confines itself to 'cognitive restructuring' alone, can give no guarantee of lasting, sustainable change. And to face the full reality of personhood and being human inevitably entails engaging with our deepest pain and betrayals in our earliest object relationships.

Scott Peck has recently written that 'much disease is actually the result of the attempt to avoid the necessary pain of living … most disease may best be defined as a failure of the healing process' (Peck, 1993: 17). If it is true that the existence of pathological belief systems is substantially the result of our extreme resistance to facing the unavoidable pain of living, then it is only by addressing directly and experientially integrating our unresolved pain (whether it be pre-, peri- or post-natal) that we will be able to evolve towards a more healthy, integrated human polity and society.

What Jill Hall has recently called 'the archetype of victimhood' in her tellingly titled book, *The Reluctant Adult* (Hall, 1993), is surely a central feature of Peck's 'necessary pain of living'. The experience of being a victim, and the desperate attempt to avoid it, seem to foment distortions of life at all levels, both within the individual person her/himself ('organic' disease, dysfunctional behaviour and belief systems, unhappy and destructive relationships, and so on), right up to the macro, societal level, in our institutions (Menzies Lyth, 1988); culture (Alford, 1989); politics and international relations (Wasdell, 1991a); the operation of global capitalism (Wasdell, 1991b); the environmental crisis (Wasdell, 1991a), and so on.

From a humanistic and depth-psychological standpoint, the task of changing our dysfunctional belief systems is unavoidably experiential in nature. It is only when we have been able fully to face up to and integrate our own deeply personal 'necessary pain of living', and to transcend our deeply entrenched tendency to avoid, repress and deny our pain, that there can be hope for a sustainable future for our species (Grof, 1988).

Conclusion: implications for practice

> There can easily be a smell of grandiosity about the idea of a [cultural critic] .... It is not on the whole favourable to making an effective intervention in debates in the public sphere to have as a major premise that, to put it crudely, we are living in a madhouse.
>
> (Richards, 1994: 22, 160)

It is crucial to consider the constraints that are likely to be encountered by anyone attempting to raise the questions addressed above in their working environments. The fundamental point here is that there will tend to be enormous resistance to these ideas, both at the individual and the institutional level, precisely because they touch the deepest, most vulnerable and potentially most shaming places in all of us.

Wasdell (1989) argues that there is a 'social transference' reaction to the psycho-social analyst, such that there is a desperate attempt to repair the breach in the social defences occasioned by the psycho-social analyst's analytic breakthrough, with the analyst being identified with the repressed precipitating traumata which generated the now deeply repressed and denied psychotic levels of anxiety, against which the defences of the social system were subsequently reified (p. 3). In other words, the denied elements of the 'common unconscious' are projected on to the psycho-social analyst, and progress in the psycho-social field tends to be 'slow, painstaking and exhausting' (p. 4).

The taking of an awareness of these questions into our work cannot but help have an effect in raising the general level of understanding of these crucial issues, and at least as important is that we practitioners make an ongoing and open-ended personal commitment to work with *our own* 'reluctance to become adults' and 'psychic pain of living', such that we minimise the extent to which those with whom we relate in our professional and personal lives are constrained in becoming aware of these issues by *our own* resistance to integrating this most difficult and challenging material.

I am aware that I have risked 'the smell of grandiosity' by setting out the foregoing arguments in such stark terms. Yet as all of us who have explored our personal histories in therapeutic settings will surely testify, the 'work' of fully facing and integrating the reality of our deepest pain and betrayals is a hugely challenging task, and one which is at times subject to the most intractable denial, evasion and resistance. The task of our individually and collectively evolving towards a world in which policy-makers, managers and researchers are able to make 'healthy' decisions and adopt fully humanistic methodologies, rather than perpetrating ideological actings-out from unconscious and repressed psychopathology, is indeed an enormously daunting one.

References

Alford, C. F. (1989) *Melanie Klein and Critical Social Theory: An Account of Politics, Art, and Reason Based on Her Psychoanalytic Theory*, New Haven, CT: Yale University Press.

Castoriadis, C. (1995) 'The new wave of criticism of psychoanalysis', paper presented to 'The End of Psychoanalysis?' conference, University of London Union, Psychoanalytic Forum with Institute of Romance Studies, 25–6 March.

Fahy, T. and Wessely, S. (1993) 'Should purchasers pay for psychotherapy?', *British Medical Journal*, 307 (4 September): 576–7.

Grof, S. (1988) 'Modern consciousness research and human survival', in S. Grof (ed.), *Human Survival and Consciousness Evolution,* New York: State University of New York Press, pp. 57–79.

Hall, J. (1993) *The Reluctant Adult: An Exploration of Choice,* Bridport: Prism Press.

House, R. (1984) *The Geography of Public Finance in the UK: Conventional and Radical Formulations*, Norwich: unpublished Ph.D. thesis, University of East Anglia.

House, R. (1995a) Review of Hall, 1993, *Self and Society,* 23 (1): 52–3.

House, R. (1995b) 'Love, intimacy and therapeutic change', *Self and Society*, 24 (1): 21–6.

House, R. (1997) 'The dynamics of professionalisation: a personal view of counselling research', *Counselling,* 8 (3): 200–4; reprinted as Chapter I.5, this volume.

Keat, R. and Urry, J. (1975) *Social Theory as Science*, London: Routledge & Kegan Paul.

Lasch, C. (1979) *The Culture of Narcissism*, New York: Norton.

Lather, P. (1992) 'Postmodernism and the human sciences', in S. Kvale (ed.) , *Psychology and Postmodernism*, London: Sage, pp. 88–109.

McGill, V. J. (1954) *Emotions and Reason,* Springfield, IL: Charles C.Thomas.

Maguire, M. (1995) *Men, Women, Passion and Power: Gender Issues in Psychotherapy,* London: Routledge.

Menzies Lyth, I. (1988) *Containing Anxiety in Institutions: Selected Essays, Volume 1*, London: Free Association Books.

Moustakas, C. (1994) *Phenomenological Research Methods*, Thousand Oaks, CA: Sage.

Peck, M. S. (1993) 'Salvation and suffering: the ambiguity of pain and disease', *Human Potential*, Summer: 15, 17, 24–6.

Richards, B. (1994) *Disciplines of Delight: The Psychoanalysis of Popular Culture*, London: Free Association Books.

Rowan, J. and Reason, P. (eds) (1981) *Human Inquiry: A Sourcebook for New Paradigm Research*, Chichester: John Wiley.

Solomon, R. C. (1976) *The Passions: Emotions and the Meaning of Life*, Notre Dame, IN: University of Notre Dame Press.

Spinelli, E. (1994) *Demystifying Therapy*, London: Constable; reprinted by PCCS Books, 2005.

Storr, A. (1966/1968) 'The concept of cure', in C. Rycroft (ed.), *Psychoanalysis Observed*, Harmondsworth: Penguin, pp. 50–82.

Wasdell, D. (1989) 'Constraints encountered in the conduct of psycho-social analysis', London: Unit for Research into Changing Institutions [Meridian House, 115 Poplar High Street, London E14]. http://www.meridian.org.uk/Resources/PsychoSocial_Analysis/Constraints.htm

Wasdell, D. (1990) 'The roots of the common unconscious', London: Unit for Research into Changing Institutions, Meridian Monographs, 1. http://www.meridian.org.uk/_PDFs/Roots.pdf

Wasdell, D. (1991a) 'The psychodynamics of war and religion', London: Unit for Research into Changing Institutions. http://www.meridian.org.uk/Resources/PsychoSocial_Analysis/WandR2/index.htm

Wasdell, D. (1991) 'The pre- and perinatal ground of capitalism and the free market economy', London: Unit for Research into Changing Institutions (Meridian House, 115 Poplar High Street, London E14). http://www.meridian.org.uk/Resources/PsychoSocial_Analysis/Capitalism/contents.htm

Winnicott, D. W. (1986) 'Cure', in *Home is Where We Start From: Essays by a Psychoanalyst*, Harmondsworth: Penguin, pp.112–20.

A Case to Answer | 7

Richard Mowbray

All that is necessary for evil to triumph is for good men to do nothing.
(Edmund Burke [attributed])

Introduction

Following the 1993 transformation of what had been billed as an annual series of 'conferences' into the impressively entitled UK Council for Psychotherapy (UKCP), a fatalistic malaise seemed to descend upon the world of psychotherapy and associated activities in the UK. Given the prevailing wisdom that statutory registration was inevitably coming, sooner or later, not least to comply with forthcoming EC requirements, whether they liked the idea or not, training organisations and practitioners scrambled for a place on the soon departing 'registration express' – all aboard!

However, for those who were not too deeply mesmerised, there were also two significant signs of active dissent to this scramble: The announcement and subsequent publication of *The Case Against Psychotherapy Registration* (Mowbray, 1995) and the formation of the Independent Practitioners Network (IPN).

The oppositional stance evident in the title of *The Case Against Psychotherapy Registration* and some but not all of its content was deliberately explicit – the idea that a 'case against' might exist at all was in itself a novelty at the time. Opposition to registration is not to my mind 'negative', as some have maintained. As indicated by the subtitle of the book, *A Conservation Issue for the Human Potential Movement*, I personally see opposition to the register-building activities of UKCP, BAC/UKRC, BPS, BCP et al. as being the equivalent of an ecologically aware resistance – a Greenpeace-type action to preserve part of an old growth forest rather than merely engaging in a debate about what type of structure should be built on the 'clear-cut' site, whilst the clearing continues.

Although the development of these registers is usually presented as virtuous and believed to be so by many, the collective action involved in these moves does not respect a need for evidence of benefit. It is not in fact rooted in altruism, truth or love, and Burke's admonishment fits the bill.

Assumptions challenged

I think it is fair to say that since publication of *The Case Against Psychotherapy Registration* (referred to hereinafter as *The Case*), the ground of awareness has shifted, and assumptions about the benefits of professionalisation and registration in the fields of counselling, psychotherapy, psychology and personal growth in the UK, which were formerly taken for granted, are now matters for debate, discussion and substantiation. These formerly unassessed assumptions can be summarised as the assumption of *inevitability*, the assumption of *necessity*, the assumption of *benefit* and the assumption of *preference*:

a. The assumption of *inevitability*
The assumption of inevitability is in many ways the most powerful of these assumptions, since it has the capacity to become self-fulfilling – misinformation can have its day and get a bandwagon under way. Professor Clyde Miller, founder of the Institute of Propaganda Analysis, has 'bandwagon' as his seventh principle of propaganda: 'Everybody is doing it and so should you'. This assumption is derived in part from the following contributory assumptions:

1. That statutory registration is required to meet requirements of European law.
2. That the impetus for statutory registration originates from within governments.

b. The assumption of *necessity*
The assumption that the incidence of harm resulting from these occupations is so large as to warrant remedial action.
Even though the matter of registration is now subject to debate, much of the argument is downstream of this particular assumption. That is, it proceeds on the basis of 'something must be done, but

what?', rather than starting from the question 'does something need to be done?'. Because some instances of harm can be cited, it has been taken for granted that the extent of risk involved is so high that something ought to be done about it. A less rational assumption that may also be implicit is that any degree of risk is unacceptable. Like it or not, however, a degree of risk is inherent in human activity – being alive is a risky business, and though we might aspire to it, a perfectly safe and predictable life would in all probability make for a life not worth living.

c. The assumption of *benefit*
The assumption that professionalisation protects the public and is therefore a good thing.

d. The assumption of *preference*
The assumption that, assuming there is an unmet need for public protection, professionalisation is the best way of providing it. That is, if additional measures are needed to provide an adequate level of client protection, then professionalisation is preferable to the other means available.

Since publication of *The Case* in 1995, evidence that challenges all of the above assumptions is now readily available for those who are willing to acquaint themselves with it. The book has been widely received, provoking debate and controversy and inspiring others to take action in defence of the UK's uniquely open milieu.[1] Two years on, despite some 'huffing and puffing' and resort to personal invective, the arguments and evidence I assembled have not been refuted nor even credibly challenged.[2] Moreover, a number of other books have since emerged (including the current volume) which, from differing perspectives, add further weight to the view that registration and professionalisation are not necessarily beneficial for the fields of counselling, psychotherapy, psychology or personal growth.[3]

Whether the organisations concerned (and their registrants – whose fees after all enable the whole process of registration) are willing to seriously address the uncomfortable information now readily available *and to act accordingly* is another matter which I will address below.

The elusive case for registration

Whilst the issue of registration may now be up for debate, whether by way of response to *The Case* or otherwise, no 'case for' of comparable cohesiveness has yet been made by any of the organisations currently pursuing registration in the UK (or elsewhere for that matter).

For example, in a letter to *Self & Society*, Digby Tantam, Chair of UKCP, argues a case for registration (albeit stating that his comments are not UKCP official policy) (Tantam, 1996: 39); however, the arguments that Tantam puts forward in favour of registration are similar to those that I have comprehensively addressed in *The Case* and found to be without much substance when applied to fields such as psychotherapy. There is the familiar citing of other professions as precedents and the presumption of their altruistic motivations. There is the argument that if gas boiler installers are registered, why not psychotherapists? There is a harking back to the Sieghart Report (Sieghart, 1978) for validity, and there is the assumption that the customers of psychotherapists are particularly vulnerable to exploitation and that registration will enhance their protection. He acknowledges that UKCP has no definition of psychotherapy as yet, but regards this as a virtue rather than a problem.

Alan Law, Registrar of the UKRC, tries to justify the establishment of that register with an array of the usual catch phrases designed to evoke the assumptions of necessity and benefit: 'protect the public', 'anyone can call themselves a counsellor', 'meet high standards', 'the hallmark', etc. However, as usual no substantiation is provided (Law, 1997: 9–11).

No doubt the organisations concerned are endeavouring to gather evidence to support their positions in favour of registration. However, such evidence would be intended to justify positions already adopted and structures already created, just as in 1982 a 'Task Force' of the American Psychological Association deemed it imperative to 'assemble a body of persuasive evidence' to justify the educational and training prerequisites for practice that were *already* being required of licensed psychologists (Dawes, 1994: 106). Such *ex post facto* evidence should therefore be regarded with appropriate circumspection since the organisations are 'rolling merrily along in the absence of such findings' (ibid.: 108–9).[4]

In the interests of providing an aid to scrutinising any more substantial arguments and evidence which the organisations involved may subsequently present, there follows an outline of what would constitute the essential elements of a *valid* case in favour of registration.

A well-substantiated case in favour of statutory registration in this area would in essence amount to a validation of the argument that registration would be good for the client – the 'protection of the public' argument. I take it for granted that a sound 'case for' should be ethical in nature – that is, arguments based on practitioner self-interest would be inadmissible in this regard. This would require a thoroughgoing refutation of the material presented in *The Case* and elsewhere,[5] most of which is as applicable to counselling as to psychotherapy as to psychology since there is no accepted unambiguous dividing line between them.

Firstly, the evidence for the negative side effects of registration in general would need to be refuted; or if the reality of these are accepted, then the 'case for' would need to demonstrate why these harmful side effects of registration in general would be outweighed by the alleged benefits in the particular cases of counselling, psychology, psychotherapy or personal growth.

It would also need to be shown that it is appropriate to regard counselling and psychotherapy as 'professions'. Typically, a member of the professions is someone who has the status of an expert agent acting on behalf of a client, and whose effectiveness derives from an elaborated body of professional knowledge. In the case of counselling and psychotherapy this does not seem to be so. Practitioner effectiveness here seems to be more a function of personal qualities, particularly the ability to form a working alliance with the client.

In the case of statutory registration, the activity for which legal privilege is being sought would also need to be defined in a way that is sufficiently precise to make sense in a court of law. In particular, the limits of that legal privilege would need to be explicitly outlined. Avoidance of this process by only pursuing a legal protection of title at the outset will not do because of the ease with which such a basis for registration may be converted to the control of practice at a later date, once any political opposition has died down (Hogan, 1979: 371).

It is difficult to draw any clear-cut boundaries between counselling, psychotherapy, psychology and personal growth work. This is an indication that none of these occupations are really 'mature' in a professional sense and should therefore be left to evolve rather than be inappropriately structured by the establishment of legally significant but undefined titles.

Proof of benefit of the proposed prerequisites for registration would need to be presented. For example, where stringent training requirements such as long courses with substantial academic content are demanded, I would like to see evidence that this is a necessity for basic competence – that is, the level of competence necessary to ensure a reasonable level of safety. Endeavours to establish standards beyond that level, whether or not they are proven to enhance competence, are not really a matter for legislative involvement that has protection of the public as its rationale.

Empirical evidence of the harmful impact of counselling, psychology or psychotherapy would need to be presented. All too often this matter is addressed in the media and elsewhere by reference to anecdotal evidence – the presentation of individual instances of harm, whereas the crucial issue is the incidence and severity of harm and hence the risk factors.

Resources for the making and administration of laws are not unlimited. In order to justify the notion that counselling and psychotherapy et al. deserve special legislation, it would need to be shown that the degree of risk for the public is significantly greater than that involved in the many other activities not regulated by specific legislation.

Also, a causal relationship between the practice of counseling, psychology or psychotherapy and the harm in question would need to be established. In the light of the indefinite limits of the area of activity in counselling and similar occupations, it is invalid to assume that all those who seek such services are necessarily vulnerable individuals. This assumption is particularly difficult to endorse if, as at present, work of a personal growth nature is not clearly differentiated from that of a remedial nature (see 'Too Vulnerable to Choose?', Chapter I.3 of this volume).

Evidence would also need to be presented which indicates that registered/licensed practitioners are on average significantly less harmful to clients than those who are not registered, given that, as Daniel Hogan has put it: '… [an] array of horror stories could easily be assembled about highly credentialed psychiatrists and psychologists, all of them licensed' (quoted in *The Case*: 105). This is particularly important since, as I argue in Chapter I.3 of this volume, there is good reason to believe that in this area of activity at least, registration/licensing actually *increase* the risk of harm.

Registration/licensing systems applicable to this area are common in other countries, but this prevalence does not in itself constitute sound evidence of their publicly beneficial nature. This is the more so, given the well-documented history of how professions have acted as special interest groups, and the generally poor record of effectiveness of their disciplinary procedures as documented in my book. Ironically, the current situation for the activities in question under UK law provides one of the few remaining unlicensed working environments still available to provide the basis for a comparative study.

In sum, in order to support a sound case for professional registration in this area, it would need to be shown that there is a significant incidence, severity and hence risk of harm from the practice of counselling, psychotherapy and associated occupations. It would need to be demonstrated that this risk is ascribable to factors that can be causally related to criteria which are measurable by a licensing/registration system (such as length of training). It would also need to be shown that statutory registration would ameliorate this situation and would be the least harmful way of doing so.

Voluntary registers and *de facto* power

One approach to the absence of a sound case for the pursuit of statutory registration is to evade the whole issue. Some seek relief from the need to present such a case by adopting a position of support for and participation in 'voluntary registration' whilst claiming to be opposed to statutory registration. This is a position that has been adopted by the Association of Humanistic Psychology Practitioners (AHPP) to justify their involvement in UKCP (and, they hope, in UKRC) since the publication of *The Case* (*Self and Society*, 1997: 50). The AHPP Board claims to have maintained this position all along. However there seems to be little evidence to support that view and plenty to the contrary (Kalisch, 1997: 49).

The above stance does not concur with the history nor the official policy of the registering bodies. UKCP officers, at least, have been explicit about their statutory ambitions.[6] However, pending the hoped-for arrival of political circumstances which offer an opportunity to establish the statutory basis to which they aspire, these 'therapy bureaucracies' can be expected to focus their resources on endeavouring to establish their voluntary registers as the *de facto* equivalent of the statutory. The establishment of such voluntary registers cannot be assumed to be of a benign nature, since many of the arguments against statutory registers apply to the voluntary variety as well. Although lacking the force of law, so-called 'voluntary' registers can nevertheless have a major impact, so much so that in situations where they are able to establish a degree of monopoly power in the market, a situation of *de facto* registration can occur. Job advertisements, for example, may specify accreditation and membership of such registers as required qualifications. The addition here of statutory privilege amounts to the legal cherry on a pre-existing cake of dominance. Even in countries which do have statutory controls, *de facto* powers may be the main way in which restraint of trade is actually effected and dominance exerted (*The Case*: 146–7).

These voluntary registers are usually intended to be precursors of a statutory form (indeed, the notion of a register intended to remain 'voluntary' is something of a contradiction in terms). The organisational titles that are chosen also usually reflect the statutory aspiration. The United Kingdom Council for Psychotherapy and the United Kingdom Register of Counsellors sound like national, official bodies which are fully representative even if they are not, and less well-informed members of the public may be misled into believing that they are so.

The prospect that such registers may eventually receive the statutory backing they seek tends to undermine any sense of voluntariness that practitioners may feel about participation in them. This may be reinforced by bouts of misinformation about the inevitability of legislation. In consequence, practitioners frequently act on the basis of a fear of being 'left out in the cold' and adopt an 'insurance' mentality. Meanwhile, their fees finance the activities of the registering organisations, including campaigning for legislation.

Like statutory registration, nationally oriented voluntary registers are held out as being systems established for the public good, as ways to foster practitioner competence and client protection. Those who participate in such registers are in essence making a statement of 'us not them'. To employing agencies, the message is: 'employ us, not them'; to clients: 'work with us, not them' and 'you're safer with us than them'.

This creates its own momentum. Through gaining a dominant position in the marketplace, such organisations may be able to establish the requirements for practice that they favour. These do not necessarily correlate with practitioner competence. The market then becomes distorted through the introduction of misleading factors into the selection of practitioners. The health service and other employing agencies, insurance agencies and private clients may be persuaded to accept these 'false qualifications' as necessary prerequisites for practice when they may have very little validity as such.

As to the disciplinary systems of such voluntary registers, I do not believe they will be any more effective than professional disciplinary procedures have been shown to be, and for the same reasons, since the same factors apply – professional disciplinary action usually correlates more with the impact of the offence on the public image of the profession than with the ethical salience of the charge (*The Case*: 80–4).[7] As the current UKCP Chair admits: 'removing some, but not too many, names [from our register] will be what convinces people, unfortunately' (Tantam 1995: 2). If the evidential and ethical underpinnings of the whole enterprise are deeply flawed, one can hardly expect justice to win the day in its 'courts of correction'.

Like a voluntary roll call, a voluntary register that is intended to stay voluntary is something of a nonsense. Moreover, 'voluntary' is not really voluntary if a prospect of statutory endorsement still exists and where oligopolistic structuring of the market is under way, as at present. Just as title protection is frequently the thin end of the wedge for a practice act, so 'voluntary' registration serves as the thin end for an involuntary situation in a similar fashion.

This process of a 'voluntary' monopolistic 'takeover' is also being reinforced by the attempted creation of European-level equivalents. Thus, the Training Standards Committee of the European Association for Psychotherapy (EAP) is sponsoring the development of a European Certificate of Psychotherapy (ECP), a qualification with requirements which again bear little relationship to what is known about the bases of practitioner effectiveness.[8]

A stance in favour of voluntary but opposed to statutory registration such as adopted by AHPP and other supporters of UKCP and BAC, in lieu of a substantiated case in favour of statutory registration, is not therefore a position with much validity, and does not preclude an obligation on the part of these organisations and their participants to address the case against registration.

Walk your talk

The question of registration may now be subject to debate, though as we have seen, the register-building organisations concerned have not presented a substantiated case to support their actions. More particularly, *they have not seen fit to suspend the development of their registers until they can be justified on the basis of sound knowledge*. Despite their claims to the promotion of ethical practice, they do not appear to regard their own actions as being contingent on a need for ethical and evidential validation. I regard it as unethical for them to continue to establish registers, even so-called 'voluntary' ones, without a sound basis for doing so, more particularly in view of the evidence that the public interest is actually harmed thereby (see *The Case*). In this light, both participation in voluntary registration and the pursuit of statutory registration are unethical, and the rationales used as justification are at best misguided, at worst fraudulent.

Where organisational and individual vested interests are concerned, it is unwise to underestimate the capacity to ignore unpalatable information which threatens them. With power and financial well-being at stake, or in order to avoid cognitive dissonance and anxiety, ignorance may well be regarded as bliss.[9] Fortunately, however, cognitive serenity is not entirely within the gift of those interests since, now that the assumptive basis for their actions has been publicly challenged, the act of ignoring such information is visible to third parties, not least the clients – whose benefit registration is supposed to serve – and the government.

If the actions of the registering bodies are seen by such third parties not to be founded on sound evidence nor graced with ethical justification and intellectual respectability, the credibility of these would-be professions is at risk. Where a non-ethical basis is revealed for actions that purport to be rooted in ethics, cries of 'hypocrisy!' would not go amiss.

As and when clients and the public at large wake up to the fact that the rush to register is not in fact for their benefit, the credibility of individual registrants is also on the line through their participation in, and funding of, the process. After all, it is the fees of registrants (and their training organisations) which provide much of the economic basis for the registering bodies, including funds for political lobbying for statutory registration. For the individual practitioner, 'everybody is doing it', and fears of exclusion and economic detriment may justify expedient participation, but such justifications can hardly be paraded before clients as an altruistic and ethically sound rationale for being a registrant. At the very least, the common expectation that 'therapists' as a group have 'worked through their stuff' and are 'more together' and therefore less prey to the usual temptations than the rest of us, will be revealed to be illusory.

This is a 'real life' challenge for practitioners which exposes to public scrutiny, personal qualities – or their absence – which may not be readily apparent to clients in the seclusion of the session room. David

Kalisch has compared this situation to a 'giant Milgram-style experiment into practitioner compliance' (Kalisch, 1996: 48). This is not an insignificant matter, given the importance of the personal qualities of the practitioner in the outcome of work with clients. For human potential practitioners in particular, this situation presents an especially jarring incongruity and potential for shame. The prospect of 'humanistic warriors' (O'Hara, quoted in Rowan, 1995a: 39) running for cover while keeping their heads down and practising CMA[10] does not make for a very pretty sight.

A 'health professions' act?

The election of a new Labour government in May 1997, with an overwhelming majority, has altered the political prospects for registration in the UK, but in ways which at the time of writing are still unclear. Whether or not the Blair government will be more amenable to statutory aspirations on the part of BPS, UKCP, BCP and UKRC remains to be seen. Early signs are that the new government will be no more enthusiastic about the statutory endorsement of their stand-alone registers than was the previous administration.[11] However, no doubt these organisations will be undertaking fresh lobbying initiatives in any event, meanwhile promoting the status of their 'voluntary' registers as described above.

It also remains to be seen whether the new government will pick up on the review the Professions Supplementary to Medicine Act 1960 initiated by the previous government (J. M. Consulting Ltd., 1996). Any replacement for this Act might provide an opportunity for the inclusion of psychology, counselling and psychotherapy.

Although the Professions Supplementary to Medicine Act has hitherto only applied to certain occupations such as chiropody within the context of the NHS, the review proposals involve replacing it with a 'health professions act' that not only substitutes a common umbrella register for the individual ones that currently exist, but also extends its coverage to those other 'health professions' whose inclusion can be justified on the grounds of public protection – with an expectation that the number of relevant professions will grow (ibid.).

It was also proposed that 'common titles' should be regulated by the new act, thus bringing the private as well as the public sector under its provisions (ibid.).

The status of a 'profession supplementary to medicine' (rejigged as a 'health profession') and a place under the common umbrella may not be as appealing as an autonomous statutory register to those who favour the professionalisation of counselling and psychotherapy, but it may be what government is willing to consider. The British Psychological Society, for example, was apparently invited by the last administration to examine this as an alternative to the stand-alone statutory register for psychologists to which it aspires.

Bad laws

The practice of counselling, psychotherapy, psychology or personal growth is already subject to those general laws, such as laws of contract and breach of confidence, that regulate the provision of any service. Moreover, improvements in general consumer legislation could provide benefit here as elsewhere (see 'Too Vulnerable to Choose?', Chapter I.3 of this volume). I have argued in *The Case* that statutory professional regulation of such occupations cannot be justified on the grounds of client protection, and would actually be detrimental rather than beneficial. This conclusion is as relevant to a 'health professions' act as to stand-alone registers.

Inappropriate legislation and the consequent curtailment of freedom of choice and rights to practise in this 'realm of the psyche' are particularly sensitive issues, given the imprecise boundaries of these activities and their overlap with education and religion as well as medicine. The civil liberties implications may be even greater in the case of a 'health professions' act than with stand-alone registers. If such umbrella legislation takes the form that has appeared elsewhere, the process of parliamentary debate that would be entailed in separately legislating for particular occupations (and consequent opportunity for publicity and objection) can be bypassed once the 'umbrella' legislation has been enacted and decisions to include an occupation may be made quietly at cabinet level or through administrative fiat.[12]

Let us beware, lest whilst pursuing a raising of consciousness we neglect the social freedoms that facilitate it. To return to the words of Edmund Burke, 'Bad laws are the worst sort of tyranny'.

References

BBC1 Television (1996) *Watchdog,* 26 February.

Berger, P. (1997) Letter, *Human Potential* magazine, Spring.

Brown, J. and Mowbray, R. (1997) *The Case Effect: An Annotated Bibliography of Responses, Follow-ups and After-Effects of The Case Against Psychotherapy Registration*, London: Trans Marginal Press.

Dawes, R. M. (1994) *House of Cards: Psychology and Psychotherapy Built on Myth*, New York: Free Press.

Deurzen, E., van and Tantam, D. (1997) 'Developing a European Certificate of Psychotherapy', *International Journal of Psychotherapy*, 2 (1): 93–7.

Hogan, D. (1979) *The Regulation of Psychotherapists*, Cambridge, MA: Ballinger.

Howard, A. (1996) *Challenges to Counselling and Psychotherapy*, London: Macmillan.

J. M. Consulting Ltd (1996) *The Regulation of Health Professions: Report of a Review of the Professions Supplementary to Medicine Act (1960) with Recommendations for New Legislation*, Bristol: J. M. Consulting Ltd.

Jenkins, P. (1997) *Counselling and the Law*, London: Sage.

Kalisch, D. (1996) Letter, *The Therapist*, 3 (3): 46.

Kalisch, D. (1997) Letter, *Self and Society*, 25 (2), May.

Law, A. (1997) 'The United Kingdom Register of Counsellors', *Counselling in Scotland*, June.

Morley, E. (1997) 'Michael Pokorny', *The Psychotherapist* (London: UKCP).

Mowbray, R. (1995) *The Case Against Psychotherapy Registration: A Conservation Issue for the Human Potential Movement*, London: Trans Marginal Press.

Parker, I., Georgaca, E., Harper, D., McLaughlin, T. and Stowell-Smith, M. (1995) *Deconstructing Psychopathology*, London: Sage.

Pokorny, M. (1996) 'Statutory registration – the UKCP response', *The Therapist*, 3 (4).

Rowan, J. (1995a) 'The future of humanistic psychology', *Self and Society*, 23 (4), September.

Rowan, J. (1995b) 'An Open Letter to Richard Mowbray', *Self and Society*, 23 (4): 43–4.

Saks, M. (1995) *Professions and the Public Interest: Medical Power, Altruism and Alternative Medicine*, London: Routledge.

Scott, T. (1996) Review of *The Case Against Psychotherapy Registration, Human Potential* magazine, Spring.

Self and Society (1997) AHPP Board statement to the Editors, 25 (1), March.

Sieghart, P. (1978) *Statutory Registration of Psychotherapists: The Report of a Profession's Joint Working Party*, London: Copyright Paul Sieghart in trust for the professional bodies that composed the working party.

Stone, J. and Matthews J. (1996) *Complementary Medicine and the Law*, Oxford: Oxford University Press.

Tantam, D. (1995) 'Steady as she goes', *The Psychotherapist*, 4, March.
Tantam, D. (1996) Letter, *Self and Society*, 24 (2), May.
Tantam, D. and Zeal, P. (1996) UKCP internal memorandum to analytically oriented sections, London: UKCP, 7 August.

Endnotes

1. For a survey of responses and follow-ups etc. to *The Case*, see Brown and Mowbray, 1997.

2. John Rowan, one of the key architects of the involvement of humanistic psychology in UKCP, was critical of my proposals for SAFAA (Sufficient Available Functioning Adult Autonomy) as one of the criteria for differentiating personal growth work and psychotherapy (see 'Too Vulnerable to Choose?', Chapter I.3 in this volume), but appears to have accepted the rest of the argument (Rowan, 1995b: 43–4).

In a review of *The Case*, Tricia Scott, Board member of the Association of Humanistic Psychology Practitioners (AHPP), referred to the book's opposition to the proposed legislative changes as indicative of an 'unholistic attitude' and endeavoured to characterise me as proposing not only chaos and a 'Thatcherite free market', but also the creation of a 'super-race' (Scott, 1996: 44). In correspondence to *The Therapist* (Vol. 3, No. 4, 1996), which its editors dubbed as 'UKCP – floundering off Iceland?', Michael Pokorny, at that time Chair of the UKCP Registration Board and formerly UKCP's first Chair, made the UKCP's first official public response to *The Case*. Pokorny did his (not very effective) best to cast doubt on the soundness of the book's contents but failed to refute them. Pokorny has been described as "the creator of the UKCP" (Morley, 1997: 3). It has recently been argued that Daniel Hogan's massive four volume work *The Regulation of Psychotherapists*, which was an important source of material for *The Case*, does not have much validity regarding the current debate on the grounds that the field has moved on a long way since the publication of his book in 1979 (Berger, 1997: 13–14). However, this is not so.

The field may have 'moved on' in the UK but it has done so in a way that makes Hogan's conclusions all the more pertinent. Although *The Case* owes a great deal to Hogan's study, I also drew upon numerous other sources, including many of more recent origin. The sort of criteria now being promoted by UKCP et al. as qualifications for practice still lack the support of the 'sound scientific evidence' that Hogan called for, and neither Hogan's book nor my own appear to have been outdated by developments in our knowledge. Hogan's conclusion that psychotherapy should not be regulated through conventional licensing remains valid.

3. Howard (1996), Jenkins (1997), Parker et al. (1995), Saks (1995) and Stone and Matthews (1996) all contain pertinent new material. Although I did not come across it until after the publication of *The Case*, Robyn M. Dawes's *House of Cards* published in 1994 deserves particular mention for its powerful challenge to the already heavily licensed world of US psychology and psychotherapy.

4. Evidence was available but it lead to conclusions which were not what the American Psychological Association wanted to hear. As Robyn Dawes says: 'Why does the American Psychological Association believe that assembling "persuasive evidence" is imperative ...? The reason is not that evidence wasn't assembled, but that the evidence assembled was negative. The body of evidence at the time about psychologists in particular indicated that there was little of any value in their training and experience for their practice ...' (Dawes, 1994: 106).

5. See note 3.

6. See *The Case*.; also: Tantam, 1995 and Tantam and Zeal, 1996.

7. A recent illustration was provided by the BAC's reaction to the BAC membership of Bernard Manning, which was mischievously arranged by the BBC's Watchdog programme (BBC1, 1996). The Bernard Manning/Watchdog saga was a variation on the popular 'just anyone can practise/put up a brass plate' argument for registration, to which an appropriate response is along the lines of: 'yes, but who would actually go to Bernard Manning for counselling?' Despite protestations to the contrary, registration schemes do not generally have a very good record of ensuring the integrity of character of their members (*The Case*).

8. An ECP would involve undergoing 3,000–3,500 hours of training spread over seven years. EAP claims that 'psychotherapy is an independent scientific discipline' but appears to take little notice of the fact that there is little or no scientific evidence of a significant relationship between length of training and psychotherapist effectiveness (see *The Case*, and Dawes, 1994). The EAP Training Standards Committee is co-chaired by Emmy van Deurzen and Digby Tantam, respectively the previous and current Chairs of UKCP and familiar agitators for registration in the UK, now also operating on the European stage in pursuit of the same goal (Deurzen and Tantam, 1997: 93–7).

9. Hogan's *The Regulation of Psychotherapists* was published in 1979, three years before the first of the Rugby Psychotherapy Conferences which eventually transmogrified into UKCP. One would have thought that this book should have been required reading for those involved. Instead, an avoidance of engagement with its contents appears to have taken place. Like Nelson, they 'saw no Hogan'.

10. CMA is apparently a favoured acronym in medical circles for practitioner self-protective actions – 'Cover My Arse'.

11. It appears that the Mental Health Policy Unit of the UK Department of Health, whose advisors received a copy of *The Case*, has taken on board some of the arguments against registration (see the Introduction to this volume).

12. The Canadian province of British Columbia initiated a 'health professions' act in 1990 (see *The Case*, Appendix C).

Part II
Challenging the Basis of Professionalisation

The Myth of Therapist Expertise II.1

Katharine Mair

Psychotherapists of today are in many ways in a similar position to the physicians of 80 years ago. Their patients have faith in their expertise and expect them to say what is wrong and how to put it right. Psychotherapists' understanding of patients' problems and knowledge about how they can be remedied is, however, very much less than their patients imagine. It is also less than therapists imagine. They have been through a training which claims to give them a model by which to understand their patients, and methods with which to treat them. Physician and psychotherapist alike believe in their models and methods because they see them work. I hope to demonstrate that, although psychotherapy can be a valuable means of helping people, its efficacy is not due primarily to the models and methods that it uses (which may be as irrelevant to the patient's problems as the application of leeches was to the curing of a fever 80 years ago), and that too blind a faith in them may actually interfere with the therapist's ability to help his patient. George Bernard Shaw voiced his scepticism of the doctors of his day in his preface to *The Doctor's Dilemma* in 1911. His comments seem appropriate to this argument.

Science and the healer

> I presume nobody will question the existence of a widely spread popular delusion that every doctor is a man of science.
>
> (Shaw, 1911)

Throughout history, communities have had their designated experts in healing. They have been turned to for cure and for counsel in the face of affliction, and their authority has been accepted without question. Perhaps this is because people in distress need relief, not debate. Healing techniques have ranged from the dramatic and public rituals of exorcism to the confidential prescription of a few tablets, or the 'talking cure' of psychotherapy, and always there has been an expectation that the healer will be able to do something that will be effective.

Psychotherapists depend upon this expectation, even when they claim that they are merely enabling their patients to help themselves. They exploit the mystique of the expert healer, often to good effect, but they also assert that their achievements are due to their understanding of how people function and their skill in bringing about specified changes. Psychotherapy, like medicine, is said to be based on knowledge. Perhaps, like the medicine of 80 years ago, its true foundation is on the myth of knowledge.

Science is usually assumed to be rational, objective, value-free and open to disproof. Yet individuals who earn their living by healing must serve the needs of their communities, and must be believed. They must deal with the problems that people bring to them in a way that fits in with their expectations and their values, and they must also be authoritative. When the psychiatrist of a hundred years ago declared that masturbation was a major cause of insanity, he reflected the attitudes of those around him. He also invoked the authority of science. No one asked him to test his hypothesis and it has probably still never been scientifically tested, but because our attitudes have now changed we are certain that it was wrong.

Science enjoys prestige and power, and many psychotherapists have themselves had lengthy scientific educations. They want their efficacy to be based on their ability to relate the complaints of their clients to a body of scientific knowledge, which enables them to understand mental processes and make interventions which bring about change in a predictable way. Above all, they want to understand what is going on.

In their attempts to buttress their work with science, psychotherapists may ignore the findings of the sciences of psychology or medicine in which many of them were educated: for example, that verbal agreement between people may mask divergent thoughts, that memories and even perceptions can be distorted by wishes and expectations, and that these may be further altered in order to agree with others people's judgements; also that apparently inert substances can produce mental and physical changes in people who consume them – the well-known placebo effect. Thus psychotherapists ignore the fact that we do not really know what goes on in anyone else's mind, that people are very suggestible and that we do not understand how some of them manage to get better. These facts are disguised by a variety of elaborate conjectures about mental processes which are presented as hard data.

In presenting themselves as learned experts, psychotherapists stress that the methods they use relate to a theory of human functioning. Although some psychotherapists may sample a variety of theories, searching for the best fit with the story each patient is telling him, others will ruthlessly adapt their patients' stories to fit the one particular theory that they believe in. What is the basis for this belief? Theories of psychotherapy are often based on useful observations of the way people think and act. However, as a school of psychotherapy emerges and is promoted, these observations and conjectures can become extended and elaborated into a self-serving dogma which owes nothing to scientific inquiry.

The search for active ingredients

> Even trained statisticians often fail to appreciate the extent to which statistics are vitiated by the unrecorded assumptions of their interpreters.
> (Shaw, 1911)

The evaluation of psychotherapy is notoriously difficult, and many psychotherapists seem to find it quite unnecessary. However, as a result of a vast amount of work done over more than 40 years, evidence has accumulated of its tendency to be beneficial (Luborsky et al. 1975; Smith, Glass and Miller, 1980), and of some aspects of it being more important than others in bringing this about. Orlinsky and Howard (1986) reviewed 1,100 outcome studies, spanning 35 years, in an attempt to link the various processes in psychotherapy to its outcome. They have been able to point to five factors that seem to be related to a successful outcome of therapy:

1. *The therapeutic contract*: whether the patient was seen promptly and attended all sessions.
2. *Patient participation*: whether the patient was encouraged to take an active role in the therapy.
3. *The therapeutic bond*: whether patient and therapist both felt committed to their roles, were empathic and mutually affirmative.
4. *The patient's self-relatedness*: whether he was open rather than defensive.
5. *Therapeutic realisations*: whether some sort of catharsis or insight occurred during therapy.

None of these factors relates to any of the theories behind the therapy. The most crucial factor, according to Orlinsky and Howard, is the bond that the therapist forms with his patient, which they find more important than the therapist's interventions, since they can only work if the patient is able to be open rather than defensive. They thus support the earlier finding of Rogers, that the most important determinant for successful therapy is that the patient should be able to experience the warmth, empathy and genuineness of his therapist (Rogers, 1957); but unlike Rogers, they do not suggest that these qualities are always both necessary and sufficient for successful therapy.

Some of the assumptions behind Orlinsky and Howard's review have been criticised (Stiles and Shapiro, 1989). Psychotherapy is a lengthy interaction in which it is difficult to separate process from outcome. A patient's active participation and self-relatedness may be seen as outcomes as much as processes, though they may influence further outcomes. More importantly, if therapists gauge their interventions to the patient's need of them (for example, only prescribing as many behavioural tasks as the patient seems to need), then a zero, or even negative, correlation with outcome may mask the effectiveness of these interventions when they are used. Stiles and Shapiro argue that most of the many process–outcome studies, including Orlinsky and Howard's, try to evaluate psychotherapy as they would a drug treatment, assuming that it is possible to isolate and measure the active ingredients and that there is a linear dose–response curve (if it is any good then more should automatically be better). None of these assumptions is valid; the components of psychotherapy are interdependent and patients are not passive recipients of them; patients determine what and how much they get.

It has often been pointed out that people go to a psychotherapist when they feel bad and stay with him until they feel better. The psychotherapist then assumes that he has cured the patient. In this respect he is just like any other healer: overlooking the fact that the patient would probably have got better anyway, and enjoying an unwarranted feeling of power. Like other healers, however, he probably also overlooks the fact that any effect he does have may result not from his actions directly, but from the patient's expectations that his actions will be effective. In other words, the patient's improvement may be due to the placebo effect.

This improvement is sometimes referred to as a non-specific treatment effect, which is misleading, as Grunbaum (1989) has pointed out, because the effect itself may be highly specific. It will usually mimic the expected effects of the treatment and can produce comparable mental and physical changes. For example, placebos (i.e. supposedly inert substances) have been known to produce side effects and even be addictive when substituted for drugs which are known to have these properties (Vinar, 1969; Shapiro and Morris, 1978). When we call a change a placebo effect, what we usually mean is that it was brought about by some means other than that intended in a particular treatment.

The use of intentional placebos to test the efficacy of psychotherapy is another example of the misapplication of drug-trial methods, noted by Stiles and Shapiro (1988). In testing a drug, it is quite appropriate to try to cancel out placebo effects, which may account for an appreciable part of its action. In psychotherapy, however, the expectancy is part of the treatment. The whole point of the placebo-controlled trial is that the patient does not know which treatment is supposed to be active. Therefore he has to be persuaded to engage in an 'inert' therapy in the belief that it may help him. Critelli and Neumann (1984) point out that most of the inane procedures that have so far been adopted as psychotherapy placebos would not fool anyone. They suggest:

> At a minimum, placebo controls should be equivalent to test procedures on all major recognised common factors. These might include induced expectancy of improvement; credibility of rationale; credibility of procedures; demand for improvement; and therapist attention, enthusiasm, effort, perceived belief in treatment procedures, and commitment to client improvement.
>
> (Critelli and Neumann, 1984: 38)

Once one has achieved all that, one has created a new psychotherapy!

How does psychotherapy work?

> Nobody seems yet to discount the effect of substituting attention for neglect in drawing conclusions from the health statistics.
>
> (Shaw, 1911)

There are thought to be hundreds of different versions of psychotherapy, and many of them seem to work equally well. Does this debase the concept of psychotherapy? Is it any more than an inadvertent placebo, and does that matter? Frank (1989) neatly turns the question around by suggesting that the placebo is psychotherapy: 'As a symbolic communication that combats demoralisation by inspiring the patient's hopes for relief, administration of a placebo is a form of psychotherapy. It is therefore not surprising that placebos can provide marked relief in patients who seek psychotherapy.' (p. 97).

As long ago as 1961, when evidence of the similar effectiveness of different therapies was already accumulating, Frank first turned his attention to those factors that they all seemed to have in common (Frank, 1973). He listed four components:

1. The patient feels that the therapist, whom he respects, cares about him.
2. The setting for therapy is designated as a place of healing.
3. Therapy is based on a rationale or myth which includes an explanation of illness, deviancy and normality.
4. A task or procedure is prescribed by the therapy.

Frank pointed out that these components were shared, not only by all psychotherapies, but by all the healing arts, both magical and scientific. Compared to medicine, psychotherapy relied more on learning and was essentially a form of persuasion. The therapeutic rationale was therefore extremely important:

> The rationale of each school of psychotherapy explains the cause of the sufferer's distress, specifies desirable goals for him, and prescribes procedures for attaining them. To be effective, the therapeutic myth must be compatible with the cultural world view shared by the patient and the therapist.
>
> (Frank, 1973: 327)

Frank used the word 'myth' because the rationale for the therapy was not usually subject to disproof by therapeutic failures. This was necessary to protect the therapist's self-esteem, and hence the patient's confidence in him. For Frank the importance of the various rationales and techniques lay not in their specific contents, but in their function. The therapist emerges, in all evaluations of psychotherapy, as crucial to its success. He is not a vehicle for valuable theories of human functioning, rather, the theories are a vehicle for him. They bring him to his patients, confident that he has the expertise to help them, prepared to invade their privacy and willing to offer himself as a model, guide and friend.

Training and psychotherapy

> Bone setters make fortunes under the very noses of our greatest surgeons from educated and wealthy patients, and some of the most successful doctors on the register use quite heretical methods, and have qualified themselves solely for convenience.
>
> (Shaw, 1911)

The opinion of the United Kingdom Council for Psychotherapy seems to be that a recognised training is required in order for psychotherapists to be effective. There does not appear to be much evidence to support this opinion. Hattie et al. (1984) reviewed 43 studies in which 'professionals', defined as those who had undergone a formal clinical training in psychology, psychiatry, social work or nursing, were compared with 'paraprofessionals', educated people with no clinical training, for effectiveness in carrying out a variety of psychotherapeutic treatments. They came to the unpalatable conclusion that the paraprofessionals were, on average, rather more effective.

This review was later criticised by Berman and Norton (1985) because it included studies in which the designation of therapists into the two groups was somewhat arbitrary: some of the people labelled 'professional' had no training in psychology, and some labelled 'paraprofessional' had an academic training which could be considered relevant to psychotherapy. They considered that 11 out of the 43 studies were invalid for these and other methodological reasons. They then re-analysed the data from the remaining 32 studies and found that the advantage of the paraprofessionals was no longer apparent. However, there was no advantage for the professionals either: both groups were judged to be equally effective, both at the end of treatment and at follow up. Differential treatment effects failed to emerge when the various problems treated and methods of treatment were considered separately, and the only variables that distinguished the two groups were the age of the patient (professionals doing better with older and paraprofessionals with younger patients) and the length of the treatment (professionals doing better in shorter and paraprofessionals in longer treatments).

The success of those without professional expertise raises awkward questions about the nature of this expertise. Training gives the therapist a theory, some techniques and a professional status, but how valuable are these when it comes to helping people?

The 'paraprofessionals' in the studies reviewed above seem to have been intelligent people, given permission to try to help others with their problems. They may have had some simple instructions or guidelines, but were not trained to believe in a theory of human functioning and behaviour change: they had no model to guide them. A model simplifies the baffling complexity of all the information coming from an individual and often gives a helpful analogy: it is *as if* he has regressed to an anal level, is suffering primal pain, has learnt faulty habits, has more than one personality or has misconstrued his experiences. Part of the appeal of psychotherapy may lie in its claim to explain behaviour by a model. This has been called a 'higher order framework' (Mahrer, 1989), which is assumed to 'go beyond' or 'delve beneath' the surface confusion. The well-trained therapist may be discouraged from naively addressing himself to the problem that appears to be staring him in the face: 'We believe the tendency of many psychotherapists to ignore the traditional nosological categories and to concentrate simply on the patient's problems is restrictive and may lead to unfortunate consequences' (Beck, Rush, Shaw and Emery, 1979: 23). However, the framework itself is restrictive; it always simplifies, and may at times provide blinkers rather than illumination. Those without training may sometimes be at an advantage in having rather more to look at.

The techniques acquired by training may also be double edged. Recently there seems to have been a proliferation of manuals and 'workbooks' (e.g. Langs, 1985; Beck, et al., 1979; Luborsky, 1984) in which verbatim extracts of therapy sessions play a large part and readers are encouraged to model their responses on those demonstrated. Rogers' claim (1957) about the importance of the therapist's personal qualities of warmth, empathy and genuineness had earlier generated training methods in which students were coached to increase their 'response repertoires' and to simulate these qualities (Truax, Carkhuff and Douds, 1964). Therapy sessions were observed through one-way screens or taped, so that students could learn, not about patients, but about therapists. This assumption that the therapist needs to be told how to respond at every turn continues to be prevalent. Mahrer (1989) insists that detailed operating instructions have always been an essential component of any theory of psychotherapy: 'The theory provided a working manual of conditions-operations-consequences. If a theory did not include this component, the therapist would not know what to do, or when to do what, or what to try to do it for' (Mahrer, 1989: 50).

Perhaps this rehearsal of responses can be another handicap to the trained therapist. Individual psychotherapy is a personal encounter between two people, one of whom has the task of helping the other. An untrained person will draw on a host of perceptions and skills for this task, will adjust instinctively to the individual in front of her and proceed by a hit or miss approach until she finds something that seems to work. This strategy seems to be denied to well-trained therapists, who are expected to follow instructions and model themselves on the masters, rather than to risk being themselves. In addition to this, they have laboriously learnt how to express genuineness, empathy and warmth, only to be left with the embarrassing knowledge that his patient values these qualities only because he assumes that they are spontaneous.

The psychotherapist's dilemma

> There is no harder scientific fact in the world than the fact that belief can be produced in practically unlimited quantity and intensity, without observation or reasoning, and even in defiance of both, by the simple desire to believe, founded on a strong interest in believing.
>
> (Shaw, 1911)

At a time when a growing band of astrologers, spiritualists and 'new age' magicians are capitalising on the demand for guidance and enlightenment, most professionally trained psychotherapists vehemently distance themselves from anything that smacks of charlatanism, ignoring the possibility that unscientific practices may actually help a lot of people. There is a horror of any treatment that is 'just a placebo', however well it works. Thus, psychotherapists, unwilling to resort to trickery, must either restrict their practices to those that they believe to be theoretically sound, or must try to persuade themselves that they understand the mechanism behind those that seem to work.

In trying to maintain their position as scientific experts, psychotherapists are in danger of losing sight of their patients and the world that they live in. Psychotherapy is sometimes spoken of as though it were an end in itself rather than a way of helping people. Patients are used for demonstration purposes and treated according to therapists' need to prove themselves. There are institutions (e.g. the Centre for Cognitive Therapy, the Institute for Rational-Emotive Therapy, the Centre for Personal Construct Psychology) for the promotion of 'own brands' of therapy, where any deviation from the true design is frowned upon. Despite the movement towards integration, reputations are still built, and fortunes made, on distinctiveness. Workshops foster this, as one performer notes: 'Why would anyone come to a workshop in which I get up and say, I'm doing what everybody else is doing?' (Wessler, in Dryden, 1985: 83).

Therapists may try to convince themselves that what they are doing is in the patients' interest, but when patients fail to improve, they are more likely to try another technique or blame their original formulation, than to question whether psychotherapy is what this person really needs. Turning to friends, going to church, getting a job or simply having a rest may be far better solutions for some people. Because of this there are dangers in any ideology, whether based on science or which is frankly magical, that claims to provide solutions to the difficult business of living.

The only things people can ever hope fully to understand are those they have made themselves. Perhaps this is why, as Smail (1987) points out, most models of human behaviour are analogies with man-made objects:

> Even those 'humanistic' therapies which loudly disavow a mechanistic approach, in fact almost without exception treat human beings as if they were mechanically constructed and understandable in terms of analogies with (depending on the history of the particular theory) steam engines, telephone exchanges or digital computers. In order to belong to the 'scientific' club it is virtually out of the question for psychological theorists to characterise people in any other way, and it is impossible to belong to any other club while expecting at the same time to gain professional 'credibility'.
>
> (Smail, 1987: 39)

Doctors have the advantage of being able to observe, to some extent, the workings of the body. They have therefore made some progress since Shaw's day. The workings of the mind will never be open to the same inspection. Psychiatrists (and, regrettably, some psychologists) attempt to understand the mind in terms of its neurological correlates, thus giving themselves a medical model to justify their interventions. Like psychotherapists, they are apt to mistake description for explanation and to reify hypothetical concepts. They thus forget that the 'mental illnesses' that they successfully treat are useful analogies rather than scientific facts. Kendall's (1975) admission that 'In spite of numerous casual claims to the contrary, we have not yet established the existence of any disease entities within our territory' seems likely to remain true, but will not deter the psychiatrist from his activities. Both psychiatrist and psychotherapist are able to use their imperfect and grossly simplified models to good effect, but can become dangerous when they imagine that they have a complete understanding of their patient, and can repair him as they would a faulty engine.

If psychotherapy is seen as just one way of helping troubled people, options are increased for both therapist and patient. The challenge for psychotherapists must be to see whether it is possible to abandon some of their pretensions and still be of use to their patients. Patients and therapists alike are prey to mythical systems. Magical beliefs abound because they impose order and hope on incomprehensible and uncontrollable reality, and psychotherapy can seduce its participants into a collaboration which relieves feelings of helplessness on both sides. There are times when people can be served best by being encouraged to have less faith in experts and more in themselves. The problem is that the advice is more likely to be accepted, and less likely to be given, if it comes from someone whom they consider to be an expert.

> The true doctor is inspired by a hatred of ill-health, and a divine impatience if any waste of vital forces ... his motives in choosing the career of a healer are clearly generous.
>
> (Shaw, 1911)

References

Beck, A. T., Rush, A. J., Shaw, B. F. and Emery, G. (1979) *Cognitive Therapy of Depression,* New York: Guildford Press.

Berman, J. S. and Norton, N. C. (1985) 'Does professional training make a therapist more effective?', *Psychological Bulletin*, 98: 401–7.

Critelli, J. W. and Neumann, K. F. (1984) 'The placebo: a conceptual analysis of a concept in transition', *American Psychologist*, 39: 32–9.

Dryden, W. (1985) *Therapists' Dilemmas*, London: Harper and Row.

Frank, J. D. (1973) *Persuasion and Healing*, 2nd edn, Baltimore, MD: Johns Hopkins University Press.

Frank, J. D. (1989) 'Non-specific aspects of treatment: the view of a psychotherapist', in M. Shepherd and N. Sartorius (eds), *Non- Specific Aspects of Treatment,* Toronto: Hans Huber Publishers, pp. 95–114.

Grunbaum, A. (1989) 'The placebo concept in medicine and psychiatry', in M. Shepherd and N. Sartorius (eds), *Non-Specific Aspects of Treatment,* Toronto: Hans Huber Publishers, pp. 7–38; reprinted from *Psychological Medicine*, 16, 1986: 19–38.

Hattie, J. A. Sharpley, C. F. and Rogers, H. J. (1984) 'Comparative effectiveness of professional and paraprofessional helpers', *Psychological Bulletin,* 95: 534–41.

Imber, S. D. et al. (1990) 'Mood specific effects among three treatments for depression', *Journal of Consulting and Clinical Psychology,* 58: 352–9.

Kendall, R. E. (1975) *The Role of Diagnosis in Psychiatry,* Oxford: Blackwell.

Langs, R. (1985) *Workbooks for Psychotherapists*, Emerson, NJ: Newconcept Press.

Luborsky, L. (1984) *Principles of Psychoanalytic Psychotherapy: A Manual for Supportive Expressive Treatment (SE),* New York: Basic Books.

Luborsky, L., Singer, B. and Luborsky, L. (1975) 'Comparative studies of psychotherapies: is it true that everyone has won and all must have prizes?', *Archives of General Psychiatry,* 32: 995–1008.

Mahrer, A. R. (1989) *The Integration of Psychotherapies,* New York: Human Sciences Press.

Orlinsky, D. E. and Howard, K. I. (1986) 'Process and outcome in psychotherapy', in S. L. Garfield and A. E. Bergin (eds), *Handbook of Psychotherapy and Behavior Change,* 3rd edn, New York: Wiley.

Rogers, C. R. (1957) 'The necessary and sufficient conditions of therapeutic personality change', *Journal of Consulting Psychology,* 21: 95–103.

Shapiro, A. K. and Morris, L. A. (1978) 'The placebo effect in medical and psychological therapies', in S. L. Garfield and A. E. Bergin (eds), *Handbook of Psychotherapy and Behavior Change,* 2nd edn, New York: Wiley.

Shaw, G. B. (1911) *Preface on Doctors: The Doctor's Dilemma,* Standard Edn (1932), London: Constable.

Sieghart, P. (1978) *Statutory Registration of Psychotherapists: Report of a Professions Joint Working Party,* Cambridge: Plumridge.

Smail, D. (1987) 'Psychotherapy and "change": some ethical considerations', in S. Fairbairn and G. Fairbairn (eds), *Psychology, Ethics and Change,* London: Routledge and Kegan Paul, pp. 31–43.

Smith, M. L., Glass, G. V. and Miller, T. I. (1980) *The Benefits of Psychotherapy,* Baltimore, MD: Johns Hopkins University Press.

Stiles, W. B. and Shapiro, D. A. (1989) 'Abuse of the drug metaphor in psychotherapy process–outcome research', *Clinical Psychology Review,* 58: 352–9.

Taylor, S. E. and Brown, J. D. (1988) 'Illusion and well-being: a social psychological perspective on mental health', *Psychological Bulletin,* 103: 193–210.

Truax, C. B., Carkhuff, R. R. and Douds, J. (1964) 'Toward an integration of the didactic and experiential approaches to training in counselling and psychotherapy', *Journal of Counselling Psychology,* 11: 240–7.

Vinar, O. (1969) 'Dependence on a placebo: a case report', *British Journal of Psychiatry,* 115: 1189–90.

Training: A Guarantee of Competence? II.2

Richard House

> Sadly, the correlation between training and effectiveness as a therapist is low.
>
> (Mark Aveline, quoted in Mowbray, 1995: 132)

> A very good therapist does not get that way primarily by taking more courses or studying at a particular institution. It is not easy to measure how they get that way or who has 'it'. This is a socially and philosophically deep issue ....
>
> (Robert M. Young, 1993: 84)

> Psychotherapy transpires in the realm of meaning ... in contrast to facts, meanings cannot be confirmed or disconfirmed by the objective criteria of the scientific method.
>
> (Jerome D. Frank, 1989a: 144)

The recent publication of Richard Mowbray's controversial book *The Case Against Psychotherapy Registration: A Conservation Issue for the Human Potential Movement* (Mowbray, 1995, hereafter *The Case*) has already been met with enthusiastic acclaim from within humanistic circles in the field: thus, in an 'Open Letter' to Mowbray, John Rowan writes, 'Congratulations on your new book ... I think it is very thorough and well argued, and should make quite an impression' (Rowan, 1995: 43); and *Self and Society* editor John Button writes that 'Richard Mowbray's important and thought-provoking book should be essential reading for all current and would-be therapy practitioners ...[he] has done psychotherapy an enormous service ...' (Button, 1995: 52, 54). Thus far, however, the central arguments in *The Case* have received only limited attention within the pages of *Counselling* (see House, 1996b), yet those

---

This chapter is an abridged version of 'The professionalisation of counselling: a coherent "case against"?', published in *Counselling Psychology Quarterly,* 9 (4), 1996: 343–58.

arguments are just as relevant to the professionalisation of counselling, with the BAC's impending register of counsellors and the expressed desire of at least some in the field to introduce a legal restriction on the use of the term 'counsellor'.

I will confine myself here to just one of the nostra underpinning the conventional wisdom: namely, the view that it is possible to generate or even guarantee competent practice in this field via training and formal top-down accreditation and registration procedures. Along with client protection (see Mowbray, Chapter I.3, this volume), the practitioner-competence issue is perhaps one of the two most powerful reasons cited in support of current professionalising developments; and if it can be shown that the rationale underpinning this position is based on inadequate and erroneous reasoning, then the whole *raison d'être* for professionalisation is at the very least thrown into severe doubt.

Readers involved in the field will no doubt be aware of the dramatic changes that have been occurring apace in counselling training in recent years, with lengthening courses, ever more stringent course requirements, increasing academic content and associated moves towards the postgraduatisation of the field, and so on. For Mowbray, '*There is little if any evidence that possession of academic qualifications by psychotherapists relates to basic competence or protects the public in any way*' (p. 116, original emphasis); 'The personal qualities that are prerequisites of competence in this sort of activity cannot be "trained in"' (p. 118); and 'factors which UKCP is promoting... will not produce more competent practitioners' (p. 124). A survey of the available evidence indicates that 'the effectiveness of psychotherapy does not appear to depend upon any of the following: (1) The practitioner holding academic qualifications. (2) The length of training of the practitioner. (3) The school to which the therapist belongs. (4) The practitioner having had a training analysis' (p. 122). It is often remarked in sporting circles that the likes of Björn Borg and Vivian Richards would never have reached the pinnacles of their respective sports had they been exposed to the training techniques and principles of the prevailing conventional wisdom, and Mowbray is getting at a similar point when he asks rhetorically 'Do good mothers mother on the basis of a "developed body of mothering theory"?' (p. 140).

There is also a wider philosophical question here (cf. the Bob Young epigraph, above) regarding what, precisely, is the role of training in the development of practitioner competence. The conventional wisdom seems to contain the implicit and unarticulated assumption that there is a simple and direct causal relationship between training and competence, with training being a process that makes a person into a competent practitioner, and which they would not have been had they not trained – i.e. that it is the training *qua training* that is the crucial variable. Yet such a view is naively positivistic and is squarely trapped within what is increasingly being seen to be a grossly inadequate framework for understanding reality, from the level of subatomic physics to the levels of human consciousness and astrophysics.

In the specific case of the training–competence nexus, for example, it makes at least as much sense to reverse the taken-for-granted direction of causality, such that the crucial variable is that people are in the position within themselves to be able to choose to embark upon training, and that this is the crucial variable in competence, rather than the mechanistic view that it is training per se that somehow transforms non-counsellors into competent practitioners.

When we begin to take this kind of argument on board and problematise taken-for-granted assumptions about the causal efficacy of training, it comes as no surprise to find that, as Roberta Russell concludes in her exhaustive review of the outcome literature, 'A professional training does not appear to increase the effectiveness of the therapist; [and] therapists who have undergone traditional training are no more effective than those who have not' (1981: 7) (cf. the Mark Aveline epigraph, above). Many other commentators have challenged the conventional wisdom that training necessarily leads to practitioner competence. Here is Jeffrey Masson in characteristically robust form: 'If it is really the case [that clients benefit as much from non-professional as from experienced professional help], why then bother to have elaborate, expensive, and pretentious training institutes at all?' (1990: 227; see, for example, Strupp and Hadley, 1979). Masson goes on to quote Hans Strupp, who wrote in 1973, 'I have become increasingly skeptical that psychotherapy has anything "special" to offer, in the sense that its techniques exceed or transcend the gains that may accrue to a patient … from a highly constructive human relationship' (1990: 227).

If we accept the commonly heard view that the burgeoning demand for counselling and psychotherapy services has temporally, and by no means coincidentally, coincided with a wider cultural decline in the extended family and the influence of organised religion, together with a more pervasive cultural decline in the quality of human relationships more generally, then why on earth should we accept the view that elaborate and expensive training are required in order to discharge a societal function that has previously been effected through the quite natural medium of real-world human relationships? I am reminded here of the great Georg Groddeck, the physician-psychoanalyst-healer who lived at the time of, and had a significant influence upon, Freud (see House, Chapter IV.3, this volume). In describing Groddeck's remarkable work with his patients, Morris Robb wrote half a century ago that 'it is impossible to schematise such a [healing] process, and *to talk of training anyone else to achieve its results is absurd*, yet some approximation to a character of this sort is the only basis on which psycho-therapeutic power can be built' (Groddeck, 1951: 15, emphasis added).

As soon as we begin to question taken-for-granted assumptions about causality within the training–competency nexus, it then becomes quite natural to move away from the counsellor-centred and infantilising belief that successful therapeutic outcome is largely a function of counsellor competency, and towards the alternative, client-centred view that what matters more in terms of therapeutic efficacy is the way in which clients 'use' whatever help is available to them to effect their own healing (whether through Groddeck's 'old wive's poultice', shamanic ritual, the church confessional, placebo medication … or the most sophisticated of counselling or psychotherapeutic interventions). (I return to the change process at length, below; for a thoroughly documented articulation of this view, see Bohart and Tallman, 1996.)

On this view, not only does the erstwhile rather puzzling and counter-intuitive finding that all therapeutic modalities yield very similar success rates (Smith et al., 1980; Andrews and Harvey, 1981) make complete sense, but the basis for the view that the training of practitioners is the key factor in successful outcome is decisively undermined. It might well be, for example, that it is not the absolute level of the counsellor's personal development and technical expertise that is crucial in the healing process, but rather, the extent to which a given practitioner is congruent within him- or herself at *whatever* level of development and competence s/he has reached; or perhaps the extent to which s/he is aware of, and able fully to own, her or his limitations (these two factors are, of course, not unrelated). Such a view is entirely consistent with Russell's finding, based on a thorough literature review, that 'Paraprofessionals consistently achieve outcome [*sic*] equal to or better than professional outcomes' (1981: 7; see Strupp and Hadley, 1979).

A cautionary note from psychoanalytic theory is relevant at this point. In his brilliant 1985 paper, Howard Stein implies that what a client might subjectively experience as a true healing may not in reality be so, but may be a so-called 'transference cure' – a kind of magical flight into health that is not founded upon authentic personality change and is unlikely to sustain. Thus, for Stein, the client's receipt of a 'magic bullet' engages with the client's

> earliest mental world where gesture commands the world that is its extension. In this world there are only deeds, not people .... [T]he healer ... helps the patient to become healed or reconciled to life's irreversibility and loss's irrevocability by first declining to comply with the patient's request for magic.
>
> (1985: 189)

I do not have the space here to respond to this psychoanalytically driven scepticism about so-called superficial kinds of healing and cure; but suffice to say that it touches upon the fundamental philosophical conflict that exists between a client-centred and a theory-oriented, therapist-centred conception of what change actually consists in.

Of course, counsellors and therapists with extensive training will very likely experience themselves as better practitioners as a direct result of their training; but it by no means necessarily follows from this that the outcome from the standpoint of their clients will be more successful than it would otherwise have been: i.e. the practitioner's subjective experience of her or his own competence is logically quite distinct from the question of outcome from the client's point of view. And if it is the case, as Frank (1989a) argues, that the practitioner's sense of competence 'indirectly strengthens the patient's confidence in the therapist as a person who knows what he or she is doing' (109), such a subjectively experienced practitioner competence is by no means the sole preserve of those who have done ex(t)(p)ensive training, or fulfilled stringent accreditation standards. And yet there no doubt exists a strong and understandable urge to 'feel professional' as a way of cementing one's identity within a field which is perhaps intrinsically uncertain, a-rational, and even ultimately mysterious. But when the desire to feel and experience oneself as 'professional' is driven more by practitioner anxiety than it is by genuine, authentic concern for the clientele, then once again the danger is that professionalisation becomes practitioner-centred, rather than being in clients' best interests

… not to mention the severe doubt that must exist as to whether such acted-out and unowned anxiety can serve as a good role model for the clients we work with!

There exist a number of research findings that support the view that client efficacy in the therapeutic change process is relatively far more significant than the infantilising medical-model ontology would have us believe (for a review see Bohart and Tallman, 1996). Thus, for example, research evidence shows conclusively that 'patients' expectations concerning the duration of treatment affect the speed of their response', and 'speed of improvement may often be largely determined by the patient's expectations … as to the duration of treatment' (Frank, 1978: 45–6). In addition, there are the so-called 'transference cures', through which 'changes following brief therapeutic contact … in which little seems to have occurred beyond the arousal of the patient's faith in the therapist are sometimes deep-seated and persistent' (ibid.: 46). Further:

> the emotional state of trust and faith in itself can sometimes produce far-reaching and permanent changes in attitude or bodily states …, [such that] *the healing force appears to reside in the patient's state of faith or hope* and not in its object.
>
> (ibid.: 46, 48, emphasis added; see also Menninger, 1963: Chapter 15)

And here is Frank again: 'therapeutic success or failure depends not primarily on therapeutic procedure per se, but on the *personal qualities of the patient* which determine responsiveness to the healing properties of the therapist's personality' (1989a: 106, emphasis added).

More generally, we should not underestimate our sheer ignorance about the nature of the therapeutic experience – Frank again: 'Until more is known about the factors in the patient, therapist, and treatment situation which determine the degree and form of influence exerted by the therapist …, it is impossible adequately to isolate either factors specific to each form of psychotherapy or those involved in all forms of therapy' (1978: 55–6). And once we admit such ignorance, then the kinds of accreditation and licensing procedures that encourage the illusion of certainty in a field that is intrinsically uncertain and mysterious suddenly appear not only largely irrelevant, but actually misleadingly dangerous.

Of course, the possibility that practitioner training might be to some extent superfluous to competency is likely to be extremely uncomfortable and disquieting news for all those practitioners (which includes myself) who have spent thousands of pounds on training, and for those (which again includes myself) who have spent thousands of pounds on their own personal therapy or 'training analysis' ... not to mention appalling news for the 'counselling and psychotherapy training business' as Mowbray calls it (see Samuels, Chapter IV.1 of this volume). And yet taken together, both the available research evidence and the logical coherence of the argument strongly point in this counter-intuitive direction.

If we begin to question the taken-for-granted assumptions of scientificity and naive causal efficacy in the therapeutic change process itself, then we have yet further reason to question the very *raison d'être* of current professionalising developments. Mowbray puts it thus:

> rather than a simple Newtonian 'billiard ball' model of cause and effect which implies that a client is a passive recipient of the 'effects' of the psychotherapist, a more appropriate paradigm for looking at psychotherapy is that of 'Chaos Theory', in the light of which psychotherapy may be conceptualised as a non-linear system of mutually cueing feedback loops.
>
> (1995: 106–7)

There are echoes here of the great psychoanalyst-healer Georg Groddeck, who wrote well over half a century ago that 'because we live we are bound to believe that ... there are such things as causes and effects ..., whereas we really know nothing about the connection between one event and another' (Groddeck, 1951: 77).

It is little wonder that at this stage in the evolution of human consciousness, the ego is enormously reluctant even to countenance the view that, to quote Groddeck again, 'everything important happens outside our knowledge and control' (p. 78), and that 'It is absurd to suppose that one can ever understand life' (p. 84; see also Hall, 1993). Yet the professionalising mentality inevitably makes the normally unarticulated assumptions (1) that it is possible both in principle and in practice to assess and measure the contribution that the practitioner *qua* practitioner makes towards the we-ness and the outcome of a therapeutic encounter; and (2) that what is healing or transformative in a counselling relationship has more to do with the causal efficacy of the practitioner than it does with the way in which the client will 'use' (in the Winnicottian sense) the practitioner for her or his own healing or transformation.

I believe that in the realms of human relationship and co-created intersubjective experience (Orbach and Eichenbaum, 1994), both of these assumptions are quite simply false (and even if they weren't false, there is absolutely no way in which this could be demonstrated or proven methodologically). In sum, what I am arguing here (and cognitive-behaviourists aren't going to like this) is that the scientific mentality is singularly inappropriate in the fields of counselling and psychotherapy (cf. House, 1996a, b; Chapter I.5, this volume). Here again is Jerome Frank (1989b: 144): 'traditional scientific methods are not well suited to investigating the phenomena of psychotherapy, since they deal exclusively with facts, whereas psychotherapy transpires in the realm of meaning'.

The anxiety-driven impulse to measure, assess, control and mechanise a process that is quintessentially human, intersubjective, mysterious and quite possibly in principle beyond the ambit of rationalist scientific understanding is not only inappropriate, but actually violating of the essence of the therapeutic healing process. One of the central problems and harmful effects of didactic registration mindedness (DRM) is that it diverts attention from and distorts what is really healing in therapeutic relationships, and as a result, it will inevitably reduce the efficacy of therapeutic practice to the extent that it encourages practitioners to entertain false beliefs regarding what, precisely, is healing within a counselling experience.

Kiev has written that 'primitive [meaning "non-Western" – RH] therapies are fundamentally magical, that is, non-rational attempts to deal with non-rational forces' (1964: 10). The central underlying rationale of DRM is that of scientific rationality; yet if the ills of the human condition are intrinsically non- or a-rational, then it follows logically that it is inappropriate to apply scientific mindedness to human experience and processes that are in principle beyond the realms of scientific understanding.

If DRM is taken to its logical conclusion by those who would uncritically professionalise our field, then a quite possibly terminal damage may be done to the very essence of what is healing in the therapeutic relationship – an unwitting and unintended consequence perpetrated by those who claim, and no doubt sincerely believe themselves, to be doing quite the opposite. And that would be a truly tragic outcome for all of us, practitioners and clients alike. If it's true that the drive towards professionalisation is much more to do with acted-out, dysfunctional psychodynamics than it is to do with a healthy engagement with the dynamics of power, powerlessness and authority, then we'd better wake up to that reality pretty quickly, before substantial, and even irreversible, damage is done to our field.

Conclusion

> Licensing does not protect the public. Licensing does not exclude incompetents. Licensing does not encourage innovation. It stultifies ....
> (Will Schutz, quoted in Mowbray, 1995: 213)

Not only does there exist a formidable and compelling case against the centralised professionalisation of counselling via statutory registration; but this is as much a question of politics, vested interests and unconscious organisational dynamics as it is one of ethics and good counselling practice. If we embrace the argument that counselling is a form of healing via two interpenetrating and co-creating subjectivities rather than a mechanistic, scientific medical-model activity, then there must be very severe doubts as to whether competence can be measured, practice be successfully monitored and controlled, and capacity to practise be accredited and guaranteed in anything approaching a reliable way – not to mention in a way that honours the foundational humanistic values of our practice rather than betraying them. And if such attempts at monitoring, controlling and didactically accrediting are inappropriately foisted upon the field, then the cost in terms of the quality of the healing care that good counselling practice provides may well be an enormous one.

If we agree with Jill Hall (1993: 4) that 'Rational thought is not the most fitting mode with which to know the universe ..., and thus not a fitting mode with which to know ourselves', and with Groddeck when he argues that conscious thought is a 'tyranny' (1951: 103) leading to a fetishisation of human experience, then it is extremely doubtful whether the rationality-dominated and control-oriented form of programmatic professionalisation can have relevance to the healing orientation that counselling at its best represents. As long ago as 1990, Brown and Mowbray wrote most poignantly that 'Where there is a genuine need for structures, we should develop structures that foster our values rather than betray them' (quoted in Mowbray, 1995: 225). On the formidable arguments and compelling evidence provided in *The Case*, there must surely be severe doubt as to whether the form and momentum taken by unfolding professionalising developments are in the best interests either of clients or of the field as a whole.

References

Andrews, G. and Harvey, R. (1981) 'Does psychotherapy benefit neurotic patients?', *Archives of General Psychiatry*, 38: 1203–8.

Bohart, A. C. and Tallman, K. (1996) 'The active client: therapy as self-help', *Journal of Humanistic Psychology*, 36 (3): 7–30; reprinted in Y. Bates and R. House (eds) (2003) *Ethically Challenged Professions: Enabling Innovation and Diversity in Psychotherapy and Counselling*, Ross-on-Wye: PCCS Books, pp. 258–74.

Button, J. (1995) Review of *The Case*, *Self and Society*, 23 (4): 52–4.

Frank, J. D. (1978) 'The dynamics of the psychotherapy relationship', in *Psychotherapy and the Human Predicament: A Psychosocial Approach*, New York: Schocken Books, pp. 19–56.

Frank, J. D. (1989a) 'Discussion', in M. Shepherd and N. Sartorius (eds), *Non-Specific Aspects of Treatment*, Toronto: Hans Huber Publishers, pp. 95–114.

Frank, J. D. (1989b) 'Non-specific aspects of treatment: the view of a psychotherapist', in M. Shepherd and N. Sartorius (eds) *Non-Specific Aspects of Treatment*, Toronto: Hans Huber Publishers, pp. 142–6.

Groddeck, G. (1951) *The World of Man*, London: Vision (original work published 1934).

Hall, J. (1993) *The Reluctant Adult: An Exploration of Choice*, Bridport: Prism Press.

House, R. (1996a) '"Audit-mindedness" in counselling: some underlying dynamics', *British Journal of Guidance and Counselling*, 24 (2): 277–83; reprinted as Chapter I.6, this volume.

House, R. (1996b) 'In the wake of "Watchdog"', *Counselling*, 7 (2): 115–16.

House, R. (1997) 'The dynamics of professionalisation: a personal view of counselling research', *Counselling*, 8 (3): 200–4; reprinted as Chapter I.5, this volume.

Kiev, A. (1964) 'Introduction', in A. Kiev (ed.), *Magic, Faith, and Healing: Studies in Primitive Psychiatry Today*, New York: Free Press.

Masson, J. (1990) *Against Therapy*, London: Fontana (original work published 1988).

Menninger, K. (1963) *The Vital Balance: The Life Process in Mental Health and Illness*, New York: Viking Press.

Mowbray, R. (1995) *The Case Against Psychotherapy Registration: A Conservation Issue for the Human Potential Movement*, London: Trans Marginal Press.

Mowbray, R. (1996) 'SAFAA is safer', *Self and Society*, 23 (6): 16–19.

Orbach, S. and Eichenbaum, L. (1994) 'From objects to subjects', paper presented at the Freud Museum Conference on 'Psychoanalysis and Feminism', London, May.

Rowan, J. (1995) 'An open letter to Richard Mowbray', *Self and Society,* 23 (4): 43–4.

Russell, R. (1981) *Report on Effective Psychotherapy: Legislative Testimony,* New York: R.R. Latin Associates.

Smith, M. L., Glass, G. V. and Miller, T. I. (1980) *Benefits of Psychotherapy,* Baltimore, MD: Johns Hopkins University Press.

Stein, H. F. (1985) 'What is therapeutic in clinical relationships?', *Family Medicine,* 17 (5): 188–94.

Strupp, H. H. and Hadley, S. W. (1979) 'Specific vs. non-specific factors in psychotherapy: controlled study of outcome', *Archives of General Psychiatry,* 36: 1125–36.

Young, R. M. (1993) 'The profession of psychotherapy in Britain', *Free Associations: Psychoanalysis, Groups, Politics, Culture,* 29: 79–84.

Inputs and Outcomes: The Medical Model and Professionalisation II.3

Nick Totton

A doctor speaks

In the *Independent on Sunday* of March 17th, 1996, Dr Peter Fenwick (described as 'one of Britain's leading psychiatrists') had this to say:

> One in 10 people will suffer some mental illness at some time in their lives. The other 90 per cent are, medically speaking, mentally healthy. Yet in practical terms, the fact that these people are not actually mentally ill tells us nothing about how well they are. It gives no indication of how fulfilling they find their lives, how successfully they actually run them .... There are plenty of people who tolerate chronic, low-grade unhappiness in their jobs or relationships for years. Few of these people are ever likely to come to the attention of a psychiatrist, but their mental health is well below par.
>
> (Fenwick, 1996: 8)

This is about as extreme a statement as one could easily imagine of the medical model of human psychology. Not satisfied with the claim of medicine to handle the 10 per cent of people who get defined as 'mentally ill', Dr Fenwick makes an extended bid: 'the fact that these people are *not actually mentally ill* tells us nothing about how well they are'.

It's a nifty piece of footwork, borrowing from the discourse of holistic approaches: wellness is more than just not being ill. Very true; but only relevant to mental and emotional states if we grant the original claim, the assertion that 'medically speaking' is the appropriate way to speak about these states. And there's another discourse being touched on here: the business-oriented discourse of self-improvement, where what we do with our lives is 'run' them, successfully or otherwise. This dovetails with the practical moralism of the last phrase: 'their mental health is' – a regretful 'tut' from the crusty-but-kindly practitioner, a guilty hanging of the 'patient's' head – 'well below par'.

The psychiatrist proceeds to lay out his stall:

> But is there an equivalent of a healthy eating and exercise regime for the body to improve our mental state? I believe there is. We now know enough about how the mind works to make any necessary changes in our lives and thinking to achieve a sustained sense of what I call mental well-being.
>
> (Ibid.)

This is wonderful: psychiatrists, it turns out – the 'we' who 'know how the mind works' – are not only the people to go to if your life becomes difficult; they are also the experts on *how to live*. 'It is perfectly healthy', Peter Fenwick tells us, 'occasionally to feel sad, lonely, irritated or valueless; it isn't healthy to have these feelings constantly.' Gee, thanks, Doc.

What we have to get a grip on here is that this sort of stuff is being taken *seriously*. Peter Fenwick's article (and Dr Fenwick is generally considered a radical anti-reductionist in his own field) launched a massive series on 'The Dynamics of Change', with flags and whistles. Representatives of Freudian, Jungian and other schools wrote in, not to question the good doctor's viewpoint ('characteristically fascinating' – Anne Zachary, British Confederation of Psychotherapists – Zachary, 1996), but simply to plug their own enterprises. One hundred years of psychotherapy, and we still don't seem to have grasped that it's different from 'healthy eating and exercise'.

Professionalisation

The reason why this is being taken seriously by people who quite certainly know better is, of course, 'professionalisation'. Those who wrote in to the *Independent on Sunday* did so in order to remain competitive in the marketplace which is trying to install itself at the centre of the psychotherapy and counselling world. There are now far too many trained practitioners out there looking for work; and if the bubble is not to burst, new markets must be opened up, new punters must be persuaded that they need the product. If the state and other institutions can be persuaded to pay for it, so much the better; but for these things to happen, therapy and counselling must present themselves as *medical*.

One of the clearest opponents of the medical model in psychotherapy, oddly enough, was Freud – the man who started it off, and who in some ways loaded it with its freight of medical culture and terminology. Freud militantly opposed the idea that to be a psychoanalyst, one should be required to have medical training; in the postscript to his work on the subject, *The Question of Lay Analysis*, he says very emphatically that 'psychoanalysis is not a specialised branch of medicine. I cannot see how it is possible to dispute this' (Freud, 1927: 355).

Many practitioners *have* disputed this, however – starting with a large proportion of Freud's colleagues; and here again the clear motive has always been professional status. One result is that those seen as most highly qualified to deal with the most extreme mental/emotional states are those likely to have the *least* training in psychotherapy: psychiatrists. A more general result is the very general, almost automatic, acceptance that an appropriate venue for state-funded counselling and psychotherapy is the National *Health* Service. 'Counselling in Primary Care' has become a major specialisation in the field; and I want to consider some of the effects of this development.

I need to say straight away that I have no personal experience of working in this context; and in no way do I want to seem dismissive of those who do. One very obvious and beneficial effect is that free-to-the-client counselling is getting to a lot of people who can benefit from it. The rise of counselling in GP practices, for example, is the result of a lot of hard work by very well-intentioned people (as well as by those concerned with status and income – and often, of course, good intentions and self-interest can run in tandem), and it is undoubtedly helping a large number of clients. Having said that, though, I want to look at some rather more subtle drawbacks and disadvantages of the phenomenon, and to use what is happening in the USA with 'managed care' as an example of the potential dangers of the situation.

The medical model

The fundamental problem with working in a medical context is that you are working within the medical *model* – however much you may personally disown and ignore that model, the institution which gives you a home and provides your paycheck subscribes to it; and you cannot be immune to the effects of this on your work. For one thing, you become liable to forms of measurement of your effectiveness which may seem to you wholly irrelevant. (At first, anyway: you need a good deal of intellectual confidence to argue against this approach, and may find your views weakening.) You become subject to 'outcome research'; which is widely felt to be impossible to apply to psychotherapy and counselling, in that the *relevant* outcomes are not measurable (see, for example, Seligman, 1995). The effectiveness of your work will tend to be judged by how fast you can get rid of people, and how long they stay away.

This sort of measurement is perfectly appropriate to at least some forms of medicine. Medical practice really is more effective if someone with a chronic pain stops complaining of it and doesn't come back to surgery. (Even here there is room for argument.) In a counselling context, though, we all know that it's not that simple. Counselling may be very effective and successful if a client *starts* complaining about a lot of things that they have endured or ignored for years. It may well be splendidly effective if after six sessions someone is 'feeling much worse' – that is, owning pain that they have previously been denying. And six sessions may be all you get.

This is one of the more obvious results of working in a medical context – or, of course, any other publicly or institutionally funded context. There is tremendous pressure to finish with people quickly – that is, after six or twelve or – if you are extremely lucky – 24 sessions. An entire body of theory about 'Brief Therapy' has grown up, basically, in order to justify the operational need for short-term work. (And, of course, to provide more jobs for trainers.) Claims that this work is as effective as, or even more effective than, long-term work are fundamentally circular; because they measure 'effectiveness' in terms which are appropriate to short-term work – alleviation of symptoms, greater enthusiasm for life, etc.

Now it is well known in the therapy world that after a few sessions, people tend to *either* feel much better – because of the large amount of unconditional attention they're getting, because they're being taken seriously, because they can see new ways of starting to make sense of things; *or* to feel much *worse* – because they're opening up huge areas of pain and misery which they've been ignoring for years. These areas of pain may badly need opening up – if there's the opportunity for long-term work. But of course any competent practitioner will steer well away from such areas if they know they and the client only have a few hours to spend together. Ergo, the client feels much better. Whether any real change has taken place is a different matter.

I don't believe that structural change *can* happen in human beings through a few week's work. Of course there is always the possibility that someone will arrive to see you at just the point when change is ready to take place, and either or both of you may believe that the therapy has created the change. But to change the structures we have built up over years generally *takes* years of hard work. We may conclude from this that therapy and counselling aren't worth much. It depends what we expected in the first place! In other words, it depends on our model of the therapeutic process, our understanding of human nature and its relation to society, and many other things that are neither obvious nor simple, but which are in my view enormously important in making sense of what we're doing and what we want to do.

Managed care

We may be able to learn a lot from the US experience of 'managed care'. Howls of anguish have been appearing about this on the Internet for some time, on discussion lists for psychotherapy professionals of various kinds. The best account I have come across is on a web page run by John A. Martin, a licensed clinical psychologist from California and 'author of well over 100 published papers and public presentations in the areas of developmental psychology, clinical psychology and research methodology'. (The address of his website is http://www.jamartin.com) According to Martin,

> In the 1970s, psychologists finally won recognition by insurance companies that had until that time been afforded only to psychiatrists ... and thus became eligible for insurance reimbursement for their services. In entering into the world of third-party reimbursement, psychologists were required to adopt psychiatry's manual of mental disorders, the Diagnostic and Statistical Manual. Each time an invoice for a psychologist's services was submitted to an insurance company for reimbursement, a 5-digit diagnostic code was included [which] defined the client's problems within the disease model .... Though many psychologists were uncomfortable with using disease classifications for many of their clients, insurance reimbursement demanded it. In an effort by insurers to contain costs, most insurance companies currently hire intermediary 'managed care' companies to ... exercise control over

> how insurance money is spent for psychotherapy services. Psychologists … are under contract with the managed care companies to provide 'medically necessary treatment for mental and nervous disorders' for subscribers, that is, specifically to treat the disorders or conditions described in the diagnoses. In general, these managed care contracts set providers' fees and require providers (1) to provide treatment to any and all subscribers who are referred to them, (2) to submit detailed information about the course of treatment to the managed care company for evaluation and review, (3) to abide by the managed care company's final decision concerning whether treatment is in fact necessary, (4) to refrain from informing clients about alternative treatment options that may contradict the decisions of the managed care company, and (5) to absolve the managed care company of any legal or ethical responsibility in the event that the client believes that he or she has been harmed by failure to obtain adequate treatment.
>
> Providers are expected to design treatment strategies that help the managed care company to contain costs, whether or not the provider feels that lower-cost treatment strategies are appropriate. In essence, providers are expected to limit treatment to that which is deemed by the managed care company as being 'medically necessary', and are at risk for cancellation of their contracts if they fail to do so in a consistent and cost-effective way.
>
> Consequently, under the new managed care model, it's important to understand that psychotherapy clients are considered sick. It's also important to understand that the client–therapist relationship is not protected: clients now must sign away their right to confidentiality, and providers must give case managers who are employed by the managed care companies detailed information about their clients' lives and the course of treatment.
>
> (Martin, 1996)

All of this may be horrifying to us; but it is, of course, eminently logical and even fair from the point of view of the insurance companies. If the problems for which someone receives counselling or therapy are not medical ones – if they are not 'ill' – why should the insurance pay? Equally, it seems to me, this is the logic of primary care counselling. If the Health Service is paying, then the client must be presumed to be sick.

Guerrillas in the marketplace

At this point I want to re-emphasise that I know this is not the view of most of those doing the counselling! Taking counselling into medical settings is, generally speaking, a guerrilla tactic: an opportunistic move (in the best sense of the word) to meet a genuine need, to work with people who cannot afford the cost of private practice, and might well never find their way to it in any case. It may even be seen (for instance by Richard House, in his article 'General Practice Counselling: A plea for ideological engagement': House, 1996) as an opportunity to challenge and ultimately change the medical model itself.

I think we need to be very cautious with this sort of thinking. It used to be known as 'altering the system from within', or less enthusiastically as 'entryism'. We have to recognise, though, that while we are altering the system *it* is also altering *us*: working away subtly at our sense of priorities, our language, our style. How many of us, for example, have had the experience of applying for state or institutional funding for some project; and watching, over the months and years of the application process, as the project's radical and creative aspects are gradually whittled down to fit the bureaucratic model?

It is of course true that we all live within a capitalist hegemony; that, like it or not, we are struggling to uphold our own beliefs in an environment which is at best unsupportive of, and most of the time actively hostile to, human happiness and productivity. This is true *anyway*; and it can be argued that, therefore, choosing to work in a system controlled by the medical model doesn't make things any worse! – it only sharpens the already-existing conflict. There is clearly some force to this; but equally clearly, there has to be a limit to the argument, or else we must decide that there is no point in trying to find ourselves a good environment in which to live and work.

Actually, I am neither expecting nor hoping that if people start to think about the sorts of issues I am raising, they will stream out of the GP practices and other medical-model venues (student counselling is subject to many of the same problems I have outlined). Primary care counselling is here to stay. What I do hope is that we can recognise it to be a *site of contestation*, as Michel Foucault puts it: a place where different projects, different world-views, are in conflict with each other – and where the other side has the big battalions. We therefore need to think very hard and clearly about every detail of what we do and say in this environment.

A fair question about all this would be: What are the alternatives? If we want to reach people who (in our view) would greatly benefit from therapy/counselling, but have neither financial resources nor awareness of this sort of work, how can we do it? There is a clash of two either/or choices: medical model vs. therapy/counselling model, and private vs. public provision.

I have no easy answer. It's worth recognising a few things, though: firstly, it is not just either ignorance or poverty which keeps people away from counselling and therapy. A large proportion of people are not accustomed to studying their own inner life, don't see the point, and don't want to do it. Or they may simply have other priorities. It's desperately frustrating trying to do psychotherapy with someone who basically needs some money and a new house. Also, there are drawbacks to someone coming to counselling because they have been persuaded that it is the answer to a medical problem. Are they truly volunteers in this situation? On the one hand, they will be looking for problem-solving; on the other hand, who are we to psychologise what they believe to be a physical issue? (Thomas Szasz has a lot to say in this area.)

It is probably true, though, that there are a number of people who themselves would choose therapy or counselling, but who do not have the financial resources. I have recently initiated a network of therapists and counsellors in Yorkshire who are offering one or two free or cheap sessions in their timetable. So far we haven't been inundated with calls. We can cross that bridge when we come to it.

References

Fenwick, P. (1996) 'The dynamics of change', *Independent on Sunday* Magazine, 17 March.

Freud, S. (1927) *'Postscript to the Question of Lay Analysis'*, London: Penguin Freud Library 15.

House, R. (1996) 'General practice counselling: a plea for ideological engagement', *Counselling,* 7 (1): 40–4.

Martin, J. A. (1996) 'Psychotherapy in the 1990s', Internet address http:/ www.jamartin.com/jmphd.html. (Note: this page is now longer extant. See http:/ /www.jamartin.co./documents_Reimbursement.html. Also relevant is http:// www.psychotherapy.net/article/psychotherapy-insurance)

Seligman, M. E. P. (1995) 'The effectiveness of psychotherapy: The Consumer Reports study', *American Psychologist,* 50: 965–74.

Zachary, A. (1996) Letter, *Independent on Sunday*, 24 March: 18.

Challenging the Core Theoretical Model II.4

Colin Feltham

The British counselling world differs from much of the rest of the world in insisting not only on career-long clinical supervision, but also on identified core theoretical models in training. (I shall mainly refer to models, although the terms approach, school, orientation, etc. are also used more or less synonymously in the literature.) Although the United Kingdom Council for Psychotherapy (UKCP) differs structurally from the British Association for Counselling (BAC), it too is organised around identified, distinct models of psychotherapy. The British Confederation of Psychotherapists (BCP) accepts only traditional psychoanalytically orientated organisations as members.

For a training course to be accredited by BAC, it must in effect show that it adheres to well-established psychodynamic, person-centred or, slightly more tenuously, to a variety of humanistic, integrative or systematically eclectic approaches. There are said to be in excess of 450 theoretical models of counselling and psychotherapy and, officially at least, BAC, UKCP and the European Association for Psychotherapy (EAP) support diversity and do not discriminate against any reputable approach. In Britain, most BAC-accredited courses are psychodynamic or person-centred, a few are based on transactional analysis or psychosynthesis, or an acceptable integration of one of these and other humanistic and skills-based or cognitive-behavioural approaches.

Why a core theoretical model?

Arguments in favour of some sort of identified core theoretical model appear to run as follows:

1. It is important that trainees are exposed to at least one coherent model and its implications. The model's parts may be described in terms of

This article was first published in *Counselling, 8* (2), 1997: 121–5.

its world-view and concept of human beings or image of the person; learning, developmental and motivational concepts; conceptualisation of psychological disturbance and health; acquisition and perpetuation of psychological disturbance; treatment goals; therapeutic strategies and techniques; expected change process; limitations; etc. (Dryden, 1996; Wallace, 1986). A training should demonstrate internal consistency; that is, the core theoretical model should be reflected in theoretical seminars, skills practice, personal growth work and supervision. Failure to embrace one model in depth results in practitioners who are confused, lacking in rigour, and whose knowledge base is thin.

2. Trainees must learn and hone the practical and clinical attitudes, skills and techniques associated with a particular approach if they are to become competent practitioners. Attempts to learn a mish-mash of skills from various models result in ineffective or dangerous clinical practice by counsellors who are merely syncretistic dilettantes rather than adept at systematic assessment, technique selection, timing, and so on. Also, theoretically inconsistent counsellors risk transmitting their confusion to clients.

3. It is expected that as counsellors become mature practitioners, they will develop a personalised model or approach that maximises their skills and best meets the needs of their clients (Skovholt and Ronnestad, 1992; Spurling, 1993). They cannot achieve such maturity without first having had a thorough grounding in a coherent model. *After* this, they may choose to develop some form of theoretically consistent eclecticism (Dryden, 1991) or thoroughgoing integration of two or more models (Wilkins, 1997). Although it is widely believed that theory should never overshadow or distort the actual therapeutic encounter, paradoxically practitioners should hold strong theoretical positions (Karasu, 1992: 8).

Why are core theoretical models untenable?

A *prima facie* case for core theoretical models certainly exists. My own objections are obviously not intended to commend confusion or incompetency in training. Rather, I have come to believe that there are serious philosophical and clinical objections which lead to the conclusion that training in and support for a core theoretical model are ultimately untenable and even oppressive. This is admittedly a change from my previous position in Dryden and Feltham (1994). My objections in summary form are as follows.

1. Since the advent of multiple therapeutic theories, there never has been a clear front-runner among psychotherapies (that is, one which consensually commands intellectual or scientific respect, or popular support); nor has there been any school without its dissidents. Transiently, those schools whose leaders have made political attempts to demean or exclude their own dissidents may have appeared to possess internal solidarity. The costs of dissent are high, as Karen Horney discovered when the New York Psychoanalytic Institute demoted her in 1941 with the following curious rationale:

    > The Educational Committee is fully in favour of free and unhampered discussion of all points of view existing in psychoanalysis. Such discussions are possible and most fruitful only if the preparatory analyses and preliminary, theoretical fundamentals are such as not to prejudice the student in advance to the basic principles of psychoanalysis.
    > (Cited in Quinn, 1987: 348)

    This position of dogma preceding and disingenuously silencing free enquiry has persisted into our own professional training bodies today, of course.

2. It is difficult to defend the position that any one model, arbitrarily singled out from 450 (or even from a mainstream ten or twenty) and offered as an in-depth training, can adequately prepare therapists to help most clients referred to them. It is well known that many psychoanalysts consider behaviour therapists to hold absurd views and vice versa; indeed, the field is full of dispute. On what basis, then, is any one model to be selected as the basis of a professional training (Feltham, 1997)? Is not the field itself confused and incoherent? Karasu (1992) cites Smith et al. (1980: 185): 'Although all therapies are equally effective, one must choose only one to learn and practice.' Must one? Why?

3. There are no core psychotherapeutic models older than a few decades (classical Freudian psychoanalysis may be the exception, but even that has been largely torn into many divided schools) and none has been shown to yield consistently excellent results or to be decisively clinically superior to others (Luborsky et al., 1975; Smith et al., 1980). Some models have seen their reputations wax and wane, and some have already become virtually extinct. In his own ambitious personality theory, Gooch (1975) acknowledged that all theories are provisional and that turnover in psychological theories is especially rapid: 'The turnover arises, among other things, from the complex and peculiarly nebulous nature of psychological material, and not least from our own inevitable involvements with it' (Gooch, 1975: 527).

4. When human nature and behaviour are themselves the object of study, psychotherapists and counsellors must realise that they share the field with philosophers, theologians, political scientists, psychologists, anthropologists, historians and others. It must surely be conceded that no one appears to be any closer than anyone else in arriving at answers to radical and perennial questions about human suffering and deliverance from it (see, for example, Stevenson, 1987).

5. Insistence on a core model perpetuates a tradition-driven practice of psychotherapy rather than one based on empiricism, on listening to clients' needs and views, on research findings and rational clinical innovation. The therapy world is characterised by competing theories and practices generated by charismatic leaders, defended by enthusiastic followers and orthodox institutes. In fact we appear to insist on core counselling models without even knowing what we mean: 'There has been no thorough examination of what actually constitutes an adequate theory of counselling' (Bayne et al., 1994: 150).

6. The argument that trainees who are not equipped with particular, theoretically mediated competencies but arbitrarily and dangerously use a mixture of techniques requires examination. It has not been demonstrated explicitly what the specific skills and techniques of each model are, exactly how they are taught and how long this training must take, whether they actually differ fundamentally from the skills espoused in other models and exactly how counsellors practise

dangerously with 'inadequate' training in them. Paradoxically, a great deal of resistance exists among therapists to the systematisation of such therapy training, for example by devising and using technical treatment manuals; instead, much training seems shrouded in mystique. The possibility must be considered that proponents of each model unintentionally exaggerate the uniqueness and complexity of their skill base, and exaggerate the alleged dangers of misapplication.

7. It is quite likely that training in a highly specific model may lead the practitioner to dispense that model to all and sundry inappropriately, fitting clients to the theory and associated techniques rather than the reverse. For example, everyone gets long-term, insight-promoting therapy or non-directive therapy, cognitive restructuring or therapy focusing on ego states, regardless of the actual presenting problem, personality, circumstances and wishes. This might be particularly true of therapists in training and those who are relatively inexperienced, who are so anxious to 'do it right' that this preoccupation becomes more determining than the client's welfare. This is an especially serious problem for defenders of the core theoretical model position, because the reality often is that clients with a wide array of clinical needs are seen by trainees or beginners, or are seen in settings where a narrow, traditional approach is being used.

   Robertiello and Schoenewolf (1987: 266) discuss the case of a client abused in one such traditional setting: 'The approach taught at this institute and practised by its training analysts, control supervisors, and the like, contained a built-in resistance to emotional ventilation.' To scream was exactly what the client indicated he needed to do, but the analyst would not and could not permit it because of his training. There is a strong case for saying that each theoretical model magnifies – indeed, capitalises on – certain aspects of human behaviour and neglects others, and that a rigorous training would actually attend holistically and equally to past and present behaviour, affect, sensation, imagery, cognition, and psychosocial, biological, cultural and spiritual factors. As far as I am aware, no such training exists.

8. There is a case for saying that it is not particular core theories that have any significant effect on clients; rather, a combination of non-specific factors is responsible for successful therapy (Frank, 1974). Many of these are about the client's *belief* in the therapist, confidence

in the status of the therapist, therapist qualities (including those built by ordinary life experiences), working alliance, the protected setting, etc. Some are about simple human needs for attention, warmth and acceptant interest (Howe, 1993). Karasu (1992: 27) argues that the therapist's passionate belief in his or her theories and methods is crucial, since the aura of conviction conveys itself to clients. Conviction, not theoretical correctness, is what counts, according to Karasu's argument.

9. We might also consider that reports of advanced practitioners' reflections on their initial training tend to identify clinical work and supervision as of far more formative significance than core theory (Dryden and Spurling, 1989). Goldberg (1992: 49) interviewed master practitioners and reported a high degree of retrospective dissatisfaction with 'misguided clinical theories'. Even before training, the intuition possessed by many individuals (that therapy is essentially interpersonal and atheoretical) manifests in a reluctance to opt for and be moulded by any narrow model, but unfortunately candidates for training have little choice but to accept one circumscribed model or another. Individual clinical giftedness, so overlooked as a factor in therapy, may well be more significant than any pedagogic theory:

> Traditionally, it has been common for senior analysts to teach the kind of orthodoxy that is expected which essentially repeats the party line. They have been reluctant or unable to really articulate what they actually do in practice. Many of our most gifted clinicians are successful because of the way they actually work, not for the reasons they declare in pedagogic situations.
>
> (Corbett, 1995: 77)

10. Another argument against core models is that they are self-evidently productions of a patriarchal society. To date, all have been founded by charismatic white men, initially of mid-European origin but now almost entirely American. (Anna Freud, Melanie Klein, Karen Horney and other women contributors have been modifiers rather than founders.) The awe in which leading figures – even Carl Rogers, the founder of non-directive, think-for-yourself, person-centred therapy – are held closely resembles religious and political phenomena of reverence,

obedience and discipleship. The common aim of psychotherapy – autonomy – is belied by the reality of training institutes which demand conformity from trainees (Masson, 1990) and by psychotherapy which either mystifies clients (McLellan, 1995) or subtly converts them to belief in the tenets of the particular approach (Levenson, 1983).

Virtually all current psychotherapeutic theory reflects white, Western psychology and implicit assumptions about the universal correctness or desirability of autonomy, assertiveness, insightfulness and emotional freedom, qualities which are not in fact valued by all individuals in all cultures at all times. Core theoretical models in psychotherapy and counselling encourage monolithic, ethnocentric and patriarchal thinking, and tacitly discourage and marginalise (even forbid) any kind of anarchic (Feyerabend, 1993), personalistic (Smail, 1978), radically feminist (McLellan, 1995), politicised (Newman, 1991) and dialogical (Sampson, 1993) accounts of human functioning, distress and healing.

11. All psychotherapeutic models are predicated on the assumption that human nature and behaviour are understandable, classifiable, adaptable and even predictable. Most clinical practice operates on the assumption that the client's new insights, attitudes and behaviours will act upon his or her environment with automatic benefits. Of course, it can also be argued that our environment is often indifferent or hostile to us and that our efforts to conceptualise, control and order our lives are susceptible to constant frustration. All therapeutic models are partly fictions and inadequate because they de-emphasise or even deny the role of chance, complexity, macro changes outside of our control, and chaos generally. Perhaps inadvertently, they promote their methods as almost infallible. Beneath the promised orderliness of therapeutic Valhalla there may always be a necessarily ragged, imperfect, vulnerable and unimprovable or ungovernable self (Feyerabend, 1993; Rose, 1989; Vicinzey, 1969).

Acknowledging differences

Let me try to combine and present these arguments differently by comparing two approaches to studying and addressing of individual problems in living.

Approach number one goes like this. My own problems were greatly helped by therapy x; I have now trained rigorously in therapy x and I see daily the benefits it brings to people; I continue to study and refine my technical grasp of therapy x, which I believe to have an edge over other therapies; I don't believe researchers have grasped the subtleties of therapy x; I don't believe it can be readily integrated with other therapies; it is essential that trainees themselves have therapy x and dedicate many years to learning its complexities; it is essential that all practitioners operate from a secure theoretical base.

Approach number two goes like this. I see that people have a wide variety of problems and that society itself is hardly a sanity-generating milieu; I see that hundreds of explanations are held up and as many solutions proposed, none of which seems wholly satisfactory or unequivocally effective; I believe there is some sense and nonsense in most therapies and I strive hard to see how each individual can best be helped by the more sensible bits from each (or indeed by bits of religion, education, philosophy, etc.); I do not believe the pursuit of theoretical or technical purity and separatism is healthy or credible; I think such tendencies are tribalistic, wasteful and ultimately detrimental to mental and social health.

The first approach is quite common, and often flows from personal experiences of perceived salvation or need for certitude and ultimate meaning. Many of us cling to an ideological object, such as a particular religion, political view or psychotherapy, which we cherish and can never let go of. Arguably, all such ideologies act as opiates, and their true function is to infuse us with a reassuring but defensive sense of certainty and direction in an unpredictable and frightening world. It is comforting to think that Freud, like Jesus, heroically explored the psychic wilderness single-handedly and has passed on the hard-won answers to us lesser mortals. But why – in psychotherapy and religion especially – do we invest so much faith in such figureheads? And how can we distinguish between crazy and/or mistaken cult leaders and reputable discoverers and master practitioners (Storr, 1996)? The tendency towards emotional investment is quite evident in this approach.

The second approach is perhaps less common and is characterised by a mixture of pragmatism, restless truth-seeking, agnosticism, scepticism, and distaste for or avoidance of certainties and in-groups. Positively, this approach echoes the message of mystics and philosophers through the ages to avoid the traps of thinking that you have finally understood, and to embrace instead the *via negativa*, eliminating all illusory solutions. Negatively, those attracted to this approach may be pathologically avoiding belonging to any group, casting themselves romantically as outsiders, heroic and lonely defenders of unpalatable truths. They may simply be manifesting a naughty child/rebellious adolescent archetype, or a negative transference towards theory (Rangell, 1985). The tendency towards nihilism, cynicism, arrogance and empty relativity is obvious in this approach.

I cannot pretend to *know* that I am right about core theoretical models being untenable. Indeed, sometimes I shudder a little when I read a student's incoherent essay displaying a grasshopper-like predilection for jumping from one unrelated theme to another, or magpie-like attraction to glittering, gimmicky techniques unanchored in any solid understanding. Sometimes I read eloquent and persuasive passages in the literature of some deeply traditional psychotherapy and doubt my own scepticism. On the other hand, students who are poor writers or ill-disciplined thinkers can be very warm, intuitive and effective healers, and many therapeutic encounters remind me how ill-fitting most generalised theory is to real individuals. I find some untrained carers or supposedly superficially trained therapists more human and insightful than some highly trained practitioners who may be steeped in one or another core theoretical model.

Implications

If my scepticism about core theoretical models has some validity or interest, where might it lead? I propose the following possibilities.

1. BAC, UKCP and similar professional bodies might consider the pleas of trainers who wish to base their syllabus not on traditional core models (nor, obviously, on sloppily constructed programmes) but on a range of responsibly critical, institutional, eclectic, systemic, transtheoretical, atheoretical, interdisciplinary, dialogical or pluralistic perspectives (Samuels, 1993). This questions the widespread developmental view that a first training must treat (adult) trainees as babies to be spoon-fed traditional material (however stodgy or toxic), and that only advanced trainees or mature practitioners can handle a rich diet of pluralistic perspectives, real debate and critical analysis.

It is often said that therapists must be able to tolerate ambiguity in clients – but not in the theoretical content of courses?

2. Researchers might investigate further the comparative effectiveness of practitioners trained in conventional traditions with core theoretical models and those trained differently (experimentally, eclectically, minimally, informally, autonomously, etc.).

3. Trainers and theoreticians dissatisfied with the prescriptive positions of existing professional bodies might risk launching themselves as independent commentators, critics and creators of new therapeutic cultures and methods, thus challenging the assumption that the only alternatives to traditional models are flimsy, illegitimate hybrids.

4. Academic departments of counselling and psychotherapy might further develop the function of questioning the field and its assumptions, becoming what critical and philosophical psychologists now are in relation to classical psychology. Such study might include detailed historical and sociological analysis of the roots of therapeutic ideologies and of the ways in which therapeutic enthusiasms regularly swell and fade in their efforts to capture conceptually and clinically the elusive rhythm of human suffering, aspirations and limitation.

5. There is no reason to abandon the search for a grand unified theory of human suffering and psychotherapy. Although ambitious and unfashionably counter-postmodernist, it is possible to conceive of an overarching, interdisciplinary conceptual structure which might accommodate and reinterpret diverse therapeutic theories (e.g. Stevens and Price, 1996).

6. Continuing identification of the active ingredients of effective therapy (that is, placebo factors, relational qualities and distinctive techniques) could lead to a fruitful pragmatics of psychotherapy divorced from speculative aetiological, personality and clinical theories (Lazarus, 1990; Thompson, 1996).

Finally we might (but we won't) inject some humour and humility into our debates about training by admitting that our knowledge base is still insubstantial and our techniques pretty fallible. We might (but we won't) inject some ontological seriousness into our thinking and training, shifting the axis from received wisdom and 'conceptual imperialism' (Goldfried et al., 1992/2003) to live, urgent, owned and shared analysis of the human condition (Bohm, 1994). As still relatively young and status-hungry professions, counselling and psychotherapy are probably in no mood for any radical revision of their theories and practices. This is regrettable, since not only do they thereby defend untenable orthodoxies, but unwittingly and oppressively place an obstacle in the path of real enquiry and growth.

References

Bayne, R., Horton, I., Merry, T. and Noyes, E. (1994) *The Counsellor's Handbook*, London: Chapman and Hall.

Bohm, D. (1994) *Thought as a System*, London: Routledge.

Corbett, L. (1995) 'Supervision and the mentor archetype', in P. Kugler (ed.), *Jungian Perspectives on Clinical Supervision*, Einsiedeln, Switzerland: Daimon.

Dryden, W. (1991) *Dryden on Counselling. Vol. 1: Seminal Papers,* London: Whurr.

Dryden, W. (ed.) (1996) *Handbook of Individual Therapy,* 3rd edn, London: Sage.

Dryden, W and Feltham, C. (1994) *Developing Counsellor Training,* London: Sage.

Dryden, W. and Spurling, L. (eds) (1989) *On Becoming a Psychotherapist,* London: Routledge.

Feltham, C. (1996) 'Beyond denial, myth and superstition in the counselling profession', in R. Bayne, I. Horton and J. Bimrose (eds), *New Directions in Counselling*, London: Routledge, pp. 297–308.

Feltham, C. (ed.) (1997) *Which Psychotherapy? Leading Exponents Explain Their Differences*, London: Sage.

Feyerabend, P. (1993) *Against Method,* London: Verso.

Frank, J. D. (1974) *Persuasion and Healing: A Comparative Study of Psychotherapy,* New York: Schocken.

Goldberg, C. (1992) *The Seasoned Psychotherapist,* New York: Norton.

Goldfried, M. R., Castonguay, L. G. and Safran, J. D. (2003) 'Core issues and future directions in psychotherapy integration', in J. C. Norcross and M. R. Goldfried (eds), *Handbook of Psychotherapy Integration,* New York: Basic Books, pp. 593–616. (Original work published in 1992)

Gooch, S. (1975) *Total Man: Notes Towards an Evolutionary Theory of Personality,* London: Abacus.

Howe, D. (1993) *On Being a Client: Understanding the Process of Counselling and Psychotherapy,* London: Sage.

Karasu, T. B. (1992) *Wisdom in the Practice of Psychotherapy,* New York: Basic Books.

Lazarus, A. A. (1990) 'Can psychotherapists transcend the shackles of their training and superstitions?', *Journal of Clinical Psychology*, 46: 351–8.

Levenson, E. (1983) *The Ambiguity of Change*, New York: Basic Books.
Luborsky, L., Singer, B. and Luborsky, L. (1975) 'Comparative studies of psychotherapies: Is it true that "everyone has won and all must have prizes"?', *Archives of General Psychiatry*, 32: 995–1008.
McLellan, B. (1995) *Beyond Psychoppression: A Feminist Alternative Therapy,* North Melbourne: Spinifex.
Masson, J. (1990) *Final Analysis: The Making and Unmaking of a Psychoanalyst*, London: HarperCollins.
Newman, F. (1991) *The Myth of Psychology*, New York: Castillo.
Quinn, S. (1987) *A Mind of Her Own: The Life of Karen Horney,* London: Macmillan.
Rangell, L. (1985) 'On the theory of theory in psychoanalysis and the relation of theory to psychoanalystic therapy', *Journal of the American Psychoanalytic Association*, 33: 59–92.
Robertiello, R. C. and Schoenewolf, G. (1987) *101 Common Therapeutic Blunders: Countertransference and Counterresistance in Psychotherapy,* Northvale, NJ: Aronson.
Rose, N. (1989) *Governing the Soul: The Shaping of the Private Self,* London: Routledge.
Sampson, E. E. (1993) *Celebrating the Other: A Dialogic Account of Human Nature*, New York: Harvester Wheatsheaf.
Samuels, A. (1993) 'What is a good training?', *British Journal of Psychotherapy,* 9 (3): 317–23; reprinted in a much extended version as Chapter IV.1, this volume.
Skovholt, T. M. and Ronnestad, M. H. (1992) *The Evolving Professional Self: Stages and Themes in Therapist and Counsellor Development,* Chichester: Wiley.
Smail, D. J. (1978) *Psychotherapy: A Personal Approach*, London: Dent.
Smith, M. L., Glass, G. V. and Miller, T. I. (1980) *The Benefits of Psychotherapy,* Baltimore, MD: Johns Hopkins University Press.
Spurling, L. (ed.) (1993) *From the Words of My Mouth: Tradition in Psychotherapy,* London: Routledge.
Stevens, A. and Price, J. (1996) *Evolutionary Psychiatry,* London: Routledge.
Stevenson, L. (1987) *Seven Theories of Human Nature*, Oxford: Oxford University Press.
Storr, A. (1996) *Feet of Clay: A Study of Gurus,* London: HarperCollins.
Thompson, R. A. (1996) *Counseling Techniques: Improving Relationships with Others, Ourselves, Our Families, and Our Environment*, Washington, DC: Accelerated Development.
Vicinzey, S. (1969) *The Rules of Chaos*, London: Macmillan.
Wallace, W. A. (1986) *Theories of Counseling and Psychotherapy,* Boston: Allyn and Bacon.
Wilkins, P. (1997) *Personal and Professional Development for Counsellors,* London: Sage.

Not Just a Job: Psychotherapy as a Spiritual and Political Practice II.5

Nick Totton

The whole argument for the 'professionalisation' of psychotherapy rests on the assumption that psychotherapy is a profession – or at least, less grandly, a job. I have often argued that it would be preferable to see it as a job (e.g. like plumbing) rather than as a profession (e.g. like law or architecture). And it certainly *looks* like a job (and often feels like one): practitioners generally, though not always, get paid for what they do, they have time 'on duty' and 'off duty', they take holidays, and so on. I want to argue, though, that from a certain point of view psychotherapy only *pretends* to be a job: that in crucial ways it is something else altogether, something which is rather hard to pin down, but which can be indicated by describing it as a *spiritual and political practice*.[1]

The example of psychoanalysis

The question 'What sort of thing is psychotherapy?' was freshest for the first generation of psychoanalysts, who knew that they were doing something new. They discussed it mainly in the context of medicine: was psychoanalysis, or was it not, a sub-form of medicine? Freud very strongly believed that it was not (see Chapter II.3, this volume); but many other analysts disagreed with him – for reasons very much to do with power and status – and have continued to situate psychoanalysis within medicine. Perhaps this is a happier fate than psychotherapy's more recent one of being thrown in with the so-called 'caring' or 'helping professions', but it is really no more appropriate.

Here I can only assert, rather than demonstrate, that the whole supposed 'analogy' between physical illness, on the one hand, and emotional distress or unusual mental states, on the other, is worse than dubious: philosophically untenable, a metaphor or myth that serves as a point of purchase for techniques of social control – in much the same way as calling communism 'a cancer in the body politic'. Psychoanalysis, like psychotherapy in general, cannot be part of 'mental medicine' because there is no such valid category to be part of. As David Pilgrim writes, 'psychotherapists, despite their inappropriate and anachronistic title, do not treat illness – they struggle with distress and meaning' (Pilgrim, 1992: 231).

It has always been understood even by those committed to the medical model that psychoanalysis, as well as being a way of treating those identified as 'sick', is a way of thinking about human beings and the human situation in general. Through the so-called 'second fundamental rule', the demand that analysts be analysed – as well as through the more or less continuous informal mutual analysis in which the early analysts engaged – it soon became clear that there was a great deal of benefit in analysis for those not defined as 'sick': in other words, that it is a process of value to human beings in general. As Freud says, 'the possibility of [psychoanalysis's] application to medical purposes must not lead us astray' (Freud, 1927): astray, that is, from this crucial *non*-medical purpose of psychoanalysis.

One convenient locus for discussion of these issues is the 1927 psychoanalytic debate on 'lay analysis'. Arguing against the many analysts supporting a medical identity for their profession, Hanns Sachs, himself a non-medical practitioner and a prominent training analyst in Berlin, insisted that although

> severe recognisable neuroses are naturally far commoner among my patients than among my analysands in training, ... as the analyses proceed one observes that this fact has no decisive significance. Character-anomalies, inhibitions, disturbances in the emotional life, which in ordinary intercourse have to be accepted as troublesome but unavoidable traits, reveal their true nature only during psycho-analytic treatment – no matter whether it is undertaken for purposes of cure or not ... I have had to learn to regard the difference between 'patients' and 'pupils' ... as of merely secondary importance.
>
> (Sachs, 1927: 200)

Similarly, Robert Waelder writes that psychoanalysis

> has so far enlarged the conception of mental illness beyond the truly narrow clinical boundary that it practically includes almost everything that lives. We now speak of the 'neurosis' of a person in the same matter-

of-fact way that we speak of his 'character', 'personality' or 'abilities'. (Waelder, 1927: 275)

And Theodore Reik, a lay analyst whose prosecution by the Austrian state was an important factor in the whole debate, is even more explicit: 'Our interest in analysis would not be less if its methods, points of view and result were valid only in the sphere of the normal mind' (Reik, 1927: 242).

If we are all 'normal neurotics', then the question of non-medical analysis is – as many analysts argue in this debate – explicitly tactical: how far does psychoanalysis need the protective status of the medical profession to further its own, very different ends?

Psychotherapy as an enlightenment practice

But if psychoanalysis – and *a fortiori*, psychotherapy – is not a branch of medicine, what sort of beast is it? It is clearly a unique and specific pastime; but does it, in its undoubted individuality, stand wholly alone in the range of culture and history, or does it have membership in some sort of family or genre or genus of human activity?

I shall continue to use psychoanalysis as an exemplar of psychotherapy in general; and argue that, in a taxonomy of social formations, psychoanalysis is most appropriately positioned as an *enlightenment practice*: alongside such other practices as they occur within Buddhism, within Hinduism, within Islam, within Taoism, within Judaism, within Christianity; and in a few other settings.

I am not suggesting that psychoanalysis is identical or similar to any one of the above, any more than they are identical or similar to each other. The 'parallels' between psychoanalysis or psychotherapy and Zen Buddhism, for instance, have been described more than once (e.g. Fromm and Suzuki, 1960); I find such descriptions largely sterile and unconvincing. What I do maintain is that what I am calling 'enlightenment practices' have some identifiable features in common, which psychoanalysis – in at least some of its forms – shares: sufficiently so to be seen as another approach to the same task.

What is this task? What do I mean by an enlightenment practice? One necessary feature, it seems to me, is that an actual *practice* is involved: not just a theory or belief, but a technique or set of techniques, aimed at creating some sort of change in persons. (Several of these practices would say that there is no such thing as 'change', and/or no such thing as a person; but we will leave that to one side for now.)

The shift that is attempted can be described and conceptualised in many ways. But perhaps all the practices I am considering might agree that it involves a *radical lessening of anxiety*: a profound relaxation, which follows from a reappraisal of our situation as human beings.

Broadly speaking, the enlightenment practices all lead us to the sense that something which previously seemed hugely important and hugely difficult is now quite unimportant. The relief which this entails is enormous and life changing. Through the techniques of an enlightenment practice, we typically become aware that we experience ourselves as subject to impossible demands. We further realise that these demands *are*, indeed and strictly, impossible: in other words, that they do not really exist.

I imagine that it may immediately be clear in a broad sense that this description applies also to psychoanalysis – at least in some of its forms, and in the hands of some of its practitioners. I will say more in a moment about how the shift of perception is understood within analysis; first, though, I want to make clear that, although most enlightenment practices exist in a religious context, I am not suggesting that psychoanalysis is 'really a religion'.

This connection to religion is circumstantial rather than essential. Until recent times, by far the most convenient – and safest – place to practise this sort of discipline has been within the locally dominant religious context. In fact, there is at least one exception: Stoicism appears to meet the criteria I have outlined for being seen as an enlightenment practice, but is basically agnostic or atheist in its position. One can also quote the famous Zen Buddhist slogan 'If you meet the Buddha on the road, kill him'; and mention that, although most Sufis are Muslims, some Sufi schools, for local historical reasons, exist quite happily within Hinduism instead.

My argument is that psychoanalysis, in the different conditions of modern times, has swum within the protective sea of medicine in the same way that other enlightenment practices use the camouflage of religion. Of course, many psychoanalysts are wholly unaware of this situation – as we can see very clearly, for example, in the 1927 debate from which I have already quoted. Suitably enough, analysis is an unconscious enlightenment practice! Or rather, different practitioners have very different awarenesses of what they are about. And it's important to realise that equally within Buddhism, Sufism, etc, there is always a powerful tendency away from the enlightenment awareness, into institutionalisation, religion, superstition, even bureaucracy.

If psychoanalysis is an enlightenment practice in the sense I have described, what are its specific goals and techniques? What is it that disappears, is seen to be non-existent, through a successful analysis? Among the entities which are said by different schools to disappear, or at any rate to diminish, are: the centrality of the ego, sexual shame, Oedipal or pre-Oedipal guilt, the 'false self'. Often, of course, these entities have had to be hypostatised by the theory in order to make them disappear again! One might say that each formulation is what Zen would call 'a finger pointing at the moon': a more or less helpful indication of an experience which it cannot fully describe. Looking at the techniques of psychoanalysis may take us closer to understanding the goals.

Like other enlightenment practices, psychoanalysis works by substituting its own 'impossible demands' – primarily, the demand to free associate – for those which we experience in life in general. Like them, it does so with the effect of bringing the analysand to a realisation that other tasks which life seems to involve – for example, reparation, spontaneity, consistency – are impossible in the same sense as free association: that they are paradoxical, and finally meaningless.

In Zen there are koans, for instance: unanswerable questions which one is required to answer. In almost every tradition there is some form of meditation: where one is required to attend closely to one's spontaneous process without changing it. Free association, the 'fundamental rule', is the analytic version of this – a demand with which no one can fully comply; as Ferenczi first pointed out in 1927, it 'represents an ideal which ... can only be fulfilled after the analysis has ended' (1927: 210). In other words, as Adam Phillips puts it, 'the patient is not cured by free-associating, he is cured *when he can free-associate*' (1995: 102). It is not actually clear that anyone can free associate; or rather that, while free associating, anyone can remain 'themselves', in the sense of maintaining an experience of consistent, continuous and bounded identity. It could be argued that one purpose of free association as a strategy is to educate us in doing without such an experience.

One function of the demand to free associate is thus to highlight its *impossibility*: to make the analysand forcibly aware of resistances and inhibitions – and, more deeply, of one's *lack of title*, so to speak, in what is said, thought and felt. The simple tactic of free association cuts deeply through our illusions, and single-handedly de-centres the ego: the impossibility of 'saying whatever comes into your head' reveals the impossibility of accounting for oneself.

In Reichian therapy, my own original training, attention to breath plays a very similar role to free association. When one tries to allow the breath to happen freely *while at the same time attending to it consciously,* sooner or later consciousness and spontaneity begin to interfere with each other: resistance begins to emerge, resistance which corresponds to repression and which is embodied in the breath. Breathing is right on the interface between voluntary and autonomic function: any attempt to 'control ourselves' – which is in large part what repression is – will emerge in the breath. This seems to be at least part of the reason why many schools of meditation are centred on attention to the breath.

By working systematically through all the levels of resistance to spontaneous breath – to 'being breathed' – the therapist and client will encounter all the familiar repetition compulsion, transference neurosis and other phenomena which appear through systematic work on free association, or indeed any other sustained encouragement to let things happen spontaneously and without censorship. The demands which interfere with each other are not in fact consciousness and spontaneity, but consistency and spontaneity: the 'spastic I' (Totton and Edmondson, 1988: 17) has learned to regard consciousness as a matter of self-consistency, of a continuous self-commentary which saves appearances. Like free association, attention to breathing reveals the impossibility of maintaining both consistency and spontaneity. Or, from a slightly different angle, it reveals that we cannot *deliberately* be consistent or spontaneous – because we can never be anything else.

What 'disappears', then, is the apparent distinction between me and myself. And in true paradoxical fashion, characteristic of the enlightenment practices wherever they are found, it disappears through being made *absolute.* In Lacan's or Reich's very different usages, it is the 'ego' which is shown to be only a figure of speech, a trick of the light – a state of bodily tension or of mental attention. In Winnicott's terms, it is the 'mind' as something distinct from and over against the bodymind unity: 'In the overgrowth of the mental function reactive to erratic mothering, we see that there can develop an opposition between the mind and the psyche-soma' (Winnicott, 1949/1975: 246). 'Acceptance of not-knowing,' Winnicott says. 'produce[s] tremendous relief' (ibid.: 250): a sentence which could stand as epigraph to this paper. Any Buddhist, for example, would be familiar with these positions; and it is certainly not by mistake that the word 'ego' has been taken over as the translation of Buddhist terms.

Transference, of course, is equally bound up with demand: the demands the analysand makes or would like to make on the analyst – and also the demands the analysand experiences the analyst as making, centred on the one actual demand that is expressed, in however liberal and moderate a form: the demand to free associate. The transference relationship is a laboratory for all the impossible demands we experience in life – demands to perform in various ways, to make reparation in various ways, to be a socially acceptable personality, *to be someone*. It opens the possibility of substituting for demand, desire, which tends to dissolve any fixed someone we try to be. And this sort of intense relationship, calculated to first foster and then dispel illusion, is found in different forms in many enlightenment practices.

Take for instance the following description:

> The first stage of meeting one's therapist is like going to a supermarket. You are excited and you dream of all the different things that you are going to buy: the richness of your therapist and the colourful qualities of his [*sic* throughout] personality. The second stage of your relationship is like going to court, as though you were a criminal. You are not able to meet your therapist's demands and you begin to feel self-conscious, because you know that he knows as much as you know about yourself, which is extremely embarrassing. In the third stage when you go to see your therapist, it is like seeing a cow happily grazing in a meadow. You just admire its peacefulness and the landscape and then you pass on. Finally the fourth stage with one's therapist is like passing a rock on the road. You do not even pay attention to it: you just pass by and walk away.
>
> At the beginning a kind of courtship with the therapist is taking place. How much are you able to win this person over to you? There is a tendency to want to be closer to your therapist, because you really want to learn. You feel such admiration for him. But at the same time he is very frightening; he puts you off. Either the situation does not coincide with your expectations or there is a self-conscious feeling that 'I may not be able to open completely and thoroughly'. A love–hate relationship, a kind of surrendering and running away process, develops. In other words we begin to play a game, a game of wanting to open, wanting to

> be involved in a love affair with our therapist, and then wanting to run away from him.
>
> (Trungpa, 1987: 42–3)

I expect you will have realised that this is not, in fact, a description of therapeutic transference: it is a passage from a talk by a modern Vajryana Buddhist teacher on the relationship between guru and disciple, with the word 'therapist' substituted for 'guru' throughout.

Psychotherapy as a political practice

Perhaps by now I have established, in broad outline, why psychotherapy can usefully be considered as an enlightenment practice. I have focused on psychoanalysis, which in some ways is a very good exemplar; from other points of view, though, an equally strong case could be made for Gestalt, Rogerian work, or Process Oriented Psychology, for example. Each uses its different techniques and emphases towards the same goal of radical relaxation about the conditions of our existence.

I want now to explore the political dimension of psychotherapy; or rather, two distinct and opposed political dimensions. It seems to me that psychotherapy engages with power in two different ways: through its social role as bearer of a certain distribution of power through the psychotherapeutic discourse – and through its clinical practice, as an often inexplicit deconstruction and subversion of power relations, including its own.

The first of these engagements with power is very straightforward. Over the century of its existence, and like many enlightenment practices in their own social environment, psychotherapy has repeatedly struggled for and occasionally achieved a fingerhold on cultural hegemony – most strikingly in the USA after World War II. Psychotherapy has become, and striven to become, arbiter of what is normal and acceptable, both individually – is this person properly adapted to society? Is their difference from the norm 'sick'? – and collectively – what does psychotherapy think to be the proper policy towards single parents? About drugs? Is psychotherapy for or against nuclear arms? Racism? The EMU?

In making and claiming the right to make both sets of decisions – about individual and collective acceptability – psychotherapy is inevitably involved in continuous negotiations and tradings-off with other loci of political power. This was perhaps most brutally blatant in the Soviet Union with the incarceration of dissidents in mental hospitals; and it's important to say that bad faith was not the primary issue here: there was a serious, if misconceived, argument involved that these people were suffering from maladaptation to their society. It was the *same* argument, in fact, that was used (usually) more blandly in the USA during the same period, as ego psychology made its pronouncements about normality and abnormality, juvenile delinquents and homosexuals.

I think we have to conclude that the nature of this claim by psychotherapy to social hegemony is not in fact altered by the appeal or otherwise of the particular stance put forward. In other words, whether 'psychotherapists think' (know) that political dissidents should be given shock treatment, or that unemployed people should be given respect, the same critique applies to the discourse of expertise involved. Psychotherapists or counsellors have no more, and no less, authority on political matters than any other citizen. *To claim otherwise is to exploit the transference and projection phenomena which we spend our working lives trying to deconstruct.*

And this, of course, is my second category of political practice. Rather than simply utilising the positive transference on to the therapist, Lacan's 'one who is supposed to know', in order to change the client's experience (as Freud originally felt we should do), psychotherapy subjects the positive transference to a searching critique. It tries to help the client realise, ultimately, that the practitioner is no different from them; that the qualities of wisdom, insight and understanding which the client has found in the practitioner are *projections* – and therefore ultimately within the client themselves. (This is where other enlightenment practices aim to arrive also, but by different routes – for example, the Trickster approach.) Some forms of therapy use transference to get beyond transference; others try to elude or confront it as they go along. For my purposes here, the differences don't matter.

This critique, it seems to me, is a political one: a critique and giving-back of *power*. It has immediate and powerful implications for the client's relationship with the public world: implications which were articulated for the first time, perhaps, when Wilhelm Reich, while he was still an analyst, pointed out that his clients were tending to leave their oppressive jobs and unsatisfactory relationships – not as an unfortunate side effect, but precisely as *an expression of the success of the therapy* (Reich, 1942/1983: 175–7).

Psychotherapy tends to change our political relationships – because they cannot ultimately be separated from any other relationships. Could the slogan 'the personal is political' have come into being without the context of psychotherapy? In practice, of course, this slogan has tended to be the property of a particular, left-oriented politics. (It can also be used to suggest that *only* the personal is political, and to deny the reality of political and socio-economic oppression: a stupefying piece of empire-building in the service of ideology. See, for example, Pilgrim, 1992: 232–5.) But I am arguing that the 'inner truth', so to speak, of psychotherapy is a radical anarchism ('no-rule') of a sort which goes beyond left–right polarisations.

Psychotherapy, in other words, is political precisely *through* its status as an enlightenment practice. It is political in the same extreme, 'anti-political' sense as the *Tao Te Ching* (Feng and English, 1973):

> Do you think you can take over the universe and improve it?
> I do not believe it can be done.
> The universe is sacred.
> You cannot improve it.
> If you try to change it, you will ruin it.
> If you try to hold it, you will lose it.
> (verse 29)

> The world is ruled by letting things take their course.
> It cannot be ruled by interfering.
> (verse 48)

More and more, therapists, especially group therapists, are realising that they have a serious contribution to make to the central problem of politics: conflict resolution. But this contribution flows ultimately not from any particular skill at discriminating right from wrong. It flows from the sort of central, peaceful, non-interfering stance indicated by Lao Tse.[2] Conflict is resolved by letting things take their course.

Implications

As Reich found in the 1920s, the sorts of experiences which people have in psychotherapy will tend to make them more autonomous, more spontaneous, more aware of their own needs and desires, more empathic, less driven by compulsions of all kinds: more relaxed, in fact. This will tend to make them more tolerant of difference, less tolerant of oppression – political qualities. It will also necessarily bring them up against aspects of our collective life which militate against a relaxed, spontaneous and autonomous style. What happens then? Something difficult, unique and interesting in each case! – unless, as practitioners, we take some sort of evasive action to prevent this process unfolding, because we find it too challenging, too embarrassing, too stirring for ourselves, too undermining of our position of power and status.

If I am even roughly right in my argument – that psychotherapy, or a powerful trend within psychotherapy,[3] functions as a deconstructive spiritual and political practice rather than as a form of medicine or social work – then I would also argue that this has major implications for the 'professionalisation' debate.[4] So far as I know, there is no powerful lobby for the registration of political activists, or the establishment of effective training standards for spiritual teachers. There is, certainly, a lobby for some method of dealing with the harm caused by irresponsible or fraudulent spiritual teachers; but interestingly enough, the notion of standardised training practices has not been raised. (There is, of course, a sanction against political activists who sufficiently annoy the state: they get arrested or otherwise disposed of.)

What I am getting at is that the terms of reference of the professionalisation debate lock out of discussion some of the most fundamental aspects of the activity in question. By treating therapists as social technicians, on a par with lawyers and accountants, the proponents of professionalisation are in one sense aggrandising; but in a deeper sense, they are grievously underestimating the significance of what we try to do. (Of course, this significance is not personal to us – as soon as we claim it in that way, we become incapable of doing it properly. It is the *practice* which deserves honour, not the practitioner.)

In asking or demanding that the institutions of the state underwrite a special status for psychotherapy, the UKCP is implicitly offering something in return. It is offering that psychotherapy acts *as the servant of civil society*: that psychotherapy, in turn, underwrites the state. You don't need to be a political anarchist to wonder whether this is a devil's bargain; and whether it is compatible with the real goals of our work. To quote the *Tao Te Ching* again:

On the day the emperor is crowned
Or the three officers of state installed
Do not send a gift of jade and a team of four horses,
but remain still and offer the Tao.
(verse 62)

References

Brazier, D. (1995) *Zen Therapy*, London: Constable.

Epstein, M. (1996) *Thoughts Without a Thinker*, London: Duckworth.

Feng, G.-F. and English, J. (1973) *Lao Tse: Tao Te Ching*. London: Wildwood House.

Ferenczi, S. (1927) 'The problem of the termination of the analysis' in *Final Contributions to the Problems and Methods of Psychoanalysis*, New York: Bruner/Mazel.

Freud, S. (1927) *Postscript to The Question of Lay Analysis*, Penguin Freud Library 15.

Fromm, E. (1991) *The Sane Society*, London: Routledge. (Original work published 1942)

Fromm, E. and Suzuki, D. T. (1960) *Zen Buddhism and Psychoanalysis*, New York: Harper.

Mindell, A. (1992) *The Leader as Martial Artist*, San Francisco: Harper San Francisco.

Phillips, A. (1995) *Terrors and Experts*, London: Faber and Faber.

Pilgrim, D. (1992) 'Psychotherapy and political evasions', in W. Dryden and C. Feltham (eds), *Psychotherapy and Its Discontents*, Milton Keynes: Open University Press, pp. 225–42.

Reich, W. (1983 [1942]) *The Function of the Orgasm*, London: Souvenir Press.

Reik, T. (1927) 'Contribution to the Symposium on Lay Analysis', *International Journal of Psycho-Analysis*, VIII.

Sachs, H. (1927) 'Contribution to the Symposium on Lay Analysis', *International Journal of Psycho-Analysis*, VIII.

Samuels, A. (1993) *The Political Psyche*, London: Routledge.

Totton, N. and Edmondson, E. (1988) *Reichian Growth Work: Melting the Blocks to Life and Love*, Bridport, Devon: Prism Press (2nd edn, PCCS Books, 2009).

Trungpa, C. (1987) *Cutting through Spiritual Materialism*, Boston: Shambhala.

Waelder, R. (1927) 'Contribution to the Symposium on Lay Analysis', *International Journal of Psycho-Analysis*, VIII.

Welwood, J. (ed.) (1983) *Awakening the Heart: East/West Approaches to Psychotherapy and the Healing Relationship*, Boston: Shambhala.

Winnicott, D. W. (1975) 'Mind and its relation to the psyche-soma', in *Through Paediatrics to Psychoanalysis: Collected Papers*, New York: Basic Books, pp. 243–54. (Original work published 1949)

Endnotes

1. I am by no means the first to point out these connections: see for example Brazier, 1995; Epstein, 1996; Welwood, 1983; Samuels, 1993; Fromm, 1991; and Heron, Chapter I.1, this volume.

2. See in particular Mindell, 1992.

3. I am not referring to any particular school here, but to the implications of our fundamental techniques – implications which renew themselves and make themselves available for rediscovery in each therapeutic session.

4. Some practitioners in the USA have avoided registration issues by declaring themselves to be religious functionaries, but this is not what I have in mind!

Part III
From Professionalisation to Pluralism

The Accountable Therapist: Standards, Experts and Poisoning the Well III.1

Brian Thorne

When I write, I usually have something to say about which I feel strongly and which I believe I can articulate with reasonable clarity and persuasiveness. Indeed, much of my pleasure comes from presenting a well documented and lucid argument with passion. In this instance, however, I find myself in a rather different mood. Instead of clarity, I shall present my confusion, and in order to do that I fear I shall have to inflict a certain amount of autobiographical data upon my reader. Indeed, I have a somewhat unnerving sense that I am embarking on a process of self-therapy in public. Perhaps, though, readers will not be too dismayed at being cast in the role of eavesdroppers, even of voyeurs – legitimate snoopers into the somewhat bewildered psyche of a battle-scarred person-centred counsellor.

Essentially I have felt for some years now like a man who is in danger because he has become imprisoned in the profession of therapy. Let me attempt to explain. This summer I shall have completed 29 years as a counsellor, and that is a long haul judged by any criterion. During that time I have experienced astonishing developments in the world of therapy and counselling in our country, and in a minor way I suppose I have contributed to some of them. When I began as a counsellor in 1968 there was no Association for Student Counselling, there was no British Association for Counselling, there was certainly no UK Council for Psychotherapy. The man whom I still regard as the greatest therapist I ever met – George Lyward of Finchden Manor – possessed no formal qualifications as a therapist and put MA(Cantab) after his name in the conviction – wholly justified it seemed – that this would be sufficient evidence for any discerning person that he was wholly competent at the job. Nobody seemed to worry much that his Cambridge degree was in

---

The first draft of this chapter was originally presented as a lecture at the Annual Meeting of the Ashby Trust in 1991 and subsequently published in *Self and Society*, 23 (4), 1995.

history. There were, of course, some powerful analysts around who held mysterious court in Hampstead, and those were the days of the Tavistock ascendancy and of residential weeks in pursuit of Leadership Skills where Tavistock-trained consultants traumatised businessmen and academics alike by their sometimes impenetrable interpretations of group process and their disciplined regard for the second hand of their watches. But on the whole, those few counsellors and therapists around had only rudimentary support systems, strange hybrid trainings and little sense of belonging to a greater body of brothers and sisters. What I remember vividly, however, was the sense of dedication and of adventure: the exhilaration of being pioneers in a new world.

In 1989 I was invited to contribute to a book entitled *On Becoming a Psychotherapist*, and was confronted by the somewhat daunting task of recalling my own training and the first months in my new and, at that time, almost unknown profession (Dryden and Spurling, 1989). In fact, the writing proved to be a thoroughly enlivening experience, for it put me in touch again with the motivational energy which constituted the driving-force behind my aspirations of those days. In the first place, I did not recall being particularly excited as I set out for my training course. On the contrary, there was more a sense of being pulled somewhat against my will towards a kind of inevitable destiny. I knew that to become a counsellor meant giving up much that I loved dearly, for I was a gifted teacher and could have looked forward to a pretty successful career, I think, in the teaching profession. Secondly, I recall clearly my determination not to get sucked into a kind of psychological ghetto; I was keen, for example, to retain my literary and theological interests, and not to lose those perspectives on reality which had underpinned my life for so long. In short, I was highly resistant to any notion of a psychological framework for human personality and human interaction which would negate my understanding of persons *as essentially mysterious beings who shared in the overarching mystery of the cosmos*. I entered lectures on psychological theories of personality fortified by Wordsworth's *Intimations of Immortality*:

> Our birth is but a sleep and a forgetting: / The Soul that rises with us, our life's Star, / Hath had elsewhere its setting / And cometh from afar / … trailing clouds of glory do we come / From God, who is our home.

Fortunately for me, it turned out that my training did not constitute an assault on my previously held convictions and understandings. On the contrary, it deepened them, added to them and gave them a new coherence and potency. The good fortune, as I see it, was that I was being trained to be a client-centred counsellor in the tradition of Carl Rogers. As I read Rogers' books with increasing enthusiasm, I realised that I was not being asked to take on board a whole new perception of reality or a highly complex theory of human personality. I was not even being required to change my basic way of being with those who sought my help. Instead, I found in Rogers someone who seemed to esteem the validity of my own experience and who gave names to attitudes and behaviours which I had falteringly attempted to embody for many years. And so it was that Carl Rogers became, for me, not the new guru or source of all wisdom for the aspiring therapist, but a gentle companion who spoke of unconditional positive regard, empathy and genuineness, and this gave shape to what for me had previously been an almost instinctive and somewhat incoherent response to others in need.

The client-centred or person-centred approach not only enabled me to retain a firm hold on my own identity, but went some way towards preserving me from arrogance and from the insidious snares of psychological power-mongering. Weighty theories about personality development and complex maps of the unconscious certainly have their fascination, but they can make those who have studied them feel important and erudite. Such a training would, I think, have been bad for me, for I was only too aware that I was a powerful person, and anything that might have added to that sense of power would probably have knocked my humility for six for a long time to come. In effect, I was being trained to reject the role of the expert and to become proficient at the far more delicate task of being the faithful companion. As I look back on that training experience and as I think now of my work as a trainer of person-centred therapists, I have no doubt whatever that the whole enterprise is concerned with mutuality, with intimacy, with power-sharing, with transparency, with tapping into currents of love and creativity which are the essence of spiritual reality. The expertise, if that is the appropriate word, lies in the capacity, to quote Scott Peck's words, 'to extend oneself for the purpose of nurturing one's own or another's spiritual growth' (Peck, 1978: 199).

Over the years I have come to acknowledge that *all* of my most challenging clients have drawn me inexorably into the same terrain. They have, in fact, challenged my ability to love. It is notable that in the vast corpus of professional literature which now exists on counselling and psychotherapy, there is not much reference to this issue of love. And yet I have known for many years that, for me, offering the core conditions of acceptance, empathy and congruence, if I do so consistently and honestly, means a willingness to love my clients and the likelihood that I shall end up doing so. I would go further: my experience has convinced me that it is, in fact, essential for me to love my clients if genuine healing is to occur, and that the deeper the wound or the greater the deficiency, the more likely it is that I shall have to extend myself in love to a degree which is costly in effort and commitment. There is part of me which does not like that conclusion. There are times when I would prefer my success as a therapist to depend on my knowledge, my therapeutic skills or techniques, my experience, my years of self-exploration. But I know that I should be deluding myself to believe that. Perhaps I have now run across too many incompetent therapists who are loaded with degrees and qualifications, or have undergone lengthy training analyses. However, love which finds its expression in 'the will to extend one's self for the purpose of nurturing one's own or another's spiritual growth' cannot permit fusion or the falling in love which leads to all kinds of sexual complications. The love to which I refer, in fact, is very demanding in the discipline it imposes.

I must confess that I often find it difficult to see why a therapist without a belief in the potential divinisation of humanity and therefore in a divine source of power should submit himself or herself to such a discipline. It may be, however, that what I have described as the longing for the spiritual growth of another can be experienced as a profound and unselfish desire for a fellow human being to become fully human. For me this amounts to the same thing, but I can readily appreciate that for many therapists the change in language is important. I am persuaded, too, but less readily, that a deep and unshakable yearning for the fulfilment of another's humanity need not be linked to a belief in God, or indeed to any 'religious' interpretation of reality.

Having 'come clean' about this primacy of love in the therapeutic enterprise, I do not wish to be accused of naivete or sentimentalism. Love as I mean it in this context clearly demands the most rigorous training and discipline and levels of self-knowledge and self-acceptance, which are unlikely to be attained without effort except by the most fortunate and beloved of persons. In short, I believe that counsellors need high-quality training, regular and sensitive supervision and every opportunity to extend and deepen their personal and professional resources. Events of recent years, however, lead me to write these words with a heavy heart and with a persistent sense of foreboding. Here lies the crux of the disquiet to which I referred at the beginning. Increasingly I have found myself becoming imprisoned in a vicious circle of feverish activity as the new accountability culture permeates the world of therapy. Now, it seems, we must not only do good work but manifestly be seen to do it, and we must also seek to convince the public at large, and the government in particular, that we are worthy people, wholly reputable and dripping with prestigious qualifications which ensure our legitimacy and our continuing employability.

All this is very painful for me. As long ago as 1977, I was a prime mover in the establishing of a rigorous procedure for the accreditation of student counsellors. It was my conviction that we owed it both to our clients and to ourselves to aim for the highest possible standards, and to challenge ourselves to become ever-more open to personal and professional development. Little did I guess at that time that only 20 years later we should find ourselves caught up in an increasingly vicious circle where accountability, appraisal, evaluation, value for money, raising of standards, open competition and the like are the buzz words. Our culture has become virtually obsessed with seeing the world through the eyes of cost accountants and other measurers of human effectiveness, where 'effectiveness' often seems to mean the ability to persuade others to think and to do what, left to their own volition, they would never dream of thinking or doing – and to do it cheaply. I believe that we have witnessed a political transformation in the last two decades which has produced a society where more and more people are seeking the help of counsellors and therapists because of the stress caused by competitiveness, constant surveillance and the fear of failure. At the same time, the therapists to whom they take their concerns are themselves increasingly fussed about their legitimacy, their performance, their cost effectiveness, the approval of government or, at a more mundane level, their acceptability to insurance companies.

When someone told me a few years ago that the new Archbishop of Canterbury was also into appraisal and parish audits I experienced a wave of despair which threatened to engulf me altogether. Could it be that a priest will soon be evaluated on the quality of his sermons, the beauty of his singing, the numbers in the pews, the health of his marriage! Not so, it will be argued, for such appraisal will lead to a new level of self-exploration and a real sense of caring by senior clergy for their less experienced colleagues. It was shortly after the Archbishop's reported penchant for appraisal was made public that a Diocesan Bishop and his Suffragans informed the world that they had embarked upon just such an appraisal process, and that its benefits and fruits were wondrous to contemplate. Men in the pews, too, were only too keen to point out that they in the world of business and commerce had long since been swept up into the appraisal, accountability culture, and that it was about time the vicar had a dose of what it was like in the 'real' world.

As so often that splendid journal *The Tablet* came to my rescue. Talking about higher education, it likened what was happening there to many other areas of our national life. The universities and polytechnics had allowed themselves to become infected, said *The Tablet*, with 'the language of the grocer's shop'. As a result higher education was in danger of losing its soul (20 May, 1989). These phrases struck me as describing with disturbing accuracy much of what I experienced as a university counsellor.

For many academics and administrators, there has been an almost total transformation in the ethos of academic life, and they find themselves caught up in a competitive rat race where not only departments can be swept into internecine strife but individual worth is construed almost entirely in terms of research output or the ability to attract funds. Many staff who entered upon their careers with a genuine love of scholarship and the pursuit of knowledge find that there is no longer a place for them unless they are prepared to develop the skills and the mentality of the entrepreneur. For their part, students in such an environment can quickly cease to experience themselves as persons and become, rather, consumers of knowledge. And so it is that they come to the counsellor's office obsessed with the production of the perfect essay, or paralysed with anxiety that they may not achieve the first-class degree which alone can bolster their dehumanised self-concept. The consumerist mentality and language of the grocer's shop has so infected the personality that soul has fled, and left only a barren identity preoccupied with achievement and the concomitant fear of failure. Not infrequently now I find myself viewing counselling services in higher education as monasteries of a new dark age, for they keep alive the vision of a world where persons matter more than things, and where mutuality and understanding are more important than achievement and competition.

The danger is that the therapists themselves will collude by capitulating to the consumerist ideology and putting all their energy into ensuring that they are offering a good product, and by proving by their words and actions that they are intent on serving loyally in the brave new world of the managerial interest. And gradually and insidiously – perhaps without ever realising it – we, too, shall lose our own souls and become gloriously efficient at enabling our clients to function competently in a world devoid of meaning where all that matters is what we do, how we perform and the impressive range of our material possessions. Hence, my dilemma and my anxiety.

One of my later contributions at the end of the 1980s to the raising of standards was my Co-Chairmanship of the BAC Working Group on the Recognition of Counselling Courses. In many ways this was a wonderful experience, as for three years with a group of much loved and respected colleagues I struggled away at establishing criteria and processes for the evaluation of courses. It was stimulating and enjoyable, and what is more I felt proud of our results. But now I am aware of the agony and the heart-ache which have been caused to many trainers up and down the land who for reasons, sometimes beyond their control, can never hope to have their courses recognised. Similarly, I see the frequent adverts in the national press where applicants are required to have BAC accreditation or to be eligible for it before their candidature can even be considered. Where, I ask, is the soul in all this? Could it be that all the energy I have devoted over the years to schemes for accreditation and recognition, all the many hours spent in committee and in working parties – could it be that all this, instead of improving the quality of therapy and enhancing the well-being of both therapists and clients, has led instead to the creation of an exclusive professionalism and added anxiety, competitiveness and the fear of judgement to the lives of those who were previously lovingly and conscientiously responding to the needs of their clients? Have I, in fact, played right into the hands of those who have neurotically created this death-dealing culture of accountability and appraisal, where the basic assumption is that nobody is really trustworthy and where everyone has to be monitored and given incentives if they are to do a good job? I am genuinely bewildered by these questions, and there are times when they threaten to tear me in two.

Sometimes I feel that my own therapeutic tradition makes things ten thousand times worse for me. I am committed to my client's path which he or she alone is capable of discovering, given that I am equally committed to offering my unconditional acceptance, my empathy and my own transparent genuineness. As a therapist I am resolutely opposed to the imposition of external standards, to the passing of judgements, to the formulation of clever interpretations. By word and behaviour I attempt to convey my validation of the uniqueness of the individual, and to counter the conditioning which for so many people has led to a sense of inferiority, inadequacy or even worthlessness. And yet in my professional arena my name has – with justification – become associated with accreditation, with the application of rigorous standards, with external judgements. Even as I write, I am conscious that in a month's time I shall be attending the next meeting of the Executive Committee of the United Kingdom Register of Counsellors on which I faithfully serve.

Many years ago in an essay entitled 'Beyond the Core Conditions' I described my work with a particular client called Sally for a book entitled *Key Cases in Psychotherapy* (Dryden, 1987). The object of the book was to invite therapists of many different traditions to focus on therapeutic relationships which had proved maximally challenging and which had revolutionised their therapeutic practice. I was, I believe, particularly daring – or perhaps foolhardy – in that book, for I chose to describe a relationship with a woman who had come to see me because of grave sexual difficulties. Indeed, she herself collaborated with me in the writing of the chapter. I should like to end by quoting from the final section of the account where I am attempting to assess the significance of the relationship for my work as a therapist and for me as a person:

> In some ways, I have come to think that it was with Sally that I had the courage for the first time to test out the person-centred approach to the furthest limits. For more than a decade I had attempted to be accepting, empathic and genuine with my clients. I had also tried to trust their innate wisdom and to have faith in their capacity, given the right climate, to find their own way forward. Never before, however, had I found the courage and ability to experience and express those attitudes and beliefs so consistently over such a lengthy period of time.
>
> With Sally I could not dodge the implications of believing that I am an eternal soul, that the source of all being is infinite love, that the body is the temple of the divine, that sexuality and spirituality are indivisible, that prayer is a route into the invisible world. To be genuine with Sally meant living out those beliefs in the moment-to-moment relationship with her. Talking about them was at times important and necessary, but far more fundamental was the way in which those beliefs coloured and permeated my acceptance, not only of her, but also of myself. I had to take my own soul and body seriously and to cherish them as much as I

> cherished hers .... With Sally I dared to be whole because nothing less would do, and in the process I discovered levels of genuineness, acceptance and empathy which gave access to a transcendent world where healing occurs because the understanding is complete. In short, thanks to my work with Sally, I have come to acknowledge and to affirm that for me the practice of person-centred therapy cannot be divorced from my journey as an eternal soul ....
>
> I now believe that most existing theories of personality and personality development sell the human species short. With Sally, I came to recognise the essential mysteriousness of personality and found in this a refreshing change from theories which attempt to offer an almost complete understanding.
>
> In summary, my work with Sally convinces me that, if two people believe that love is the governing power in the universe, and that we have not yet penetrated more than a fraction of the mystery of human personality or human relating, then they may be prepared to accept and to share their weakness, vulnerability, embarrassment and ineptitude and find that it is in the apparent poverty that riches are concealed.
>
> (Thorne, 1987: 65–7)

I have little doubt that my work with this client was the most taxing and the most rewarding I had undertaken up to that point in my career. What is more, I have never felt more responsible to someone, nor more in touch with my own integrity. And yet I have a strange feeling that the courage which we both required had little to do with professional standards and responsibility as we usually understand them, and very little to do with the letter of the ethical code, and everything to do with its spirit. We were drawing pure water from the well of suffering which is also the well of life. Could it be that this is the very water we are in danger of poisoning in our zeal to become exemplary professionals with impeccable credentials and ever higher standards? The question does not go away.

References

Dryden, W. (ed.) (1987) *Key Cases in Psychotherapy,* London: Croom Helm.

Dryden, W. and Spurling L. (eds) (1989) *On Becoming a Psychotherapist,* London: Tavistock/Routledge.

Peck, M. S. (1978) *The Road Less Travelled,* London: Hutchinson.

Thorne, B. (1987) 'Beyond the core conditions', in W. Dryden (ed.), *Key Cases in Psychotherapy*, London: Croom Helm, pp. 48–77.

Counselling in the UK: Jungle, Garden or Monoculture? III.2

Denis Postle

Tight corners produce a sharpening of both metaphors and elbows. As the market for psycho-practice in the UK changes, it does indeed put many practitioners in a tight corner. How do I register? Can I register? Do I want to register? It has spawned a jostling of elbows for dominance by the register-builders, and one particular metaphor, vegetation, that I'd like to explore here.

In a recent talk to a conference at St George's Hospital entitled 'Registration: what it will mean to you the counsellor' (Deurzen, 1996), Professor Emmy van Deurzen, a former chair of UKCP, had a lot to say about counselling and registration that seems to me highly dubious. I want to review her talk here in a some detail because it furnishes a good example of the world-view that has necessitated the development of alternative ways of being accountable.

In the opening of her presentation she leaves her audience in no doubt of her dominant position in these matters by the well-known professorial/parental device of telling the audience what they think:

> You know what registration is about in practical terms. You have been told how the United Kingdom Register of Counsellors is going to work. You know the facts and you still have the fantasies. Sometimes you think that being registered would guarantee your professional status and make you feel a whole lot better about yourself. At other times you think that all this registration business will just make the distinctions between people more artificial and more definitive. You fear that you might be really penalised if you cannot obtain registration or that registration will just make everybody less interested in what they do as the profession becomes bureaucratised and systematised, perverting and distorting its original purpose.

This is a mode of address that might be thought to elbow out of the way the adult autonomy of the listeners. It supports a sense I'd previously had that Professor van Deurzen is someone who even sees dominance as natural, at least in herself, since why else would she presume to tell an audience of counsellors what is in their minds? And indeed in an interview about UKCP last year, she spoke of the inevitability of hierarchies forming.

Yet is the institutionalised dominance that counselling and psychotherapy registers represent really inevitable? Or the only choice? Isn't it at the very least, open to question?

One of feminism's sweetest gifts has been its challenge to the 'naturalness' and 'inevitability' of male dominance and therefore dominance in general, since the theorising about dominance had hitherto been in the hands of – surprise, surprise – mostly men. And isn't this, as I would suppose, a perspective that belongs in any self-respecting counselling or psychotherapy training? Is it not the case that many, if not most, clients come with difficulties that are at root to do with power, with the playing out of agendas of dominance and subjection? Since I believe that most psycho-practitioners do indeed try to work, and even live, from a 'power-with' ethical stance which responds to the damaging effects of domination, it seems reasonable to hope that the organisations which represent them should also do so.

Like a number of other practitioners I have become convinced that the UKCP is not such a body. As David Kalisch puts it:

> UKCP is a dominator hierarchy seeking to borrow power from another dominator hierarchy in order to impose its dominance .... It is not possible to canvas for pluralism and diversity whilst voting for statutory registration.
>
> (Kalisch, 1996: 38)

Professor van Deurzen went on to say that, while counselling and psychotherapy were small scale and scarce, she was happy with self-monitoring: 'Of course this freedom was sometimes abused, but there is no doubt that the advantages of creativity and diversity that it engendered on balance outweighed the negative factors.' Now, however, this has mysteriously changed. 'The situation that has now evolved with the rapid expansion of this sector has required us to check this unbridled freedom and diversity. We have needed to mitigate the creativity and individuality with quality control and accountability.' The question for me, and I guess for many readers, is – who is this 'We'?

Professor van Deurzen asserts in the conclusion of her talk that:

> When a garden has been very fertile and has been left to itself for a long period of time it is overgrown. Sprawling plants obscure each other's light and deprive each other of nutrients. It is then necessary to cut the plants back, quite drastically and carefully select the ones that one wishes to encourage and make room for, at the same time as uprooting those plants considered to be weeds.

This seems to me riddled with presumptions that domination and control are natural and inevitable. There is the presumption that the field of UK psycho-practice is a garden, and not, for example, a meadow. As Professor Yi-Fu Tuan has pointed out, gardening is one of the areas, along with pet-keeping, where dominance commonly finds expression. 'It is then necessary to cut the plants back ...'. Again, who decides? Who is it who claims to know what to cut back and what to select and which are weeds to be uprooted? On what criteria? Does Professor van Deurzen inhabit an evidence-free zone?

She is undoubtedly aware of the dangers in the pruning that she is suggesting: 'If it is done haphazardly and too aggressively the result can be a sparse, unattractive environment in which little growth can be observed for a long time to come.' However in these times of rapid growth:

> The pruning of registration and standard setting is a welcome and entirely necessary phenomenon ... as far as I am concerned: it was high time that we began to disentangle this overgrown field, for it had turned into a jungle, where some weird and wonderful creatures were sometimes doing untold damage.

Here is a professor of psychotherapy and counselling, using the word 'jungle' to represent a state of appalling and threatening disorder populated with damaging creatures. How come she hasn't noticed that 'jungle' also means 'rainforest', by far and away the richest ecological structure on this planet? One on which the whole of its climate and possibly its future depends? And one, indeed, populated with weird and wonderful creatures. Such as for example the gorilla, that along with jungle, has also been notoriously abused as a carrier of negative projection, i.e. King Kong, yet in reality is a gentle vegetarian creature.

For me, Professor van Deurzen's talk provides a narrowed, inadequate and fundamentally unreliable perspective from which to claim to know who in counselling or psychotherapy is a weed and who is not. Strangely enough, the present Chair of UKCP, Professor Digby Tantam, is also on record as hoping that registration will 'weed out unpromising, ineffective, or downright harmful innovations at a much earlier stage' (Tantam, 1996a).

Notice the phrase 'weed out'. Psychotherapy registration is not some informal evolutionary process through which valuable mutations survive and the others disappear; a register *creates* weeds. Indeed, for it to make sense, it *has* to create weeds to justify the high cost of the education of cultivars. This is a cultural and political decision, the conscious creation of privilege. I believe that it damages the interests, both of the psychotherapy client population and of psychotherapists in general. The former are likely to be denied sufficient choice to find a good match for their issues. And the latter, due to becoming locked into a culture where quality assurance is dominated by hierarchical bureaucratic control, will gradually drift towards a 'play safe', 'low risk' style of practice.

This is especially likely if this control is focused through cascades of supervisory deference (Young, 1996) or a desire to end the 'balkanisation' of therapy (Savage, 1996). As Kalisch has suggested, at the heart of bureaucratisation that UKCP represents is a desire that the wildness, iconoclasm and potential dangerousness of creative thought and imagination be tamed, anaesthetised and rendered anaemic in order to be safe for human consumption (Kalisch, 1990). Perhaps anyone who feels that creativity is not compromised by psychotherapy registration would outline how they would propose setting up from scratch a new psychotherapy training school and gaining UKCP recognition for it.

Diversity matters, and those who move to damage it deserve confrontation and resistance:

> Society is like an amoeba: it moves from the margins, not from the centre. Cut off from its margins it can only sclerotise and shrivel, become ever less responsive to change.
>
> (George Monbiot, 1996)

In seeking to understand the ecology of psycho-practice, I recommend the eloquent testimony of Vandana Shiva, in *Monocultures of the Mind*, a book about what happens when diversity is damaged or undermined (Shiva, 1993). Shiva is writing about the destruction of forests in India but her observations seem to me to apply very well to the UKCP's annexation of psychotherapy. The UKCP may argue that within their structure there is a wide diversity of practice. Local flavours there certainly are, but if we take an ecological perspective of the emergence of the UKCP as a public body, several factors combine to make it a 'monoculture of the mind'. These factors include:

- The requirement that entry and training be at postgraduate level (UKCP, 1993).
- The belief that outside the remit of the UKCP and its participant organisations there is no tradition of psychotherapy of comparable value (Tantam, 1996a, b).
- The conviction that welding together the disparate sects of psychotherapy into a profession that has the same sort of status as science or medicine is an intrinsically worthy project.
- The belief that the public needs to be protected from psychotherapists (Tantam, 1996a, b).
- The belief that the public can be protected from charlatans by the existence of adequate training standards, codes of practice and complaints procedures (Deurzen, 1996).

Shiva (1993: 7) writes:

> Monocultures first inhabit the mind.
>
> Then as a monoculture takes root, they have a characteristic relation to the world around them ....
>
> Monocultures of the mind generate models of production which destroy diversity and legitimise that destruction as progress, growth and improvement. ... [This leads to] impoverished systems both qualitatively and quantitatively. They are also highly unstable and non-sustainable systems. ... [Monocultures spread] not because they produce more, but because they control more. The expansion of monocultures has more to do with politics and power than with enriching and enhancing systems.

One of the ways in which monocultures can be recognised is through their attitude to the distribution of power. Uniformity goes hand in hand with centralisation, while diversity demands de-centered control. Resisting monocultures, Shiva argues, requires active protection of, and promotion of, diversity. Diversity as a way of thought and a way of life is what is needed to go beyond the impoverished monocultures of the mind.

Shiva's ecological overview points to another characteristic of monocultures: the inflation of one local practice into global dominance, so that, for example, a local tradition, British public school education, becomes the means by which a whole continent is subjugated – India in the nineteenth and early twentieth centuries.

Power is also built into the perspective which views the dominant system not as a globalised local tradition but as a universal tradition inherently superior to local systems. What has been a local tradition is inflated into global dominance. So that 'scientific psychology', 'psychotherapy', and perhaps soon 'counselling' are elevated from being local varieties of psycho-practice to the globally dominant. What people who overvalue control in human affairs miss is that the universal will emerge anyway, and that the ethical, technical, and theoretical corsets of UKCP will frustrate this evolution and generate new forms of iatrogenic damage in clients. As Shiva (1993: 10) reminds us:

> The universal would spread in openness. The globalising local spreads by violence and misrepresentation. The first level of violence unleashed on local systems of knowledge is not to see them as knowledge.

Knowledge (or practice and experience) that does not fit the criteria of the dominant 'universal' definition of 'psychotherapist' is inadequate, wrong or dangerous. A person claiming to practise psychotherapy outside the umbrella of the UKCP is then potentially a 'charlatan':

> The public needs ... to be protected from charlatans by the existence of adequate training standards, codes of practice and complaints procedures .... We were also disadvantaged by the fact that anybody could set up as a therapist and in some cases practice erratically and irresponsibly, tarnishing our reputation.
>
> (Deurzen, 1996)

As Shiva (1993: 10) goes on:

> When local knowledge does appear in the field of the globalising vision, it is made to disappear by denying it the status of a systematic knowledge, and assigning it the adjectives 'primitive' and 'unscientific'. One of the

> ways in which this is made to happen is through the separation of weeds and cultivars.

And Shiva also has this to say about weed-making:

> Declaring a locally useful species a weed is another aspect of the politics of disappearance by which the space of local knowledge shrinks out of existence. The one dimensional field of vision of the dominant system perceives only one value, based on the market, and it generates [forestry and agricultural] practices which aim at maximising that value.
> (1993: 27)

Digby Tantam writes of psychotherapy as a garden, attempting to offer an 'ecologically sound' image. He continues:

> Unfortunately everything in a garden is not lovely. Some plants are poisonous. Other become vectors for pests and viruses. Trees are not ideal for every situation, but neither are ground cover plants. Bulbs will mature and flower in a year, but shrubs will take much longer. Some nurseries undercut others by producing poor stock cheaply ... and so on. I am sure you can see how this metaphor applies to psychotherapy, and how it could be made to apply further.
> (Tantam, 1996b: 98)

Gardening, along with pet keeping is one of the most ubiquitous pointers to underlying attitudes of domination (Tuan, 1985). The gardening metaphor as employed above implies a 'gardener', a 'controller'. Applied to psychotherapy, the assumption is of an intrinsic right to dominate, exactly the point I seek to make here. Shiva goes on to further delineate how colonisers who succeed in inflating their local knowledge into universal dominance consolidate their gains:

> By elevating itself *above* society and other knowledge systems and by simultaneously excluding other knowledge systems from the domain of reliable and systematic knowledge, the dominant system creates its exclusive monopoly.
> (Shiva, 1993: 12)

Attempting to inflate psychotherapy, a local tradition, to that of a dominant universal, a process that will necessarily marginalise the alternatives, requires concealment. An ambitious 'dominant universal' such as UKCP requires a public face, a serviceable political fascia of 'public accountability' and 'ethical responsibility', and public protection in support of its attempt at creating a monopoly. Behind this, it can conceal its inaccessibility to 'outsiders' and, most significantly, clients. Because individual participation is impossible. Once more, Shiva (1993: 12) has a useful perspective on the process: 'Paradoxically, it is the knowledge systems which are considered most open, that are, in reality closed to scrutiny and evaluation.'

Sadly, this is what tends to be typical of existing dominant professions such as law, medicine and science. UKCP is intent on helping psychotherapists create their own customised stronghold, its own monocultural agribusiness; how long before it becomes a desert?

I thought it worth spelling out some of these incongruities and the questions that are thereby raised at length, because in many ways, they represent the factors of disinformation and hubris that have done so much to generate the climate of fear and uncertainly that registration evokes in many psycho-practitioners. However, confronting the inadequacies of existing organisations, particularly their tendency to mirror societal norms around the distribution of power, implicitly raises another question. What kind of institution would properly represent the ethics and values of the many counsellors, psychotherapists and facilitators who have seen through the command-and-control agendas of UKCP, BPS and BCP? What kind of institution would model a rainforest?

References

Deurzen, E., van (1996) 'Registration: what it will mean to you the counsellor', 5th St George's Counselling in Primary Care Conference, Keynote address, 12 June (mimeo).

Kalisch, D. (1990) 'Professionalisation – a rebel view', *Self and Society.* 18 (1): 24–9.

Kalisch, D. (1996) Letter, *Self and Society*, 24 (2): 38.

Monbiot, G. (1996) 'Campaigners become enemies of the state', *The Guardian,* 29 August: 19.

Savage, P. (1996) *The Psychotherapist*, 6: 12.

Shiva, V. (1993) *Monocultures of the Mind: Perspectives on Biodiversity and Biotechnology,* London: Zed Books. http://amorystarr.com/ad_ict4d_reader/shivamono1993.pdf

Tantam, D. (1996a) Letter, *Self and Society*, 24 (2), May.

Tantam, D. (1996b) 'The structure and formation of national umbrella organisations in psychotherapy', *International Journal of Psychotherapy*. 1 (1): 97–100.

Tuan, Y. (1984) *Dominance and Affection: The Making of Pets*, Yale University Press: New Haven and London.

UKCP (1993) *Training Requirements.* See http://www.psychotherapy.org.uk/training-standards.html

Young, R. M. (1996) *Psychodynamics of Psychoanalytic Organisations,* Online at http://human-nature.com/culture/ppo1.html

Psychotherapy and Tragedy III.3

David Smail

Increasingly, it seems to me that psychotherapy lives in a world of its own.

I'm not entirely sure why this should be. Perhaps it's just that I'm getting older, callused by the years, and less susceptible to idealistic visions. The explanation I prefer, though, is that the end of the twentieth century has yielded up a very different world for most of us than did the middle, when perhaps the real boom in therapy could be said to have got under way in earnest (when, that is, a largely esoteric set of psychoanalytic mysteries began to give way quite rapidly to a luxuriant crop of therapies widely available and understandable to non-initiates).

However this may be, the contrast between the world outside the walls of the consulting room and that within them has, for me, become so stark that what goes on inside seems to have almost no relevance any more for what goes on outside. Unless, I suppose, you occupy one of the more protected ghettos of the metropolitan middle class and/or are able to surround yourself with the excited make-believe generated by the information and publicity media of so-called 'postmodernity'.

During what Eric Hobsbawm calls the 'Golden Age' of this century, which stretched roughly from the end of the Second World War until it began to unravel in the mid-seventies (Hobsbawm, 1994), occupants of the developed Western world enjoyed a relative social and economic stability and prosperity which enabled us to believe that the *choices* open to us in the conduct of our lives were fundamentally matters of psychology. For example, if you wanted to work, you did, and, what's more, in the field of your choice. Personal relationships could be established and their continuance anticipated in a setting where the essentials of livelihood – money, housing, health care, pensions, etc., etc. – seemed to have a

---

Paper read at the J. Richard Marshall Memorial Meeting of the Psychotherapy Section of the British Psychological Society, 27 April 1996, and published subsequently in the Psychotherapy Section *Newsletter*, 20 (December), 1996: 3–13.

predictably stable future. So the *variability* in what we did – the triumphs as well as the catastrophes, the joys as well as sorrows, seemed to be more a matter of our *psychology* – our personal inclinations and understandings, our 'insight' and our 'will' – than of the influence of any factor external to us. In this setting, if things were going wrong, it seemed entirely plausible to assume that it must be because of mistakes one was making oneself; one looked inside rather than outside for the reasons for failure and unhappiness, and in that situation the assistance of psychotherapy seemed an entirely natural recourse.

However, for most people the past 15 years or so have, progressively, undermined our security. The future has become uncertain, relationships troubled. The distal economic and political influences which provided the taken-for-granted structure in which we could, so to speak, exercise our psychology have undergone incalculable and apparently uncontrollable changes. The (albeit paradoxically) stabilising cold war has given way to, at worst, chaos, criminality and nationalist genocide, and, at best, economic privation for the most vulnerable members of society, ruthless opportunism and the construction of a new morality centred entirely on the values and standards of Business. Nation-states have become relatively impotent in a rapidly globalising economy so that not only individuals but also their collective political institutions are barely able to influence events. Suddenly we are confronted with the realisation (even if dawning only slowly) that it is not we who control our lives through the personal choices we make, but powers whose operation we can often not even see, let alone understand and influence.

For many, many people the world has become bleak and cold and dangerous in ways which we would have been hard put to it to imagine 20 years ago. The psychological consequences of this are a deep and pervasive sense of insecurity; multiple crises of identity (as a person, a worker, a sex, a nationality); the disintegration of 'relationship'; an increase in the desperate opting for the reassurance of magic, religion and make-believe; a withdrawal into privatism as well as a tendency to violent tribalism. And so on.

Small wonder perhaps that psychotherapy should be a major growth industry in this context. Walking into the cosy warmth of the consulting room provides a refuge from the cold, threatening world outside which is hard to resist. Psychotherapy, certainly, could opt to become one of a number of comforting illusions which, like astrology, born-again religion, or the racial mythology of fascism, offer a corner in which to escape from the privations of a cruel world, and no doubt psychotherapists could in the process make a reasonably decent living. But if so we'd certainly have to give up any *scientific* pretensions. What strikes me most about psychotherapy in the context of the current world is, I must say, what I can only describe as a kind of deranged optimism.

For what the past decade or two show us in ways we can no longer ignore is that people are injured, psychologically as well as physically, not *essentially* by errors of their own judgement, the vagaries of their consciousness, lack of insight into their own motives or failures of their will, but by the operation of basically material powers and influences in the world around them. What really upsets the applecart and buggers up people's lives and relationships is threatening their livelihood, throwing them out of work, stripping them of social meaning, depriving them of health and education, pillaging and destroying their environment, and so on. (Note that, from the perspective of the peaceful corner of the world we occupy here, I'm not even mentioning, starving, torturing, shooting and bombing them, killing their relatives, etc.)

The idea implicit in so much of psychotherapy, that individuals can be lifted out of this context, ignore all the influences bearing down on them from the wider world and somehow work out their own destiny just no longer seems credible. The wounds people are coming to us with can no longer be seen as self-inflicted, and certainly not within their power to mend themselves. The lesson which impresses itself on the late twentieth century psychotherapist is, I submit, not so much that our clients' difficulties represent an id to be converted to ego, an existential responsibility to be grasped, or even, *pace* Freud, an 'hysterical misery' to be transformed into 'common unhappiness' (Freud, 1895: 393) . What confronts us inescapably, I suggest, is that life is *tragic*.

By this I mean that the ills which beset us are not in our own power to eradicate or control; that is to say, there is usually very little, if anything, *the individual* can do successfully to act on the forces which blight his/her life, whether these stem from powers greater than him/herself or from the flaws of his/her own character.

It is not, of course, that this is a new development, and the last thing I want to do is suggest that it is only in the last 20 years that our lives have become tragic. (From Aeschylus in the 6th century BC to Thomas Hardy in the 19th AD, tragedians have portrayed the helplessness with which the individual has so often to become the spectator of his/her own destruction.) It is more that economic and political developments over the last few years have worked to dispel the illusion that, as psychological entities, we have power over our own destiny. The author of the *Encyclopaedia Britannica's* (15th edition) entry on 'Tragedy' notes that:

> The absence ... of a great tragic theatre in the 20th century may be explained by the pantheon of panaceas to which modern man has subscribed. Politics, psychology, social sciences, physical sciences, nationalism, the occult – each offered a context in terms of which he might act out his destiny, were it not crowded out by the others .... In the dramas of Athens and England, tragedy was born of the impossibility of a clear-cut victory in man's struggle with powers greater than himself.

On a personal note, I find this vision the more persuasive since I come to an appreciation of tragedy *because of* rather than *despite* my experience of psychotherapy. For it has been wrestling with the difficulties and contradictions of psychotherapy which has convinced me that there is too often an almost fateful inexorability about people's troubles for them to be seen as 'curable', or at least as lying within their own power to ameliorate. Quite often positively embarrassed by the blandness and glibness of the verbiage of so much therapeutic theory and practice, it was with tremendous relief that I came to the pathetically belated realisation that the view I was developing of the enormous impediments to 'change' in my own and my clients' struggles with life was in some respects one that I shared with Sophocles and Shakespeare.

I'm sure I'm not alone in this. Many psychotherapists, I know, are sobered as well as moved by the plights experienced by their clients, and some, as for example Roy Schafer (Schafer, 1976), have explicitly acknowledged the tragic dimension of their undertaking. But the vast bulk of the therapeutic literature – whether 'dynamic', humanistic' or 'cognitive-behavioural' – betrays an extraordinarily facile optimism about what people can achieve by, essentially, tugging fairly hard at their own boot-straps with a bit of encouragement from the sidelines by their therapist.

There's something very paradoxical about people who sit listening to the deepest pains and sorrows of others day in and day out, and witnessing as well the all-too-frequent failure of their best and most courageous efforts to overcome them, ending up with the promotion of fatuous notions like 'interpretation of the transference', 'taking responsibility' or 'cognitive restructuring', etc., etc.

But if psychotherapy has very little to say about how people are to escape the tragic inevitabilities of their lives, it certainly provides us with endless material showing how tragedy comes about, even if the significance of this is mainly to confirm what human beings and the chroniclers of their tragedies have known from the very beginning. I'd suggest in fact that the actual experience of psychotherapy emphasises in particular the two themes which are given most prominence in literary tragedy: the unavoidable outcome of fatal flaws of character, and the inexorability of social power. Ironically, it is precisely the inevitability of these two types of adversity which psychotherapy underlines in the very process of setting out to 'cure' them.

If psychotherapists really were able to alter character, we'd surely by now be a society of clones. Contrary to the nightmares of Huxley or the daydreams of Skinner, the lesson which seems to me to be drawn from the practice of psychotherapy is that it is extraordinarily difficult for people to change the psychological characteristics which become, as they grow up, part of their embodied make-up. It is, for example, no easier for you to change your basic self-confidence than it is to start speaking Chinese. It may even be more difficult. The impress of power stamps upon us at the most vulnerable stages of our development experiences of and attitudes towards reality which – as tragedians often show so movingly – we spend the rest of our lives working out.

This kind of process has of course not escaped our attention, but rather than take it seriously as a given of the human condition, we tend to psychologise it with facile notions like 'repetition compulsion' or 'unfinished business' which carry with them the entirely unjustified assumption that past experience is a kind of mistake which can be corrected. We encourage a view of the often agonised knowledge that people acquired of the world as children as 'baggage' which can somehow be jettisoned. With the best will in the world, and having for decades struggled to realise the therapeutic dream of relieving people of their painful pasts, I can find no evidence that the possibility of doing so is anything more than wishful thinking.

When it comes to looking at the problems that beset people in the present, we do not find ourselves on very much stronger ground. (For a fuller account of the role of social power in the generation of psychological distress see Smail, 1993, 1996 and 2005.) Beyond operating as a kind of personal sponge to soak up people's distress, psychotherapists have no power to act on the social influences which give rise to that distress in the first place, and quite often are in no position even to see where it's coming from. William Epstein, in a damning critique of the claims of psychotherapy, makes the point more forthrightly than anyone so far that psychotherapy's privatising of what are in fact public deficiencies has absolutely no rational evidence to support it, and is maintained only because of its political convenience to those who want to maintain the material advantages which they already have. Psychotherapy, he suggests:

> ... is an immensely attractive strategy for a society that is reluctant to allocate substantial funds to address its problems. If it were effective, then psychotherapy would offer efficient, low-cost remedies. Yet, even apart from the issue of its effectiveness, psychotherapy still provides a useful vehicle to proselytise the ideology of social efficiency in evading more productive and expensive approaches to social problems.... The ideology of therapeutics is ... consistent with a conservative social ideology that is unwilling to accept broad-based social expenditures to provide greater social equality through government action.
> (Epstein, 1995: 6)

It is not of course that psychotherapists are politically motivated villains deliberately trying to pull the wool over the eyes of their unsuspecting clients. It is more that, sheltered by a politico-economic climate which has its uses for us, we are at present enjoying a fools' paradise. In a wonderfully funny article in *Changes* a while ago, Simon King-Spooner (1995) likened psychotherapy's position to that of the white dodo, a native of the island of Reunion in the Indian Ocean. Described by a contemporary as 'a great fat fowl of the bignesse of a Turkie, and so short-winged they cannot flie, being white, and in a manner tame', the white dodo came to grief, King-Spooner points out, because it failed to keep itself in trim to cope with the predators who, inevitably, eventually found their way to the island. Psychotherapy, likewise, needs to pay careful attention to its critics if it is not suddenly to find itself overtaken by events.

Critiques like that of Epstein are already casting very hawk-like shadows over us, and may well proliferate as the future unrolls. If psychotherapy is to avoid the risk at some perhaps not too distant point of becoming dismissed as an irrelevance, it is going to have to address itself to the contradictions involved in claiming to be a 'treatment' for ills which are in fact the result of societal pressures far out of our personal reach to influence.

In my view, therapeutic psychology has at the end of the twentieth century to make fundamental adjustments to the philosophy it instituted at the beginning of it. In a fascinating passage in one of his *Introductory Lectures*, written, interestingly, only a year or two before the outbreak of the First World War, Freud chides Sophocles for the 'amorality' of his treatment of the Oedipus legend. I've often wondered how Freud managed to derive his version of the 'Oedipus Complex' from Sophocles' tragedy, since, apart from the name, there is so little resemblance between the two. But this passage makes it plain: Freud simply dismisses the tragedian's concern with the relation between Oedipus and powers (the gods) greater than and outside himself, and wrenches the structure of the work into a form which will support his own, entirely contrary notion of internalised will and unconscious morality. Completely disregarding the fact that Oedipus is overtaken by his fate despite the best efforts of all to avoid its coming to pass, and tries, desperately and unsuccessfully, to discharge his duty by obeying the dictates of superior power, Freud maintains instead that there is a 'secret sense and content of the legend' to which the auditor reacts.

> He reacts as though by self-analysis he had recognised the Oedipus complex in himself and had unveiled the will of the gods and the oracle as exalted disguises of his own unconscious. It is as though he was obliged to remember the two wishes – to do away with his father and in place of him to take his mother to wife – and to be horrified at them. And he understands the dramatist's voice as though it were saying to him: 'You are struggling in vain against your responsibility and are protesting in vain of what you have done in opposition to these criminal intentions. You are guilty, for you have not been able to destroy them; they still persist in you unconsciously.' And there is psychological truth in this. Even if a man has repressed his evil impulses into the unconscious and would like to tell himself afterwards that he is not responsible for them, he is nevertheless bound to be aware of this responsibility as a sense of guilt whose basis is unknown to him.
>
> (Freud, 1917: 374)

What is particularly interesting about this, I think, is its demonstration (to be found throughout Freud's work) of the out-and-out *moralism* of the man who, in his 'scientific' guise, is so often credited with the invention of 'psychic determinism'. What we witness in passages such as this –

portraying the repression of 'evil impulses' for which 'we like to tell [our]selves afterwards that [we] are not responsible' – are not scientific observations, but precisely the laying of the foundations of the 'conservative social ideology' of which Epstein writes. Indeed, so far from maintaining scientific detachment, Freud has positively to mutilate Sophocles' play in order, like a cuckoo, to install within it his own brain-child.

Freud was quick to see – if only unconsciously! – that the *raison d'être* of psychotherapy as the treatment of private individuals would be very hard to maintain if patients were not to be seen as at least in some sense responsible for their predicaments and able, once id had been transformed to ego, to will the appropriate changes to their conduct. As with Sophocles, so with the individual patient: the *tragedy* had to be taken out of life and replaced by *responsibility*. It is with the reversing of this reversal, I submit, that psychotherapists should now concern ourselves if we are not to waddle off dodo-like into extinction.

The best hope of rescuing a life from tragedy – certainly of the 'flawed character' variety – may well be the exact opposite of attending to and working on its origins within the private individual. Once character has been fatefully impressed upon us as relatively powerless infants by the overwhelmingly much greater powers around us, there is not a great deal to be achieved by our trying to turn ourselves inside-out in a desperate attempt to reconstitute ourselves as other than we are, by trying to replace the forces that created us by optimistic but impotent myths, or by rejecting the truths we have learned about life for falsehoods we would prefer to believe.

Much more to the point might be trying collectively to create a world which could *receive and make sense* of what we have learned about it. Suffering is a form of knowledge. It tells us what is wrong with our world. But society is more willing to listen to some messages than to others. The kinds of things people whose distress takes them to psychiatrists and psychotherapists have to tell us are often exactly what we are least willing to hear. What happens in these circumstances is that the voice of suffering is simply ignored, treated as without meaning, or as a 'personal problem' for which the person him/herself has to 'take responsibility'.

There will always be suffering, for some things which are wrong with the world are just inevitable and some, such as our biological mortality, are even necessary. The tragic element cannot be escaped. But that does not mean that we should not struggle to provide a world which makes use of what people have to tell us. What may rescue the most tortured or damaged private existence is, ideally, finding meaning within a public world which acknowledges and makes use of the experience of pain.

If the worst comes to the worst, we could compensate for personal privation and disadvantage by treating people as more than mere psychological entities (more, that is, than the sum of their private experience) and as having a possible *function* in public space. Increasingly in the world as it is, people are just *reduced* to their private selves, so that there is no possibility of their escaping the ravages of their past by being able, not to deny it or erase it, but to *overcome* it. In this way, if we're not careful, the principal contribution of psychotherapy becomes to inflate the importance of private experience and help imprison people within it.

What I'm suggesting, then, is turning from the inner to the outer. Precisely the opposite of Freud's manoeuvre. In many ways this is a matter not for psychotherapy, but for politics. And indeed I do think, as I have argued for many years now, that the best hope for improving the lot of 'ordinary people' – psychologically as in every other respect – is through the building of a re-dignified politics. There is precious little sign of that happening at the present time. But, if we started to take seriously the view that what damages people are the powers of a social world which bear down upon them, and if the influences of childhood all too often constitute the tragically unalterable casting of dice, where does this leave the practice of psychotherapy?

I must admit that I don't think the implications of this view are all that encouraging for psychotherapy, but neither are they disastrous. They are least encouraging for those who would hope to make the case for psychotherapy – whatever the particular brand – as constituting some kind of, if not cure, then technical recipe for change to be achieved through the knowledge of the therapist as professional expert. The most that a therapist who aspires to this kind of role can hope to achieve, I suspect, is to engage with patients in a kind of strategic review of the options open to them to make a difference to their lives. This assumes of course that the patient has options.

No doubt most of the patients who formed the clientele of the originators of the principal therapeutic schools were pretty well-resourced individuals whose material advantages afforded them a range of choices in the conduct of their lives. Certainly, what little research there is in this general area suggests that psychotherapy is indeed most effective with

YAVIS patients (young, attractive, verbal, intelligent and successful: see Schofield, 1964). In any case, psychotherapy on this view has to relinquish any claim, explicit or implicit, to the *transformation* of its clients, and becomes merely a procedure through which their assets and liabilities are audited. There is of course no shame in providing such a service, but it is unlikely to be of use to anyone whose assets are strictly limited.

Psychotherapy may also have quite a useful role in *demystifying* its clients about the origins of their distress. Although I think psychotherapists often perform this function unawares, it is not on the whole a conscious and deliberate part of their purpose. The (not-always-stated) aim of most approaches to therapy is to confront patients with the unconscious intentions or faulty attitudes, etc., through which, supposedly, they create and maintain their problems. In fact, on the other hand, quite a lot of the work in therapy of clarification of the causes of distress may well concentrate on the past and present circumstances which gave rise to it and which were in fact in no way attributable to the patient's agency.

If this could become a deliberate and central, rather than an accidental, feature of psychotherapy, it might certainly have its uses in relieving some of the distress which goes with people's feeling *responsible* for their own predicament. To draw people's attention to the noxious structure of social power in which their troubles are generated could thus be a possibly comforting and mildly subversive activity, but it wouldn't of course change anything at all basic. Psychological pain might be slightly the less painful for having an accurate explanation attached to it, but it is certainly not eradicated thereby, and the actual causes of distress still lie well beyond the therapist's sphere of influence.

But if therapists can't solve their patients' problems, at least they can offer their sympathy and their solidarity. If to suggest that we cannot 'change' people may be seen as a defeat for the therapeutic enterprise, we may yet come to see the converse – that we accept people as the characters they inevitably are, without diagnosing or pathologising them – as one of its principal potential strengths. An existence already marked by tragedy is rendered the more intolerable by suggestions that, either morally or aesthetically, the person *could* or *should* be otherwise.

The nature of the relationship between therapist and patient has of course been a matter of intense concern throughout the past hundred years, with just about every shade of opinion being represented, from the advocacy of the therapeutic aloofness of orthodox psychoanalysis, through the emphasis on warmth, empathy and genuineness of the Rogerians, to the unabashed avowal of therapeutic love (the most eloquent expression of which probably being Ian Suttie's – Suttie, 1960).

I think it is in fact extremely difficult to escape the conclusion that the most potent aspect of psychotherapy is the solidarity afforded patients through their relationship with someone taking an intense, ongoing interest in their welfare. Having someone on one's side makes a genuine, material difference to one's ability to do battle with the world. This, indeed, is what 'relationship' is all about. But this is an uncomfortable notion for psychotherapists to accept, and it is little wonder that they regard it as uneasily as they do, for the questions to be asked are obvious.

If, after all, the most useful thing therapists do is offer patients their support, what distinguishes them from anyone else in this respect? How could the provision of solidarity in this way justify professional training and status? What are the ethics of providing, in essence, love for money? What limits should be placed on such support? What about issues like 'dependency' and so on? Wouldn't such an approach lead to the provision of open-ended 'therapy' which would simply defeat its own object by rapidly becoming unavailable on any significant scale?

Perhaps, as much as anything, it is the democratisation of therapy which has embroiled us in these paradoxical tangles. For therapy on the original analytic model of five-times-a-week for as long as it takes comes very close to constituting the purchase of a kind of personal confidant who really does become a significant figure in the individual's landscape, someone who can share with him or her the unavoidable tragedies of life, offer consolation and attempt to give them meaning. There would be little point in trying to persuade the few who can afford that kind of attention that the theoretical ideas underlying it didn't hold water. It would be a bit like telling an octogenarian billionaire that the beautiful 20-year-old he'd just married didn't really love him for himself – the entirely understandable answer would probably be 'so what?'.

But psychotherapy has now become a technicised industry in which throughput has become a central aspect of its processing of people in distress, and we are, if anything, more wary than ever of acknowledging that our principal and most potent function lies in accepting people as they inevitably are and providing solidarity in the face of tragedy. That would be a modest aim indeed, and certainly wouldn't change the world. But neither, surely, would it be dishonourable.

References

Epstein, W. (1995) *The Illusion of Psychotherapy,* New Brunswick and London: Transaction Publishers.

Freud, S, (1895) *Studies on Hysteria*, Pelican Freud Library, Vol. 3, Harmondsworth: Penguin Books.

Freud, S. (1917) *Introductory Lectures on Psychoanalysis,* Pelican Freud Library, Vol I, Harmondsworth: Penguin Books.

Hobsbawm, E. (1994) *Age of Extremes. The Short Twentieth Century 1914–1991*, Harmondsworth: Penguin Books.

King-Spooner, S. (1995) 'Psychotherapy and the white dodo,' *Changes,* 13: 45–51.

Schafer, R. (1976) *A New Language for Psychoanalysis*, New Haven and London: Yale University Press.

Schofield, W. (1964) *Psychotherapy: The Purchase of Friendship*, Englewood Cliffs, NJ: Prentice-Hall.

Smail, D. (1993) *The Origins of Unhappiness*, London: HarperCollins.

Smail, D. (1996) *How to Survive Without Psychotherapy*, London: Constable.

Smail, D. (2005) *Power, Interest and Psychology*, Ross-on-Wye: PCCS Books.

Suttie, I. (1960) *The Origins of Love and Hate*, Harmondsworth: Penguin Books.

The Making of a Therapist and the Corruption of the Training Market III.4

Guy Gladstone

Please allow me to introduce myself –
I'm a man of wealth and taste.
I've been around for a long long year,
Stole many a man's soul and faith …
What's puzzling you is the nature of my game.
('Sympathy for the Devil', The Rolling Stones, 1968)

Overview

This chapter is written by a practitioner who became a therapist prior to the new dispensation of accredited training and psychotherapy registration. Without being asked I was later 'grandfathered'[1] into a club which needed members in order to thereafter regulate entrance. So I have it both ways and am free to shoot from the hip. Oh, how the radical and aberrant are gathered back into the bosom of recuperation! This is an essay that with pleasure will avoid the style and tone of the psychotherapist writing for the learned journal. There will be no studied modesty, no deferential review of the literature and no conjuring up of an initial impression of significant dissent which, upon further reading, evaporates. Instead, expect forays into your sensibilities from the trickster, and to have your head banged by the polemic of the agitator.

The main argument here is that becoming a mature practitioner is an outcome of a series of apprenticeships to people worth learning from in a variety of settings, an idiosyncratic process that escapes the market-driven logic and production lines of the institutionalised therapy training industry now emerging. I would also argue that experiential groups should be the essential matrix out of which some will self-select to train as practitioners. Such a model is at odds with the trend towards rapid amassment of trainees for marketed university-associated courses. For trainers, safe training is safe trading. However, normal university intake age and course timespan are incompatible with the unpredictable time needed for the foundational preliminary of in-depth personal work without a training agenda.

My colleague at The Open Centre, Richard Mowbray, has published *The Case Against Psychotherapy Registration*, subtitled most aptly, 'A Conservation Issue for the Human Potential Movement'. Jacob Moreno, the originator of psychodrama, a modality I work with, spoke of the 'cultural conserve', meaning those forces in society that foreclose upon the spontaneity of the individual. Thus the Playpower of the sixties has given way in the field of psychotherapy to the power plays of the nineties. Practitioners of Humanistic Psychology in particular, once part of the promisingly creative third wave in psychology (Psychoanalysis and Behaviourism being the first and second waves), are now labouring under the societal legacy of the eighties and early nineties – conformity, respectability and accountability. The first sign that a humanistic soul has sold out on their countercultural forbears is the display after their name of 'UKCP Registered'. Of course if this habit becomes pandemic enough it will lose any USP (unique selling point) value it ever had.

The last 15 years correspond both to the period of my life in which I have practised as a psychotherapist and the period of promotion by Conservative governments of the ideology of free-market individualism. This has been a time in which a malign view of human beings has consolidated institutionally. Trainings today are mostly so heavily marketed that many counsellors and psychotherapists only begin a personal therapy because it is a course requirement. However, the home ground of my involvement in this work is several core modalities of the Human Potential movement:[2] Bioenergetics, Encounter, Gestalt and Psychodrama. Excited by all these as a client and group member, I later crossed over to become a therapist. In retrospect I greatly value the time spent in personal therapy, when I had no idea I would become a therapist.

Thus, in this essay I'd like to start by acknowledging those influences on my development as a practitioner that, with benefit of hindsight, I would stand by as worthwhile. These are the influences which, were it possible to design such a training, I would want to see included by some means to ensure a humano-ecological variety, a conservation of the quick, rather than a conserve of the dead. The roots of my work are in the counterculture of the sixties and seventies. Like many adventurous middle-class people in the sixties, I chose disposable jobs like dish washing and work on building sites rather than foreclose upon my search for a personally meaningful place in the world. Such a place would include being paid to do what I would love and value doing anyway.

I believe the route to competence as a therapist passes through vagaries and vicissitudes that can not be legislated for. Even the Association of Humanistic Psychology Practitioners, a group I have belonged to and been accredited by for over ten years, has all but forgotten its declared values, so hypnotic and insistent has the pressure from the register builders (UKCP et al.) become to perceive professionalism as an outcome of an academic–bureaucratic model. For the record, I quote from the AHPP's brochure for prospective members 15 years ago:

> *AHPP stands for:*
> Professionalism based on self-direction and self-regulation.
> High standards of practice and ethics which are defined and monitored by practitioners individually and collectively.
> Inclusive professionalism – any route to professional competence is acceptable.
> Regular reassessment of competence.
> Creativity, spontaneity and experiment.
>
> *AHPP is against:*
> Professionalism which tries to deny skills to those outside a closed circle.
> Professional boredom when practitioners fail to develop their skills.
> Professional conservatism which keeps out novel ideas and practices.
> Rigid categorising and labelling of persons and processes.

Already well-tried and proven routes to competence, such as experiential learning communities, open learning systems and apprenticeship to experienced practitioners, are being eclipsed or at best have lip service paid to them. Through registration ('voluntary' but planned to be statutory), trainers of counsellors and psychotherapists would set the seal upon their commodification of narrowed training options. We can now look forward to the next generation of counsellors and psychotherapists, NVQ'd, hatched at carefully conserved factory farms from which they will appear tagged BAC/UKCP/BPC/BPS. This will be the kiss of death for the evolution of creative praxis.[3] The naturalisation of academically acquired therapeutic citizenship entails a discounting of experiential learning. An ersatz competence, essay writing, can be substituted for deep engagement with personal issues. Intellectual window-dressing shields a training from excessive drop-out arising out of the going getting too rough for those facing themselves for the first time. Lectures, seminars and tutorials sanitise the prevailing confusion of educational and therapeutic supports.

Presenting my personal route into the work I do today and some parts of my life that balance an engagement with the inner world will serve, on the one hand, to exemplify a road now less travelled (to adapt M. Scott Peck's metaphor), while on the other hand it may explain why, as a character in William Burroughs' *The Naked Lunch* put it, 'I ain't innarested in contracting your horrible condition'.

Personal development before training

My very first contact with therapy was 26 years ago through almost leaderless groups held in a PNP (People Not Psychiatry) household. I progressed to my first formal therapy, three years of weekly group and individual sessions with Glyn Seaborn Jones. This was preceded by a launching period, a three-week intensive of daily individual sessions during which one withdrew from all usual work and social distractions. With the help of his eclectic bodymind approach, the stiff-upper-lipped public school boy began to let down into his feelings and lose the benign sixties gloss acquired through meditation and esoteric studies. I recovered an emotionally expressive body. Some years later the PNP link took me into an involvement with the Atlantis commune in Donegal. There, through a volatile cocktail of Janovian Primal and rough-house Encounter referred to as 'jungle therapy', feelings were discharged between residents at a level of intensity that made most Bioenergetics look and sound like a vicar's tea party. The more psychopathic survived, paranoia was massive and some disintegrated. This experience taught me more about the holding functions of the group psychotherapist than years of formal training could.

In those heady days I was interested in literally taking therapy out of the privy closet of the session room and into everyday life. This quest led me into co-counselling and the residential peer self-help therapy fortnights at Laurieston Hall Community. I was particularly fascinated by the area between Reichian therapy and theatre and had begun training as a mime. I became interested in communities with a therapy-based praxis developing intentionally utopian alternatives to couple relationships and the nuclear family. Inspired by several visits to the Austrian AAO commune at Friedrichshof and its offshoots in Berlin and Geneva, in 1981 I joined with others to form a short-lived London group. The European communes were extraordinary examples of a stable cohesive and uniquely secular experiment in twentieth-century tribal living, studied by anthropologists. From these experiences I developed a capacity to play with my inner world in public and the knack of accessing the therapeutic potentials of the mischievous clown. But perhaps more importantly, living in a commune impressed me with the relativity of social structures. The white male English heterosexual therapist may benefit from immersion in a radically different cultural formation. The theory and metapsychology of most schools of psychotherapy carry forward normative assumptions (e.g. that people grow up in nuclear families) that no longer correspond with the experience of many who will come into contact with psychotherapy or counselling as clients.

Training as a therapist

In the early eighties I began formal training, at first through the Institute for the Development of Human Potential (IDHP) with its rich mix of humanistic workshops and peer-determined learning structures. Soon after I trained with the Institute of Psychotherapy and Social Studies (IPSS) which, in those days, with R.D. Laing on the staff, unabashedly connected therapy and politics, whilst encouraging a fusion of psychodynamics with humanistic and existential approaches.

Repeating fruitless patterns of relating and a good measure of unhealthy narcissism made it imperative that I return to personal therapy, this time to many years on the couch. I was slowly able to face the most dreadful emptiness, the feeling of being only a hollow shell of a person. Attacking my analyst for the bodymind splitting of his therapeutic culture was just one more defence against feelings of personal ruin. I left psychoanalysis more truly at home with my fantasies, able to think with feeling and feel thoughtfully. The therapists I have found most helpful, personally and professionally, have all modelled a genuine availability for the receipt of the full range of negative transferential feeling. It's OK to hate and it's OK to be hated. The New Age premium on love, like its religious antecedents, interferes with a proper recognition of human ambivalence.

Once again my personal changes organically moved my professional interest along a further track of learning, this time towards integrating the action methods I had first experienced as a client within a psychodynamic frame, now that I had also experienced therapy as an analysand. I was able to arrange for myself and some others exactly the further training I was now ready for. A five-year cycle of learning ensued with two of Alexander Lowen's former international trainers, Sander Kirsch and Jacques Berliner, who had resituated body psychotherapy within an analytical frame.

The further reaches, the nether world

Periods of search have taken me through Zen sitting, Vipassana meditation retreats, some 'direct experiences' through the invaluable vehicle of the Enlightenment Intensive and, preceding all personal therapy, membership for several years of a Gurdjieff group. These are all forms of spiritual work for the psychologically minded. However, devotional religion and its New Age derivatives, such as the Sanyas of Bhagwan Shri Rajneesh, have always repelled me. I believe that mixing therapy and religion is mostly as unhelpful as mixing therapy and friendship. In my book, the assignment of the psychotherapist is quite distinct from the task of a teacher of students or a minister to devotees. Whatever clients try to make of one – and there is often a pressure to tell them how to live – an important part of therapeutic work is to positively not lead anyone up a path, garden or otherwise, but to get out of their way as others may not have done. As the millennium approaches there will almost certainly be a resurgence of narcissistic wishes and corresponding impostors. If there is a purpose underlying therapy in general, at least as I apprehend it, then it is something truly subversive of much in our society. It is the discovering, often painful, of an individual identity, finding a way to be most fully one's self in the world, with a minimum of preconceptions. Paradoxically, this project can only be achieved through deep and sustained engagements with others, both in and out of therapy. A good benchmark by which to assess a training is whether it supports or obstructs that process of discovery.

The function of life experiences in the making of a therapist cannot be conclusively assessed and hence nowadays tends to drop out of view where training is concerned. I am doubtful whether the concept of APL (Accreditation of Prior Learning) has any substantive relevance to what I'm talking about here. (It appears to be bandied about when a training needs to broaden its recruitment base.) The contribution of life experience is twofold. There is the childhood contribution which the mature therapist will have researched in an extended personal therapy, a vital precaution against contaminating counter-transferences. There is also the equally elusive significance of much adult life experience in preparing a person for the role of therapist, enriching their work as it progresses over the years, and most of all in renewing the therapist in an occupation that, to put it crudely, can suck the juice out of you. (Question: which role offers more openings for vampires, therapist or client?) In truth this is an implausible profession.

The occupation of psychotherapist imposes some peculiar and often unforeseeable stresses on the individual who chooses it (or is chosen for it!). Personally I have been to some crazy places, not understanding at the time that I was reliving trans-generational experience that, properly speaking, was not my own, yet from which I could not, for far too long, extract myself. William Blake's dictum 'If the fool would persist in his folly he would become wise' holds true in my experience. Through my particular folly, literal in so far as I enacted ruin and attributed reality to a clever simulation, I came to understand the tragedy that has haunted my family of origin. From this experience I am inclined to believe that it is especially important for therapists to discover the often unconscious root and route of their dedication to this strange occupation. Some 50 years ago, without knowing it as such, I was apprenticed to my mother and grandmother, experts in the splitting, projection and denial of feeling and emotion. This was my first training. I have learnt to never hesitate to seek extra help if I realise I am out of my depth in dealing with my life or work. And I expect such enactments are a more common experience amongst practitioners than is generally admitted.

The nearer reaches, the wider world

It is my perception that too many therapists live their lives too little away from their work, and thus easily ignore its 'as if ' nature. By the same token it is vital to develop areas of one's life that have no direct connection with the activity of therapising, zones of experiencing which none the less may be very therapeutic in a healing sense for the therapist concerned. Some by no means exhaustive personal examples of involvements before, beyond and outside the therapeutic setting should illuminate what I mean.

Experiences that have been particularly meaningful for me and have extended my horizons and capacity for empathy have often involved travel, particularly outside Europe – in North Africa, in Indonesia and in Madagascar. Before I learnt to drive I hitchhiked everywhere and learnt to listen, hearing many strange tales, a prelude to the witnessing and wondering of my future occupation. After I had learnt to drive, owning a variety of period cars, I connected with my childhood through a 1951 model, and with my teenage through the 1960s models, materialising personal nostalgia zones. Only more recently has it become clear to me how much unbearable distress these cars served to contain. An unconscious preparation for work in cathartic and movement-based therapies was nine years' experience as a furniture remover, emptying houses (extensions of clients' bodies) of their contents and transporting these across London, across England, across Europe, then emptying these contents out of my pantechnicon (extension of therapist's body). It can be instructive to reflect on what one has carried, and for whom, in all aspects of one's life. Other lives and lives past are the peculiar province of the therapist, as for the novelist.

Growing up in the country, I couldn't wait to get to the big city. But before I was 30 I felt an urge to reconnect with my roots in a watery and mountainous region of England, and acquired a derelict cottage in the same terrain but by the sea and in another country, restoring it over the years as a place of retreat and renewal. Water continues to be an especially important element in my life. I would class my first experience of scuba diving (in the Maldives) as a spiritual experience, a profound admission to a world of wonder and amazement below the planet's surface, the ocean corresponding topographically to the world's deep unconscious. Ecstasy for me is swimming with dolphins and whales, windsurfing is a close second, and a good third on dry land is the flow of jive dancing. The fate of the natural world that cannot speak on its own behalf preoccupies me deeply. Accordingly I am a Frontline Supporter of Greenpeace and subscriber to the Environmental Investigation Agency. I can readily imagine that, were it not for those pressing determinants from my family of origin, I would have found that personally meaningful place in the world in this other theatre, the work of non-violent direct action on behalf of the environment. Both ontogenetically and phylogenetically, human life begins in water, our bodies are in a large percentage composed of water, and many forms of healing have a long association with water.

Concluding this review of key experiences in the making of one therapist, with its focus on determinants, values and recreation, I would note that the first cluster of examples given involves movement, and the second cluster involves the element of water. Together, movement and water are symbolic of the grounding of life in sensations and emotions that is axiomatic for me as a body psychotherapist.

The Maverick Factor

There is a necessarily traditional line of transmission of learning in psychotherapy, as in many professions. A therapist's initial main training is the vehicle for this, and in my view this should be broad-based and eclectic rather than restricted to a single modality (cf. Feltham's Chapter II.4, this volume), even if a particular modality is emphasised. Similarly, and of at least equal if not greater importance, there is a line of transmission for personal formation and self-examination. A therapist's personal therapy is the vehicle for this. Thus I value spending nine years of an unmentionable number of times a week with an analyst whose therapeutic great-grandparents were none other than both the Founding Father, Freud, and the Horrid Mother, Klein. That made me a great-great-grandchild, so to speak, which certainly appeals to my grandiosity now that it is behind me. But the important point I want to make here is that it is the additional influences to the two main lines of transmission already acknowledged that ensure against therapeutic inbreeding and eventual sterility.

Crucial to the making of a therapist is the exposure to, and infection with, what I shall term the Maverick Factor. The Maverick Factor depends upon the opportunity to form trial identifications with advanced independent practitioners or groups (who almost certainly have no 'approved' credentials, and indeed barely give that matter a thought). It will become increasingly difficult to meet this species within the confines of accredited trainings, as mavericks will tend to avoid the company of hacks and factory farmers. However, the species is still available to learn from through personal encounters, through a supervisory arrangement and of course through group or individual therapy. Within this species are the beggars, buffoons and barbarians that an evolving therapist can really learn something from. Whereas in a mainstream training a trainee is led by the nose, the Maverick Factor is acquired solely through the individual practitioner following his or her nose, before, during or after that training. The Maverick Factor cannot be institutionalised or accredited, else some arsehole would have found a way to market it by now. It can only be cultivated through a series of informal apprenticeships, staying true to the original model of learning in the field. Maverick is a compound of marginal influences and off-beat potentials, and as such is extraordinarily resistant to corruption. A further property of the Maverick Factor is the capacity to combine dissimilar viewpoints into a productive synthesis. Like the formation of the self this tends to be a long and at times laborious process, characterised by many upsets and false starts along the way. It is the very opposite of the farcical application of the NVQ trajectory to counselling and psychotherapy; the results cannot be predicted or tabulated. Indeed, I only formulate the Maverick Factor with benefit of hindsight, as I discern the helpful internalisations that speak through me in moments of therapeutic stress, moments when I am at my edge as a practitioner. The Maverick Factor is to be found here or it hasn't been acquired. To give this concept some specificity I will cite six of my own apprenticeships, each 'M'-ed to honour their contribution to the Maverick.

From the Magician I learnt about the group as a metaphysical theatre, a Faustian interplay of alchemical forces. From the Miner I learnt to tunnel outside of transferences, in the common area of psychoses, surfacing from the unspeakable with news from the foetal. From the Mediator I learnt to discern societal impact in characterological terms, both at the level of professional politics and the level of personal formation. From the Mobiliser I learnt the value of the animated human grimace for mimicking the mask itself, and as a necessary subversion of the modelling towards inertia perpetrated upon clients by stuffed dummies of blank screen neutrality (no one is ever neutral, not even psychotherapists). From the Madhouse of so-called 'jungle therapy' (in the Atlantis commune), I learnt how the wild discharge of real feelings interpersonally favours the fittest emotional athletes and disintegrates the more vulnerable. From the Materialisation of communal free sexuality (in the AAO communes), highlighting the love affair with the breast, anal exhibitionism, urethral aggressions, and rivalry for the leader's affections, I learnt of the relativity of the nuclear family, the pervasiveness of sado-masochism and the fragility of civilisation.

The Maverick Factor permits the assimilation of both dubious and kosher ancestors.

Power over, power with

By now you the reader may either be nodding in agreement or shaking your head in dismay. The remainder of this chapter will focus on the corruption of the training market. I promised at the outset to bang some heads.

The new dispensation under which most training takes place greatly increases a trainer's 'power over' a trainee. The trainer now has the power to block entry to registered practice, thereby nullifying a large part of a trainee's increasingly heavy financial investment towards qualifying. By contrast, a well-facilitated personal development group gives its members a profound experience of 'power with' their peers. 'Power with' is the antidote to and alternative to 'power over', and provides people with an independent space and the confidence necessary to problematise the trainer's resort to 'power over', and, ultimately, the will to deconstruct all hierarchical power relations. By distributing the power to help amongst their members, groups ensure representation of more than one helping viewpoint, thus curbing excesses of dependency on 'power over' forms of authority. Any transference analysis of a trainee's difficulties with the authority of a trainer which dissembles or fudges the reality of the trainer's 'power over' is an emotionally and politically abusive analysis.

The NVQ episode

The history of markets is a history of rigging, suppressed inventions and a retrograde bias towards the lowest common denominator, the homogenous outcome, the mass product with the widest sales potential. In this regard, an episode that nicely reveals how the training business blows with the wind, and therefore has to cover its arse, concerns the National Vocational Qualification bandwagon. Despite the irrelevance of NVQs for an occupation aiming at postgraduate status (you see we can theorise/we can think), the preposterous project of NVQing psychotherapy has been taken on board by the UKCP. The logic of the market dictated the move. The BAC, UKCP's numerically powerful poor cousin and predecessor in the field having already committed itself to NVQing counselling (you see we can practise/we can do), it was feared that UKCP trainees would find themselves disadvantaged in the job market. From the point of view of the trainee, NVQs are actually a

Procrustean bed. This method of descriptive analysis of skills is wholly performance-oriented and requires a disconnected intellect to speak on behalf of a mute body, feelings and spirit. The Gadarene rush to get NVQ'd will be recalled in the history of psychotherapy as a spectacular instance of capitulation to the Spectacle. The Spectacle is the form into which all appearances must be organised under advanced capitalism. All angles have to be covered where public relations are concerned, and in this instance the future intake of trainees had to be ensured.

Recruitment ploys

I was recently invited to sit on a one-afternoon panel to academically accredit a counselling course situated within a university, that was already in existence but deemed to need revamping to make it more competitive and in keeping with current models for the delivery of counselling training. It was argued at the validating panel that personal therapy could not be made obligatory because this would result in virtually zero recruitment to the course. Personal therapy or counselling preliminary to the course was not even mentioned. Once candidates of the course had completed it, then it was hypothesised they would be better qualified to apply for that (elusive) counselling job, having gained which then they might (conceivably) be able to afford that personal therapy, and then they might (just conceivably) opt to complete that minimal requirement set by the BAC of 40 hours of individual counselling! Within such a framework of priorities, dictated largely by costings and resourcing issues, the question of personal readiness to work with people and their personal issues was almost an afterthought. There was discussion of the possibility of a trainee counsellor having a breakdown or putting their clients on a placement at risk. This was a sorry example of closing the stable door after the horse has bolted.

The course document I was invited to peruse catalogued columns of skills to be demonstrated. But who would buy from it? The language, e.g. 'On almost all occasions manage [*sic*] own physical, mental, emotional and spiritual life', made hairs rise on the back of my neck and my diaphragm contract in a spasm of nausea. Couched in 'service provider lingo', the document was replete with metaphors of feeding, as befits the late twentieth-century consumer capitalism within which counselling and psychotherapy find their place of adaptation.

In this matter of the necessity or otherwise of personal therapy it suits training institutes to maintain an essentially spurious distinction between certificate- and diploma-level qualifications. Certificate-level courses allow the training institute to substantially widen their recruitment base, using such courses as 'feeders' for a higher-status diploma-level course. The distinction is spurious because what happens when two more or less consenting adults get together in private is not governed by the qualification one has acquired. What happens is more likely to be a function of who they are and who they have become through working on themselves rather than one of them working for an exam.

Faced by a profitable but already saturated market, the business-minded who are moving into the field to manage it (let's talk 'target groups and 'trainee turnover), will see potential for expansion in the generation of specialisms through repackaging. The academising trainers are already co-operating through the charade of setting trainees largely concocted 'research' projects. Practitioners should bin their questionnaires.

Would a union help?

On the day of the recent General Election, a client remarked during his session that therapists don't have unions. What he meant was that there is no collective representation of the specific interests of the individual practitioners and trainees. The registering organisations represent the interests of trainers and their institutes, though they would have it seem otherwise. The individual tied to a training institute is as isolated as children tend to be in their separate nuclear families, and just about as powerless as children at school. The absence of any collective bargaining power for the trainee is vividly illustrated by the following development. In some areas, lo and behold a market in placements for voluntary counselling has developed. No job ahead without a CV showing prior work experience means that even an unpaid placement becomes a commodity to be traded. On top of fees paid for training, a would-be counsellor may have to buy a placement as the only way to get the experience to get the diploma to get that accreditation to get that work promised at the end of the rainbow. Thus, the dead hand of the commodity economy wags the shitty tail of the training dog, while at its other end the beast salivates over the unsuspecting trainee.

Symbiosis and projection of authority

Psychotherapy and counselling are essentially activities of individuals functioning as autonomous agents. If the politics of the field are to be consistent with the essential activity, this would entail from-the-bottom-up practitioner-based models of organisation as the predominant organisational form. Actually the field is dominated by training institutes working on a from-the-top-down model, hierarchical and elitist. This contradiction is obscured from view by the generally apolitical consciousness of most therapists. The success of the denial of anything contradictory is founded on the maintenance of a symbiotic relation between trainer and trainee. In a symbiosis, both sides maintain an unspoken contract that each knows the other's needs and is meeting them without need for discussion. Trainers can readily maintain a myth of disinterested service on this basis. When in-house personal therapy is obligatory, the trainee's identifications with their therapist will be much harder to resolve. But this assists a training in cloning itself, the more the merrier for the market. And giving senior trainees junior trainees as clients to cut their teeth on legitimises therapeutic inbreeding.

Survival needs (economics) and other personal needs (for therapy, personal development and friendship) may be especially hard for therapists to tease apart, the work itself so often being oral and nurturant. But the archaic emotional level needs constant differentiation from here and now social and economic reality, as Reich demonstrated in his analysis of fascism in the 1930s. The possibility of psychotherapists having a social and political impact beyond the session room is predicated upon a capacity to differentiate, a capacity to transcend the symbiosis just described. Few prospective trainees will be in a position to seriously put into question the visible options for their future training. Most often the trainee endows his chosen trainers with a projected authority. It is very unsettling to occupy the common position of childhood, that of not really knowing what is going on. The counterpart of the anxiety that neither oneself nor anyone else necessarily knows, is the desire to believe that someone in a position of authority, i.e. a parent/trainer, does know. Trainers and training institutes benefit from a good measure of both transference and wishful thinking. A copy in the hands of each prospective trainee of this volume or its forerunner, Richard Mowbray's ground-breaking book, well ....

Conclusions

Thus the independence, integrity and future evolution of practitioners will depend in large part on whether collegial associations such as IPN, that are independent of training organisations, can maintain an alternative centre of gravity, counterbalancing the monopolistic hegemonies formed by members of the trainers' club, and acting as guardians of a space for countercultural values. Contrary to the image being fostered by the register-builders, psychotherapy, especially depth psychotherapy, but also much personal development work occurring both within and outside what were once known as growth centres, remains an inherently countercultural activity. The image-building efforts of the registering organisations are at cross-purposes with the very nature of the work for which they claim to be providing support. Unless, of course, the work is really about the legitimation of a false adaptive self. If the role of a therapist includes being able to act as a free-speaking witness, functioning as an outsider who can represent the underworld (psychic and social), then a practitioner should not be too concerned with being respectable.

Impulses to create a discredited sub-class or out-group are a profound and a recurrent feature of the human psyche. The consolidation of accreditation procedures into the hands of trainings associated with registers can always draw on this regressive dynamic for support. An economic and perhaps future legal split into an OK class and a NOT OK class of practitioners is founded on, maintained by and acts to reinforce a psychic split. Bureaucratic, academic and commercial structures are variously antagonistic to the making of a therapist, and will jointly further the corruption of the training market.

Endnotes

1. It should be noted that there are a number of great-grandparents hiding within the inner recesses of the UKCP. They constitute a club within a club, the trainers club. These figures, who have never even undergone the training the 'grandparents' received, are invariably keen proponents of registration.

2. I would not align myself with the so-called New Age movement, which has to some degree appropriated the term Human Potential, just as psychotherapists have largely vacated it. That movement is headed up mainly by airheads who promise plenty but can rarely deliver.

3. 'Praxis' has a meaning of 'the practising of an art or a skill' (Concise Oxford Dictionary, 1990). And with its Marxist connotation of collective intentional action

for social transformation, the term 'praxis' is a good deal more appropriate for the group worker with a human potential agenda than the more usual term 'practice', the quasi-medical aura of which, alas, is precisely its attraction to many therapists.

Uncovering the Mirror: Our Evolving Personal Relationship with Accreditation III.5

Sue Hatfield & Cal Cannon

For both of us, our engagement with the dynamics of accreditation began years ago, around the time we entered the education system – how many stars did you get this week? Our personal responses to accreditation are a reflection of each of our personalities, our basic historical responses to life, our issues around fear, self-worth, authority, control, etc.

Although for one of us there was always discomfort and unease with the implicit comparisons inherent to the system, as young people we both accepted that the system's criteria determined our status, in our own eyes and in the eyes of others. This message was affirmed by our culture, our families and our schools. The whole set-up encouraged us to make judgements based on external criteria, and led us inexorably away from our own innate authority and desire to self-reflect. It effectively put a cover over the mirror, forcing us to look in one direction only. We lost any sense of our relationship with the process, with our own wisdom, and with the living wisdom of others, and put meaning into one-way relationship with qualifications, pieces of paper, rules, and representations of external authority (The Board of Education, The Royal Academy, etc.).

Our journeys in relation to accreditation have been very different, but have brought us to a similar understanding of the issues, and common ground from which to take forward our evolving ideas. We present our two stories here.

• • •

Sue's story

I was a model school student. I thrived on competition and success, being the best in the class, passing tests, pleasing teachers. At school I was happy and proud of myself. That happiness came from the self-esteem of academic success: school was the one place in my life where I felt OK.

I went off to university, believing in myself. I went with my northern accent and working-class manners to a world peopled by the southern middle classes, who drank wine and who ate lunch at dinner time and dinner at tea time. I thought I was somebody because I had all these pieces of paper that said I was clever, and I felt like nobody – I couldn't even talk properly. My world fell apart; I simply did not know how to be.

I groped my way through the first two terms, had a nervous breakdown, picked up the pieces, closed my eyes to my pain and struggled on. I found safety once again in academic achievement.

From there I went on to work as a librarian, and then to study for a diploma in librarianship. This led to an interest in teaching and so once again I embarked on a course of study. In 1978 I found myself facing a class of five-year-olds feeling as if I had no idea what to do. I learned my craft in practice, alongside other teachers: one of the most creative aspects of my learning came through team teaching, with colleagues to challenge and support me, and enable me to reflect on my practice.

By now I had collected five bits of paper, proof of some kind of identity and status. I had succeeded in building a life where I was apparently successful, but my existence was governed by the constant searching for images. I thought that if anyone really knew what I was like inside then I would be cast out from the world of decent society. But I had these bits of paper and at least some 'proof' of my OKness.

Then my world fell apart. The end of a long-term relationship left me alone, lost and feeling like there was no point in going on. I dragged myself through a year of intense despair, barely managing to sustain my work, hiding, pretending, trying to keep the mask intact. Eventually it cracked.

That point marked the end of one stage of my life, the end of one road I had travelled and the indication that it was no longer the way to go. I found myself one cold November night sitting opposite a therapist taking the first tentative steps into my inner world.

I learned things about myself, and slowly began to realise that the problem lay not in myself but in my relationship to life. I took a major step that was to return me to myself at a deeper level and lead me to the point where I could not avoid facing and finding a way to deal with my deep fear of life.

I sold my house, enrolled on an MA course, and moved to a beautiful flat that became over the next three years a sanctuary. I began the MA in the autumn, studied furiously, went off at fascinating tangents into the realms of knowledge and power, discovered a vast area of thought that began to relate to my own experience. I talked myself right out of being a teacher, burnt myself out mentally and came to the limits of my tolerance of learning within an academic context.

I gave up the course at Christmas. Over the next three years I worked very little, wrote profusely, painted through many nights, and continued my journey of self-discovery in therapy. I did a course in intuitive massage, but never got the certificate because I was away on the date of the final exam. It didn't seem to matter, but it did really.

Alongside individual therapy, residential therapy groups became an active experiential learning environment for me. In groups I was able to witness others who were on a similar journey, and to see how their process, their stories were so often the same and yet each utterly unique. I learned an enormous amount about group facilitation simply being part of these groups intensely for many, many hours and witnessing facilitation in action. I still consider that it was in these groups that I learned more about 'therapy' than anywhere else. They constituted an extremely rich training, a brilliant example of apprenticeship learning.

Quite naturally I became interested in working in this field. It was as rich food to a long-neglected plant. I began to grow – as they say. I did a one-year counselling course and then decided I wanted to be a therapist. I had no particular reason 'why', no desire to 'help' people; I just knew it was what I wanted, a logical step, a continuation of the journey. I chose what I felt was a 'good' course, one that carried some prestige in the therapeutic world; I wanted to be a 'good' therapist. The fact that my intention was to be a great therapist, a perfect therapist, a special therapist, that I would have this brilliant training that would set me up a notch above other therapists, I chose to cover in a mist so that I could not see too clearly. I sort of knew, but didn't let myself know that I knew.

During that time I began a two-year training in group facilitation and group process. Over time the group became interested in the issue of accreditation and the dynamics which generate the impulse towards that. They spent a lot of time working on this, clarifying their personal and group responses. Involvement in this issue began the process of confronting my fear in relation to external authority and my lifetime dependency on approval from others and bits of paper to prove my self-worth. I began to realise that no number of bits of paper would confer the sense of self worth I wanted.

Yet here I was, doing this 'proper' training that would give me a piece of paper at the end of it. The outcome of this process was a decision to leave the course at the end of the second year. It was not an easy decision but one I knew I needed to make. I wanted to make my own way as a therapist, make my own map, one that was based on learnings from my own journey, that made use of what I knew of myself as a human being; not one that was determined by criteria set by others.

The decision was an enormous relief. I continued my personal learning in various contexts, and a year after leaving the course I began working as a therapist. I did so with the full support of senior colleagues who knew me and knew the quality of my experience and understanding of the therapeutic process. I was part of a peer-support group and had regular supervision; referrals came from colleagues. I always had far more supervision than my workload required, considering it part of my learning and training. As well as looking at my work with individuals, much of my supervision involved looking at myself in relation to this work, asking which aspects of my own story I was living out in doing this work, and how this affected my work; what it meant to be responsible in this work, and how to ensure that my work was in the best interests of the people I met.

I acted responsibly, was supported, and somewhere in me knew I was OK, and had the skills and understanding necessary to begin this work. Being part of an experienced peer-support group acted as a natural control on the work and ensured that I only took on what I was ready for. Looking back over the four years I have now been working, I see how I have been engaged in an apprenticeship for the work alongside senior practitioners.

In theory I had no difficulty with the path I had chosen. In practice it was another story. I was surrounded by articles in the press and in professional literature that espoused the necessity of proper qualifications and accreditation. Here I was without a single piece of paper to prove I was qualified, despite what I might know about myself, and what colleagues affirmed about me. I was terrified. It keyed right in to a deep fear of being a fraud, and I had actually put myself in a position where I couldn't avoid the fear. I feared being 'found out', I wasn't a proper therapist, I had no right to practise.

I had ten years' intensive involvement in therapy, a year on a counselling course, two years on a psychotherapy course, two years on a group process course and a few hundred hours participation in experiential group therapy: I knew I had potential to be an excellent therapist; I knew I had sufficient depth of awareness to stay within the limits of my ability and to work clearly and responsibly. Still I hooked into the fear. For a long time I felt that what I needed to do was to put aside all reasoning and just do a one-year diploma, get a qualification, drop all this stuff about not being qualified and get on with it. But I knew also doing that would make not one bit of difference to my fear.

About two years after I began working I heard about the Independent Practitioners Network (IPN). Details of an inaugural meeting came to members of my peer-support group. They all felt enormously heartened by what they read, particularly the commitment to working as a group and standing by each other's work. For me it felt like a homecoming, to be part of an organisation committed to good practice and rigour, within the context of peer groups who undertook responsibility for self and peer assessment, and for monitoring each other's good practice. I felt my chosen path was at last recognised and I could be part of something which would support my commitment to creative responses to the journey of becoming a therapist.

One of the issues which from time to time raised its head was around the concept of accreditation and particularly the use of the word. I felt strongly that it was not appropriate for people to say that they were accredited by IPN, since IPN as such was not a single body but an organic collection of interlinked groups. Nor did I wish to see the Network take on the functions of an accrediting body. I had a 'thing' about people using IPN as an alternative route to being able to say they were accredited therapists. Quite how big a thing became apparent during a discussion with an IPN colleague one day. The colleague felt easy with people taking on the word 'accredited' as one of several possibilities, and I was adamant that we must find other ways to talk about our competence and credibility, since current developments within the profession filled this word with assumptions. What was surprising was that I became quite distressed. On the train journey home from the meeting I pondered on why I was so churned up about this issue.

I didn't want anyone in the Network to say that they were accredited by IPN, nor indeed that they were accredited, since for me the whole point was to get away from this notion of accreditation as being some fixed thing that conferred credibility on practitioners, and a means of telling people that they were OK as workers. In some sense I didn't want anyone to use the word since I would not allow myself to use the word.

It was in discussing this with my peer group a few days later that the dynamics underlying my response became clearer. I had tipped into very black-and-white thinking on this whole issue. I had spent my life seeking external validation, acquiring bits of paper to prove my worth. Having given that up I had polarised to the other extreme. Having rejected the external authority I had relied on all my life, I now saw that I had to be able to believe in myself, know for myself my credibility as a therapist. I had to be able to 'prove' I was OK, and no one could give that to me, neither IPN nor the peer group. I had put myself very firmly in the position of having to 'do it myself', and if I had to, then so did everyone else! I had, in effect, re-created the same dynamic. I had made my peer group a 'they': even if they weren't conferring accreditation on me, I had to prove to them that I was conferring it on myself.

There is a big flaw in this line of reasoning! We are not alone in the world, and do not work in isolation. In life and in work we are in relationship. I am part of a peer group of people engaged in the same work. Their commitment, like mine, is to good practice, to working with integrity. I am already accredited, my credibility, my validation, my affirmation is already there. I have chosen to work alongside a group of people for whom I have enormous respect; I know their work since I have witnessed them at work in many contexts. I have no doubt of their ability and fittingness to work as therapists. These people have chosen to work with me. I know that I would not work with them if I did not respect them as people and as workers, so could it be that they might also not chose to work with me if they didn't in turn respect me as a worker? Part of my estimation of them is that they would not stand alongside anyone whose work they were not willing to affirm.

There is a clear paradox that I had utterly failed to see. I do not have to prove anything, it is not about proof. It is the framework of proof and external validation itself which is unfitting, and as long as we are trying to operate within that, it will be very difficult to find new and creative responses to this issue. The framework as it stands, and as it is increasingly growing and rigidifying, is one that says that credibility is something that can essentially be 'proved' by certain criteria, something knowable as a fact. To move out of that framework is to see credibility as a living process in relationship with self, peers, clients; knowing that not as fact but as a lived experience. It requires an ongoing commitment to the process. We are never finally accredited, it is essentially meaningless; we are always in the process of being accreditable. The very word has limitations, it implies some final proof; the term 'accredited' is past tense, it is something that has happened. I much prefer the notion of credibility; to say that I am credible refers to now, it is present tense. I am credible now, I may not have been credible yesterday, I may not be credible tomorrow. Sometimes we are credible, sometimes we are not. Being a therapist is not about perfection.

At a recent gathering of IPN someone new to the Network asked about safeguards for clients; it was in the moment so clear that the best safeguard for any client is the knowledge that a practitioner does not work in isolation, that there are other people who know their work; people who care about them, and who care about the quality of their practice.

The wheel turns full circle. My engagement with accreditation has been a reflection of my personal story, my unique response to life. It has brought me to a point of deeply understanding my relationship to this work in a way that I doubt I would have, had I followed conventional routes. In my family of origin I had no adequate mirror by which to know myself; the distortion was extreme. My unique response to that was to conclude that I had got something wrong. So I shut myself away – since I was obviously faulty – and relied on the outside world to create my self-image. The therapeutic encounter was a return to myself and learning to find a self-image based on inner reality. My engagement with the issue of accreditation has been about bringing together these two aspects. I can only know of myself through my relationship with myself in relation to others: if I cannot see others then I cannot clearly see myself, since my self is created in the intimate dance of I and thou.

• • •

Cal's story

I rebelled, having gone through the education system to degree level believing until rather late that there were no alternatives – or at least not for people within a certain social framework whose innate intellectual abilities had been nurtured from birth at the expense of any other abilities.

So I left university with a degree, a husband much older than myself, and no ideas at all as to what I might now do. Having rejected the law as an option, and not being skilled in the sciences, so that medicine was out, I could not think of any other possibilities. So I 'dropped out', and went to live abroad, where nothing was fixed, nothing familiar, and I had to create a lifestyle and an income of sorts. This was relatively easy, though spartan, but I liked that. It was different. What I did well I was praised for, and nobody ever asked me about my background or qualifications. I built up a good business teaching languages to anyone who wanted to learn for whatever reason – and the fact that I myself had only learned Spanish out of sheer necessity did not seem to be a disadvantage. I could still teach it to the many ex-pats who could not master it themselves.

I became confident and proficient, which was clearly affirmed by the progress of those I taught, and their recommendations to others, and was never short of work.

However, when I became pregnant with my second child, and my marriage had hit rock-bottom, I knew I must return to England. This was eight years later. I had my old degree, no proven work experience, no other paper qualifications and no one to write references for me.

Four years later, now in a new marriage with a third child, I had decided to train as a therapist – or counsellor – or facilitator. There did not seem to be much distinction made in the Humanistic movement with which I had found myself involved, and which felt appropriate for me. It seemed to be a matter of choice, since most training courses did not define distinction either. But, there were few training courses anyway, and only one local training, which was financially beyond my means.

However, I had found a job in the mental health field, and having become part of a group of colleagues working in the broad Humanistic field – the Norwich Collective – I felt that I would receive all the supervision, support, challenge and ongoing training I would need from these experienced practitioners. So I found a training a little distance away, which was cheaper because it was attached to a university and was subsidised. For this reason I could also get partial funding from the Statutory Service for which I worked; so although it did not look very exciting, and its staff were primarily academic, I did it. I did it because I wanted to work with people as a therapist, and had heard that it was beginning to be difficult to work in this field without a structured training, which is what many of the older practitioners had done. They had devised their own ongoing trainings, identifying areas of need, areas where further work was needed, and taking responsibility for their own ongoing professional development, had formed groups and networks to enable themselves.

But I was a little too late. Apprenticeship models were already being replaced by structured trainings, often in academic institutions, and the changing cultural climate was affecting the 'growth movement' as well as everything else.

The concept of external accreditation first raised its head while I was still in training. The UK Standing Conference on Psychotherapy had just been convened, and there was much discussion in the Norwich Collective about the long-term implications of its agenda on practitioners and clients. One of its members was sent to check things out, and a letter was written to ask about membership. The Collective was horrified by the reply, which laid down criteria for membership that were entirely inappropriate for this group, which was not a business, but a peer group of independent practitioners from various disciplines, all of whom shared an adherence to Humanistic principles.

And then the landslide towards accreditation and registration really began to gather momentum. There were articles in all the journals, BAC was independently involved in its own moves towards procedures, the differences between counselling and psychotherapy were beginning to be defined by some, and counter-defined by others, and training courses began neurotically changing their structure in mid-course so as to meet ever-changing criteria for approval (accreditation) from either BAC or what was now UKCP. Students were being introduced to the notion of accreditation by BAC or UKCP as if these were immutable milestones in the professional lives of counsellors and therapists – and procedures had not even been fully devised. The whole thing was chaos, but those with investments in the process were pretending it was smoothly and unquestionably predetermined, natural and obvious.

As someone lucky enough to be alongside experienced and skilled practitioners of many years' standing, but mostly *sans* accreditation (because it did not exist) and as a new practitioner firmly believing in the importance of the personal relationship as the medium of therapeutic movement, I was acutely uncomfortable with the situation. I felt strongly that integrity, empathy, compassion, respect and openness were more important than the ability to account for oneself in writing, devise constitutions and write case studies in the practice of counselling or psychotherapy), and I felt that these qualities were basically non-quantifiable through the means of externally devised and imposed criteria.

I began from a position of outright rebelliousness (mirroring my flight into marriage and southern Spain at 20), moving quite quickly into a more mature mode, through discussion and exploration which took place within the Norwich Collective and in a group that had formed as part of ongoing training which was named the Group Process group. It was initially led by Jill Hall and Robin Shohet, but became a peer group, and it was in this group that the idea for the first conference on the Dynamics of Accreditation (held in Cambridge in 1991) was born.

The group had identified fear as the underlying, unconscious driving force leading inexorably down the road of professionalisation, registration and accreditation. We thought that offering opportunities to make this fear conscious would help us devise ways of evaluating our work according to our principles, instead of rushing headlong into structures in many ways antithetical to humanistic principles.

The conference was successful, drawing many people from the field, and generating a lot of interest and dialogue. We were not at that stage wishing to evolve alternative methods, feeling that this would increase the polarisation already happening, and place us again back into a 'rebel' position. We genuinely wanted to invite an exploration of the dynamics. Inevitably there was some tension, with people there who strongly wanted to come away with alternatives, and others who wanted to champion the system that was rapidly being developed. We held another conference the following year (in Cambridge, 1992), which was a heartening experience, and found many people who shared our misgivings, and wanted to network.

However, it was another couple of years before Nick Totton and Em Edmondson circulated an invitation to the Founding Conference of the Independent Therapists Network (now the IPN – Independent Practitioners Network) in November 1994. At last a structure was beginning to emerge, the aim of which was 'to provide intending clients with a context of basic security, within which they can make their own decisions about which practitioner is valuable for *them*'. The structure was to be that the unit of membership 'will be a *group* of at least five practitioners who *know and stand by each other's work*. ...[E]ach group will also have cross-linkages to other groups.'

I have been involved with the IPN since its inception, and although a bumpy ride at times, requiring a great deal more from me in terms of commitment and time than would a five-yearly application for BAC accreditation, for example, I feel that its structure contains and upholds its aim. I also know, and know quite well through the process of the meetings and gatherings, practitioners from all over the country whose work I would now feel able to recommend to clients. And my own work is subject to ongoing scrutiny, both in supervision (obviously) and in my IPN member group, and with their link groups.

And my own experience is this – that I have been in practice for ten years, worked privately and in both the Voluntary and Statutory Sectors as a counsellor and therapist, have never applied for BAC accreditation or to be UKCP registered, and when questioned have said why. I work in a Primary Health Care setting, now managing a Counselling Service for a group of GP Surgeries, where I was once the sole practitioner. I also work for a Voluntary Agency, co-ordinating a team of ten counsellors who work with young people. Although the job specification when I applied stated that they required an accredited counsellor, a personal explanation of my choice not to be accredited by procedures I do not trust sufficed. I am in the fortunate position of having a credible history and ten years of practice, and hope that my experience of not being frightened into applying for an accreditation or registration that does not match my professional orientation, and which I suspect is more likely to offer practitioner protection than client protection, might be helpful to newer practitioners who may not have realised that BAC and UKCP are neither compulsory nor the only organisations working to improve the practice of counsellors and psychotherapists.

• • •

The whole process of the move towards accreditation and professionalisation in psychotherapy and counselling has been driven by fear. It becomes a brilliant feedback loop, where what is apparently set up to protect *clients* – who are more vulnerable than ourselves, we think – is in fact increasingly designed to protect the *practitioner* (as are most professional structures). We deny our own vulnerability, and this very act of denial propels us into unconscious acting out, creating defence mechanisms to hide our disowned vulnerability. We are following the lead of other 'professions', where lengthy study gives access to a body of specialist information and knowledge. This is not so in counselling and psychotherapy, where, although there is a body of information and knowledge, successful practice is increasingly shown through research to depend upon the (unmeasurable) quality of the relationship between people.

When we identify only with external structures, perceiving them as the sole reality against which to measure ourselves in terms of status, self-worth and success in the world, we necessarily frighten ourselves. Having turned away from our relational wisdom, we depend on these impersonal, one-sided structures as if for our entire well-being. No wonder we then terrify ourselves into thinking we need even more structures and rules to live our lives by.

For both of us our journey has been towards uncovering the mirror again, rediscovering our connection with the 'whole story' – relationship to what lies within as well as without, relationship to process as well as product, to our innate wisdom as well as received wisdom, and to self as well as to other. The issue of accreditation has acted as a beam of light, bringing into focus the one-sided nature of our engagement with the world, enabling us gradually to realise a bigger picture. Through this process we are each, in our own ways, rediscovering what we had forgotten, a relational wisdom which is inclusive of fear – fear is just a part of life.

Part IV
Philosophy of Pluralism and Self/Peer Regulation

Pluralism and Psychotherapy: What is a Good Training? IV.1

Andrew Samuels

Politics of/and psychotherapy

Psychotherapists can learn a good deal from politics as it is practised and theorised these days. Much of what I have to say about pluralism and psychotherapy is taken directly from political theory and praxis. One political theme that seems to me to be very relevant is what the political philosophers call the 'identity/difference theme'. This means that, in some ways, every psychotherapist or counsellor is identical, and in some ways different. Now, there are no votes in such an unsexy formulation. But I invite my readers to consider it at the outset for its very complexity and ambiguity.

The professional concerns raised in this chapter are directly connected to my own ongoing work in the psychology–politics field. I am attempting to bring a psychological perspective to the political issues of the day, and to a re-invention of the political itself. I was a founder of Psychotherapists and Counsellors for Social Responsibility (PCSR) and of Antidote, the psychotherapy-based think-tank.

On a more clinical level, I am involved in working out the details of what I call the 'politicisation of therapy practice'. Everybody these days says they want to work with the political and social dimensions in therapy. It has become a kind of cocktail-party truism or slogan. Yet there are absolutely no detailed texts on how to do this. So I am trying to write such detailed texts that explicate the political person as he or she appears in the clinical situation (see Samuels, 1993).

My interest in pluralism and psychotherapy dates from the publication of *Jung and the Post-Jungians* in 1985. In that book I commented that it was not easy to find one's way around in the contemporary Jungian world. This was because very little had been written on the various competing

---

This chapter is a much extended version of the paper 'What is a good training?', *British Journal of Psychotherapy,* 9 (3), 1993: 317–23.

schools of analytical psychology that have grown up. The book and my whole approach rest on a fundamental paradox – that by concentrating on debate, dispute and difference, we can get the best possible conception of what psychotherapy as a whole really is.

Traditionally, the ways in which one defines a field involve looking for that which everybody agrees with – the consensus approach. These core values and core practices are usually regarded as defining the field. This is old-fashioned thinking. We need, instead, to think of a radical way of defining the field by reference to the differences of opinion in and around it. What defines the field of psychotherapy in my view is dispute. How does this actually work in experience?

If some psychotherapists, of whatever orientations, are having an argument about what psychotherapy really is, and you have some idea what they are talking about, and you are in some way stirred by their argument, then you are in a sense in the field. The field can be defined by the emotional ripples its arguments generate. This is a very complex and difficult idea that lies at the heart of much that I shall be proposing in this chapter. We should start our profession-defining work at the outer limits of the envelope. We should stay with dispute, argument, disagreement, miscommunication, misunderstanding, betrayal and onslaughts on the other, rather than staying with the core, the centre, the consensus. The philosopher A.N. Whitehead put this beautifully in a nutshell when he said: 'A clash of doctrines is not a disaster, it is an opportunity.' But first you have to find the clash, and use the clash to define what you are doing.

There is a cultural change to consider here, as well. I want to mention this, lest my stress on dispute sounds like an exclusively male perspective. I do not like the term, but there is what could be called a 'feminisation of knowledge' going on in the West today involving a boundary blurring between disciplines and within disciplines. There is a new valuing of subjectivity and intuition even within the hard sciences, and certainly within the social sciences and the humanities. It is my belief that altering the angle from which we define the field to one of difference and dispute, and away from one of consensus and agreement, is in an unexpected sense aligned with such new approaches to knowledge.

So, what is 'pluralism'?

On pluralism

Pluralism is an attitude to conflict which tries to reconcile differences without imposing a false resolution on them or losing sight of the unique value of each position. Hence, pluralism is not the same as 'multiplicity' or 'diversity'. Rather, pluralism is an attempt to hold unity and diversity in balance – humanity's age-old struggle, in religion, philosophy and politics, to hold the tension between the One and the Many. My use of the term 'pluralism' is also supposed to be different from 'eclecticism' or 'synthesis'. As the chapter unfolds, the distinctions should become clearer. Here, at the beginning, I would merely say that the trademark of pluralism is competition, and its way of life is bargaining.

We need a psychological working out of the idea of pluralism and, in order to do this, I will make two suggestions.

First, on a personal level, each of us is faced with the pluralistic task of aligning our many internal voices and images of ourselves with our need and wish to speak with one voice and recognise ourselves as integrated beings. So it is an issue of intense feeling. But it is also an issue of thinking – for psychological theory also seeks to see how the various conflicts, complexes, attitudes, functions, self-objects, part-selves, sub-personalities, deintegrates, internal objects, psychic *dramatis personae*, areas of the mind, sub-phrases, gods – how all of these relate to the personality as a whole. The extent of the list demonstrates the universality of the problem and its inherent fascination.

My second suggestion is that a pluralistic approach may be of immense help in dealing with issues of unity and diversity as they affect psychotherapy, with its massive ideological differences. By 'psychotherapy' I mean all psychological endeavours which seek to help individuals and small groups. We need a term which refers to the social context of the whole field – psychoanalytic, Jungian, integrative, humanistic, body, family and marital, cognitive-behaviourist, etc. – and, at the same time, to the divisions within the field. Of course, we should not forget that the field itself is composed of individual psychotherapists.

The fragmentation and dispute within psychotherapy, as each group fights for the general acceptance of its viewpoint, seems, on the surface, to be the very opposite of what is usually regarded as pluralism. However, as I said earlier, this competitive aggression is at the heart of any attempt to build up a pluralistic approach. The idea of unconscious compensation (in Jungian terms) or the idea of reaction formation (in

Freudian terms) suggests that we should look a little more deeply into the war-like situation. If we do so, then it is possible to see psychotherapy as struggling, and as having always struggled, towards pluralism. As Heraclitus put it, 'that which alone is wish both wishes and does not wish to be called Zeus'. What seems like a flight from pluralism may also be a yearning for it, and an acceptance at some level of a pluralistic destiny for psychotherapy.

A pluralistic attitude can hold the tension between the claims of and tendencies towards unity and claims of and tendencies towards diversity. Psychotherapy as a cohesive discipline with right and wrong approaches – and psychotherapy as containing a multiplicity of valuable approaches. It would not be pluralistic, as I understand it, to assert that there are many diverse truths but that these are but aspects of one greater Truth. In that religious and elitist approach, entry into the greater Truth, which would do away with all the lesser and seemingly contradictory truths, is reserved for the elect. This is not pluralistic, it is condescendingly casuistic. From a pluralist standpoint, Truth (with a capital T) and truth have to compete. Sometimes passionate and aggressive expressions of, and adherence to, the Truth can (even should) be the right way to live and function. But sometimes we need a more partial and pragmatic vision, equally passionate and aggressive in its way. Aggression, which is so characteristic of debates between psychotherapists, often contains the deepest needs for contact, dialogue, playback, affirmation.

Now, many psychotherapists are probably committed to dialogue, but the psychological difficulties associated with maintaining a tolerant attitude cannot be minimised. Psychotherapists, being human, will continually fail to be as tolerant as they would like to be. In part, this is because of their passionate devotion to their own psychological approach, to their own particular vision, or 'personal confession'. But where is a programme to combine passion and tolerance in psychotherapy? We know about and concentrate on the opposites of tolerance – envy, denigration, power, control, and so forth. But we usually pathologise these. My intent is to do something positive and realistic with the incorrigible competitiveness and argumentativeness, mining the envious shit for the tension-rich gold it might contain. Competition that is open, competition that is brought into the open, and into consciousness, competition that is psychologically integrated and valued, could lead to a new tough-minded tolerance. My approach is psychologically realistic here, staying close to and trading off what Jung called the shadow – the thing each of us has no wish to be. To paraphrase Lacan, if the unconscious is indeed structured like anything, it may be structured like an argument!

Through competition and argument with others we may come to know ourselves and our ideas better and more deeply. This is an example of the importance of the mirroring other whose presence glimmers in so many dialectical psychologies – Jung's, Winnicott's, Neumann's, Lacan's, Kohut's. This other is a creative other and needs nurturing. What is more – and I mention this as an example of the realism of pluralism – you cannot annihilate the other who is your opponent. He or she will not go away. The opponent is omnipresent and indestructible. The opponent resists the false way in which we all try to describe him or her. Sure, you can describe your opponent as narcissistic, religiose, mechanistic, idealistic, transference-bound, badly trained – but he or she will bounce back, rejecting that distortion and returning to the argument: *la lutta continua*. Like it or not, the dialogue and confrontation go on, as they always have in psychotherapy. And, amidst the seemingly ridiculous institutional splits, a kind of exchange is constantly being crafted. Let us not forget that when we project on to an other, it is often the good or positive things about ourselves that are projected (for whatever reason). Re-collection of projected contents is vital for the health and integrity of the self.

Psychotherapy is a social phenomenon which, viewed over time, has shown itself able to withstand clashes and splits and generate new ideas out of them. This capacity lies alongside the far better-known tendency for the splits to become institutional and concrete, and hence somewhat unproductive. Psychotherapy continues to be desirous of entering a pluralistic state, but lacks the ideological and methodological means to do it. It could even be possible that we are all pluralists but the prevailing ideology in the world we live in forces us to deny it. The tendency towards multiplicity and diversity is as strong – and creative – as the search for unity or a striving for hegemony.

As we proceed, we shall see again and again how these two suggestions of mine are really the same suggestion. That is to say, the experience of the One and the Many in relation to one's own psyche and personality, and the argument about the One and Many in relation to disputes in the professional area of psychotherapy are, in a sense, the same thing. However, the vicissitudes of psychotherapy as a cultural movement, the splits, plots, alliances, gossip and power struggles – all these reveal that, in their professional lives, therapists are participating in a mighty projection of the objective psyche. For, when therapists argue, it is the psyche that is speaking. Differing points of view reflect the multiplicity of the psyche itself. And when therapists recognise what they have in common, often through discussions of clinical experiences, then it is psyche in its monistic, unified vein that is revealed.

My point is that when therapists look at themselves – and they should always be looking at themselves – how they think, feel, behave, organise themselves, they are, perhaps without knowing it, also gazing at and participating in the world of the psyche.

Similarly, the books that therapists write, and candidates and colleagues read, are not what they seem to be. Texts of psychological theory can constitute for us what alchemical texts constituted for Jung. A deconstruction of psychotherapy parallels his of alchemy. Just as the alchemists projected the workings of the unconscious into chemical elements and processes, becoming caught up in the pervasive symbolism of it all, so the texts of the psychotherapists, taken as a whole and understood psychologically, may unwittingly provide us with documents of the soul. I think this is a radical re-reading of what books on psychotherapy are about. What was intended to be about psyche is *of* psyche. The conscious aim may be to plumb the past for its truths, or to connect past and present, or to reveal the workings of cumulative psychopathology. But what gets revealed, according to this analysis, are the central characteristics of psyche itself. This is where clashes between theories are so useful, because the actual clash itself contains the definitive psychic issue, not the specific ideas which are in conflict. Not psychological dialectics, but psyche's discourse given dialectical form. The warring theories and the particular points of conflict speak directly of what is at war in the psyche and of what the points of conflict might be therein.

Now, sometimes it is claimed that differences of opinion could not have such deep implications because they only show differences in the psychological type of the disputants. I agree that some therapists will tend constitutionally to prefer, see and search for multiplicity and differentiation. Others will be more inclined to favour and to find integration and unity. But this typological approach contains the seeds of its own contradiction. For, as with typology, to become truly himself or herself, the psychotherapist cannot 'belong' to one school alone. There is an interdependence, with all possible manner of divergence and convergence.

Pluralism is a perspective in which various therapists or the various schools of psychotherapy have to take note of each other, without necessarily having unity as a goal, a modular, conversational approach in which different world-views meet but do not try to take each other over.

When theories and fantasies of the psyche are in competition, what attitudes are possible? None seems really satisfactory. We can choose between theories – but that may lead to blind partisanship and possibly to tyranny. We can synthesise theories – but that may lead to omnipotence and an avoidance of the hard edges of disagreement rather than to transcendence. We can be indifferent to the dispute, but that leads to ennui and a subtle form of 'clinical' inflation in which the relevance of theory is denied. Of course we could be pluralistic – but that leads to fragmentation and anxiety (as we shall see). It is hard to act upon, this idea of pluralism!

Political thinkers and philosophers have addressed many of the questions we shall try to answer, and we can learn from that. Later, I will use pluralistic political thinking as a metaphor to further our understanding of psychological processes and of the social organisation of psychotherapy.

Let us consider how pluralism conceives of the state. This will be a useful model for a subsequent discussion of the role of national or trans-national umbrella psychotherapy organisations. Many people see the state as the container of everything in a society. But it is not. A state may also be regarded as a special interest group within society. Political process in a single society consists of arguments, competitions, bargaining, between the various interest groups in society, and perhaps the state has a regulatory role. But the regulatory role of the state itself also constitutes a special interest. The state may indeed be special when we are talking about regulation. But when we are talking about other things – art, trade, maybe education – then the state does not necessarily have a particularly special place. What I am trying to communicate is a vision of the state in which what we usually think of as the unifying factor, the container, the core, the regulator, is also one of the parts. In human psychology, the ego (and even the self), often regarded as fulfilling the functions of 'the state' for an individual, is, as many theorists have pointed out, nothing more than one part of the psyche competing with the other parts. In modern societies, increasingly, the state has to argue for its place in the sun. The state can be as vulnerable to competitive pressures as any other interest group in a society.

Pluralism and the organisation of psychotherapy

We can move this argument on or over to the question of psychotherapy organisations I referred to earlier. In the case of organisations like the United Kingdom Council for Psychotherapy, the implication of what I have been saying is that the organisation as a whole, with its central committees, is not in fact only a container or regulator of everything going on in it. They (the organisation and its central committees) are special interest groups. The centre ('ego') of UKCP is only a special interest group! The Annual General Meeting, supposedly the container of everything, is only a special interest group. There is a paradox here. What looks like the big thing is only in certain respects and at certain moments the big thing. For much of the time the big thing is only one of a number of little things. This is political pluralism applied to our understanding of umbrella psychotherapy organisations.

The manyness – the sections, the organisations, the individual psychotherapists – and the oneness – the UKCP as a whole – are in a competitive relationship. It is important to re-imagine and re-vision the centre or the conference as a whole also as parts. The centre, the Governing Board, the Registration Board, are not above the fray. They have their own state-like interests at stake. They, too, are involved in the bargaining process – as parts relating to parts, not as a whole relating to parts.

I think what I want us to do is to get beyond either maternal or paternal models for our professional organisations. In the maternal model, the big thing, the UKCP as a whole (to continue with the British example), 'holds' everything else in it. Holding as in Winnicott's idea of maternal function. In the paternal model, the UKCP sets standards and guidelines, makes regulations which everyone has to adhere to. A pluralistic model moves beyond the family altogether to try to find a new way to approach this organisational problem, which everybody is worried about: the relations between the organisation as a whole (and its central committees) and the rest. By this simple and yet oh-so-complex device of reconceiving the whole as a part, we can at least make a psychologically valid beginning in working out new models – pluralistic models – for psychotherapy organisations.

Can diversity be analysed so as to reveal its special requirements and guidelines? And can we develop a vision of diversity which makes a place for unity? For, as I have said, pluralism, as I use the term, does not simply mean diversity or multiplicity, not just the Many.

We know from politics that freedom does not guarantee diversity, for freedom can lead to a part of a system expanding to take a tyrannical hold over the whole. If I am free to do or be what I like, this will produce an unequal state of affairs between you and me. To make sure that does not happen, we may be required by political consensus or law to be more equal in some or all respects. But then an inhibition has been placed on my freedom. Exactly the same conundrum faces the psychotherapist today. If I act on, live out, hold dear, fight for my ideas, what am I to do with the differing points of view of which I am aware? I can't just deny that these points of view exist! My freedom to have a particular point of view may lead to an unhelpful, destructive denigration and abandonment of other people's ideas to the ultimate detriment of my own position and personal psychological well-being.

Equality doesn't guarantee diversity either, for equality may lead to the perils of indifference and boredom stemming from an unreal and infinite tolerance that lacks passion, is flat, bland and mediocre. This ennui can be seen in the attitude some practitioners have towards theoretical differences: they don't matter when compared to clinical inevitabilities. This myopic, clinical triumphalism overlooks the fact that everything in one's practice is suffused with theory (and, hopefully, vice versa). But if all views are considered to be of equal worth, what is to become of the freedom to feel a special value attaching to one's own view?

So, surprising to psychotherapists, perhaps, but not to political theorists, neither the freedom to think nor an egalitarian approach to thought can be said to guarantee diversity in a way that permits a unified view to coexist with it. Perhaps there is a problem with the way I have formulated things, and so I want to make a most radical suggestion. Instead of advancing pluralism as a desirable state or goal, let us begin instead to use it as a tool or instrument whose purpose is to make sure that diversity does not lead to schism and that differences between particular points of view are not smoothed over. Pluralism can function as an instrument which monitors the mosaic of the psyche or of the psychotherapy profession, rather than as a governing ideal.

One last brief point concerns pluralism and clinical practice. It seems to me that we have to start thinking in terms of what I call 'plural interpretation'. Plural interpretation is not the same as offering the patient a kind of multiple-choice interpretation, letting them choose the interpretation they fancy or think is right. Plural interpretation makes the existence in the therapist's mind of competing alternative interpretations a central plank of some interpretations that he or she may want to make. As we all know, it is often the case that there are a number of different ways in which material can be understood. These exist simultaneously in the mind of the therapist and often all of them have an equal, or nearly equal, weight. I would advocate that questions arising from the idea of plural interpretation, whether it is adopted as a technique or not, should be being discussed with any good-enough training, especially within the supervision situation, which carries this particular burden of multiple understanding.

Pluralism and psychotherapy training

Now – I hope we are in a position to use pluralism as an instrument or tool to help us look at the topic of dispute and disagreement in psychotherapy. This subject is, I suggest, of the greatest importance to anyone concerned with the training and formation of the psychotherapists of the future, seniors and candidates alike.

A pluralistic approach to psychotherapy, as I have explained it, means that a person interested in any particular area of knowledge should seek out the conflict and, above all, the competition between practitioners and ideologues in the discipline. The main implication is that even a so-called beginner should try to discover what the contemporary debate is all about. This approach differs fundamentally and profoundly from the conventional, linear style of training and education in psychotherapy. There, one is supposed to start 'at the beginning', and when the 'basics' have been mastered and one is 'grounded', exposure to more grown-up disagreements is permitted. The point I am advancing, backed up by a good deal of teaching experience, is that starting at the beginning is no guarantee of comprehension. However, if a person were to focus on the up-to-the-minute ideological conflict, then he or she cannot avoid discovering what has gone before; book learning is replaced by a living process. In a way, this is an educational philosophy derived from psychotherapy itself. In therapy, the focus of interest is where the internal 'debate' is at its most virulent; and in therapy the participants do not follow a linear 'course'.

The debates within psychotherapy give it life. They also serve to define the discipline generally, as I suggested earlier, and act as access routes for those who want to learn. What is important is not so much whether people are right or wrong, though it is vital to have views about that, but whether you know what they are talking about. For it is really rather hard to be completely wrong in psychotherapy. Or, as Kafka put it, 'the correct perception of a matter and a complete misunderstanding of the matter do not totally exclude one another'.

I am suggesting that, instead of searching for one guiding theory, we consider several competing theories together, and organise our training around such theoretical competition using papers and books written with polemical intent. Actually, if you think about it, that includes a high proportion of the literary output of psychotherapists! What holds these theories together is that the subject – the psyche – holds together; just as for modern sub-atomic physicists, their subject, the universe, holds together. In this viewpoint, passion for one approach is replaced by passion for a plurality of approaches.

Problems of pluralism

Let's consider now some of the problems with pluralism. For all manner of psychological reasons, it is very hard to get worked up about being tolerant, to be a radical centrist in psychotherapy, to go in for what has been called 'animated moderation'. Does pluralism condemn us to losing the excitement of breakthrough ideas, which are more likely to be held with a passionate conviction? My view is that such a worry rests on a misunderstanding and an idealisation of the cycle of creativity. So-called 'new' ideas emerge from a pluralistic matrix and are re-absorbed into such a matrix. As Winnicott put it paraphrasing T.S. Eliot: 'It is not possible to be original except on the basis of a tradition' (Winnicott, 1971: 117). Ideas do not come into being outside of a context; nor does the new necessarily destroy the old but often coexists with it. So, what looks like inspirational conviction arises from a plural *mise en scene* but it is convenient for the debt not to be acknowledged. And before we hail the man or woman of vision, let us not forget Yeats's words: 'the worst are full of passionate intensity'. The well-known clinical benefits of having conviction in one's ideas can still be available, but together with open communication, and the chance to learn from diversity.

This is not a dry or woolly perspective; passion abides in dialogue and tolerance as much as it does in monologue and fanaticism. The psychotherapist has never been able to work in isolation from others in the same field who have a different viewpoint. That's the conclusion I draw from the history of splits and struggles. People have to fight with one another because they cannot ignore one another. Leaving aside the never-settled question of whether any one clinical approach is more 'successful' than the others, the arrogance of isolation was never a viable option. The rows within psychotherapy cannot be ignored in a serene, Olympian fashion.

Even those who feel uncomfortable with pluralism, and seek to render it inaccurately as 'eclecticism', need to recall that their own theories arose from a pluralistic matrix and from a competitive diversity of views. For instance, Hillman's archetypal psychology was not a single, time-bound, unchallenged, piercing vision of the future of Jungian analysis. This was also something Winnicott noted in relation to Melanie Klein. In November 1952 he wrote her a remarkable, long and agonised letter protesting strongly against 'giving the impression that there is a jigsaw of which all the pieces exist' (Winnicott and Rodman, 1987: 35).

Psychotherapy's secret desires

So far, I have been trying to establish that pluralism can be seen as an extremely useful metaphorical approach to the interplay of the One and the Many in the psyche and in psychotherapy generally. I have also suggested that pluralism can keep diversity alive in the face of threats from both tyranny and ennui or boredom. I have tried to show that pluralism enables us to harness the competitive and aggressive energy trapped in theoretical dispute and competition. My overall position is that psychotherapy wants to become, needs to be, and, ironically, already is pluralistic.

In spite of all this, pluralism is threatened and under attack from all manner of entrenched interests. I would almost say, thank God that pluralism is under attack, for what would pluralism be without its opponents? There are several branches to this attack which it is possible to identify. First, holism, which tends to impose a false unity on our thinking, ignoring diversity. Second, numinosity, which forms the unavoidable heart of intolerance, for we become overwhelmingly fascinated by our own ideas and correspondingly threatened by other people's. Third, hierarchy, which sets up selected categories as pre-judged good things or goals. But the enemy of pluralism upon which I want to focus is consensus.

Clearly, for there to be any communication at all, some assumptions have to be permitted and agreed, though consensus can become like airline food – just acceptable to everyone but truly pleasurable to none. However, blandness is not what I perceive as problematic with consensus – for consensus is not really cuddly, cosy, friendly and bland at all. It can be quite violent. In psychotherapy, and perhaps even in science as well, personal allegiance and power dynamics play a part. Orthodoxy, heterodoxy and heresy come into being. I do not see us as being able to get rid of vested interests, but I would like us to do something creative with the vested interests we have.

This highly politicised state of affairs can be seen most vividly in relation to training for psychotherapy, and therefore lies at the very root of psychotherapy as a social institution. Though the candidate is an adult, a degree of regression seems inherent in the training situation due to the continuing entanglements of the candidate's personal therapy and supervision/control work. It has been claimed that the training posture actually fosters regression in general and persecutory anxiety in particular, and that this is exacerbated by a confusion that often exists in the trainers' mind between therapy and training. My concern is different. It is that the whole range of careful, thoughtful experiences most therapists have been through in their training might inadvertently have removed the creative sting. I am thinking of syllabi, seminar themes, reading lists, feedback sessions and so forth. The more integrated and professional the training programme, the greater the denial of pluralism.

I think that the denial of pluralism has contributed to the formation of cult-like bodies within our little world of psychotherapy. Being in a cult implies obedience. There may be too much obedience in psychotherapy. There is a serious danger that training programmes will become obedience cults, and that this will be rationalised by reference to the advantages of practising on the basis of a system in which one has conviction. It is striking how many of the groups which are active in psychotherapy today either are, or were in the recent past, dominated by leader figures. The leaders may be remarkable people, with a comprehensive vision, which would partially account for the tendency, but I think there is more to it than that. I do not think this pattern results from conscious fostering, but would argue that its effect is to shield the candidate from the stress and anxiety of pluralism. And then the benefits of pluralism are lost as well. The need for strong leader figures has a lot to do with the desire to avoid the anomalous. The leader sorts things out by arranging competing ideas in a hierarchical schema of acceptability, protecting or advancing his own ideas in the process. The desire to avoid anxiety and confusion when confronted with something which feels strange and new strengthens the tendency of groups to select leaders as a combination of leader and safety-net.

Perhaps it is a case of taking it in turns to be the dominant theorist, accepting that, in some ways and in some situations, the other person has a more utilisable (more 'correct', from a pragmatic viewpoint) theory. Then we may make bilateral and multilateral agreements to sing each other's song – not the same as agreeing to disagree and different, too, from eclecticism. For eclecticism means singing selected verses only. Eclecticism ignores the contradictions between systems of thought, whereas pluralism celebrates their competition. Eclecticism is intolerant, in that parts of a theory are wrenched from the whole. In a pluralistic approach, the whole theory is used, as faithfully as possible, and together with other theories, until inconsistencies lead to breakdown. Then the breakdown itself becomes the object of study.

What is a good training?

My short answer to this deliberately naive question is: a good training is an open training.

I want to talk about openness as a criterion for a good training under a number of different headings. These are: (a) sexual orientation, (b) gender issues, and (c) socio-economic factors. These can contribute to a discussion on what constitutes a good training.

First of all, sexual orientation. Here is a brief vignette concerning a patient of mine (who has given permission for publication). The patient, in his mid-thirties, who is homosexual, was interested in training at the Institute of Psychoanalysis in London. This man was, perhaps, a little naive. Prior to his analysis with me, he had been to see a very distinguished training analyst to discuss the possibilities. Not only was the patient given the information that there was no chance at all, but he was given a whole bundle of gratuitous interpretations about the infantile origins of his homosexuality in terms of the dynamics of the relationship with the father. Now, I think it is very important, if we are considering a good training, that we assert that a training cannot be a good training if it is not open in the area of sexual orientation, given that depth psychological theorising about homosexuality has been shown to be, for the most part, compounded of prejudice, fear and ignorance (Lewes, 1988).

The second criterion for openness concerns gender issues. Again, I am going to illustrate this with a very brief vignette which I have permission to publish. A patient of mine was being interviewed for admission to a training course in psychotherapy. She had two interviews. She had a baby who was at the time about six months old; she herself was 40 years old. At the first interview she was asked about her child-care arrangements which happened to utilise a child-minder. She was asked the following questions: Is the child-minder you have employed qualified? What is the size of the group the child-minder has in her house? How much do you pay? At the second interview, when she explained her child-minding arrangements, the interviewer said: 'Ah, so you've found a mother for her.' Now, obviously, this account has been filtered and maybe distorted through the analytical situation. However, I believe it is justifiable to introduce such material so as to illustrate that there is a really oppressive issue here concerning openness which must be addressed. A training cannot be a good training if it is not open in the area of gender issues.

The third aspect of openness is founded on socio-economic issues. Here is another vignette which I have permission to publish. This particular patient left school at 15 and was, to be frank, not particularly literate. So he had enormous trouble in writing the course paper. (I am not intending to raise the more general question about whether or not there should be papers to indicate that a therapist has achieved a certain level of intellectual development.) Here was somebody who, through no fault of their own, for socio-economic reasons was simply not able to manage what was involved in writing the paper. Yet the patient was apparently getting pretty good reports from supervisors and seminar leaders. On the basis of accounts like this, I think there is a crucial question concerning openness that needs to be examined in socio-economic terms. I am not forgetting racial and ethnic factors as issues of special concern over and above economics, and I discuss ethnicity in/and psychotherapy elsewhere (Samuels, 1993: 299–312).

I would not want these ideas about openness to cease to be applicable once admission to training has been achieved. It is a far more important matter than a mere admissions policy. My vision is of the production of psychotherapists who have the values and perspectives I have summarised under the rubric of 'openness'. Let us try, in our quest for a good training, to turn out socially and politically aware psychotherapists who can bring a sense of openness to what they do and how they think about it. Matters of sexual orientation, gender issues and socio-economic factors should be addressed during the training and after graduation, as well as in connection with admission to training.

Concluding reflections

To summarise again: I have outlined what I mean by pluralism and suggested that we use it as an instrument. I have suggested what psychotherapy can learn from political theory. An ideology and a methodology for the organisation of the profession are beginning to emerge. Some problems with pluralism have been discussed, and 'consensus' has been attacked.

The general impression I have of psychotherapy is that there was a golden age that is now past. The broad outlines of the enterprise are firmly drawn. If that is so, then the fertilising challenge presented by the arrival on the scene of all-inclusive theories, forcing a person to work out his or her response, has been lost. If our generation's job is not to be restricted to 'professionalisation', institutionalisation or historical recovery of the happenings of the earlier days, it is necessary to highlight the one thing we can do that the founding parents and brilliant second-generation consolidators cannot. This is to be reflexive in relation to psychotherapy, to focus on the psychology of psychology, a deliberate navel-gazing, a healthily narcissistic trip to the fantastic reaches of our discipline; a postmodern psychological outlook, redolent with the assumption that psychology and psychotherapy are not 'natural', but made by psychologists and psychotherapists. After that, but only after that, we can turn towards the world.

I will conclude with four proverbs. These are crafted aphorisms which are the result of an internal dialogue between C.G. Jung and myself about some of these matters. Some words are his and some words are mine.

> The art of psychotherapy requires that you be in possession of avowable, credible and defensible convictions.

Too much agreement spells onesidedness and desiccation.
We need many theories before we get even a rough picture of the complexity of the psyche.

Behind every fanaticism lurks a secret doubt.

References

Lewes, K. (1988) *The Psychoanalytic Theory of Male Homosexuality,* New York: Penguin.

Samuels, A. (1985) *Jung and the Post-Jungians,* London and Boston: Routledge & Kegan Paul.

Samuels, A. (1989) *The Plural Psyche: Personality, Morality and the Father,* London and New York: Routledge.

Samuels, A. (1993) *The Political Psyche*, London and New York: Routledge.

Samuels, A., Shorter, B. and Plaut, F. (1986) *A Critical Dictionary of Jungian Analysis,* London and New York: Routledge & Kegan Paul.

Winnicott, D. W. (1971) *Playing and Reality,* New York: Penguin.

Winnicott, D. W. and Rodman, F. R. (1987) *The Spontaneous Gesture: Selected Letters of D. W. Winnicott,* Cambridge, MA: Harvard University Press.

The Teaching of Psychotherapy IV.2

Peter Lomas

> Unless we purposely turn our eyes to look at something that interests us as individuals, we shall literally see nothing in the world, and we shall understand nothing in the real world unless we remember that we freely choose the direction in which to look.
>
> (Stuart Hampshire)

Our views on how psychotherapy is best learnt and taught are inevitably influenced by our philosophy of education in general. Do psychotherapists, as a group, have a particular line on this? One clue to this is the way in which psychotherapists try to influence their patients – that is to say, in what way should a person attempt to give a needed insight to another?

The tradition in which those of us work who have been strongly influenced by Freud is to place interpretation at the centre of our attempt to influence. In other words, we are not didactic. We do not say to the patient 'This is what you must think; this is what you must believe'. We try, using our knowledge and privileged position, to understand what the patient wishes to convey to us of what is most profound in them, and inform them of our impression. It is, by and large, a permissive method, allowing the patient much freedom of expression.

In practice, however, there is often less freedom than the theory suggests. Freud emphasised the prevalent resistance against interpretation and the amount of determination and persistence necessary to overcome the patient's denials. In Freud's conception of psychoanalysis it is the practitioner who has the truth, who knows what the patient should learn, and who has a body of knowledge and theory at his disposal unavailable to the patient. The fact that Freud eschewed blatant didacticism like the plague and developed a method which gave the patient incomparably

---

This chapter was first published in *Personal Disorder and the Family* by Peter Lomas, Transaction Press, 1997.

more freedom to express themselves than had hitherto been possible in psychiatry is a paradox which, I believe, inhibits our ability to see the one-sidedness of his conversations with patients. Nevertheless, in recent years, due to rigorous scrutiny of Freud's work, we are now in a better position to see the degree of coercion he imposed upon them. If we focus on this element in Freud's method (in particular, as it appears in some of his case-histories), it begins to look rather like a didactic form of education.

Since Freud formulated his ideas, the patient has increasingly come to be conceived by psychotherapy as a unique being capable of developing creatively, if given the space to do so as free as possible from the preoccupations and counter-transference impediments of the therapist; in other words there has been a shift, albeit a partial one, from the idea of a technique imposed on the patient towards the provision of what Winnicott refers to as a 'medium for growth' or 'facilitating environment'. This move, expressed so vividly by Winnicott, is also to be found in the work of several other thinkers, notably the existential psychotherapists, and words and phrases such as encouragement, holding, self-actualisation, person-centred therapy, empathy and negative capability have become part of our professional language.

Although there is a wide variation in the exact stance which psychotherapists take on this issue, an increasing number of therapists – of whom I count myself as one – are inclining to the view, present in Freud and now emerging more clearly, that the patient should be given respect as a being who is never completely knowable, cannot be fitted into any formula and needs to be encouraged to present his or her uniqueness, and that the therapist is more aptly considered as a midwife than a container of insights to pass on to the patient. We are, in a sense, becoming less confident.

If our theory of education in the consulting room has always been, and is increasingly so, slanted towards the autonomy of the patient, how does this attitude stand in relation to theories of education in general? The philosophy of education has, with a few exceptions, focused almost exclusively on the teaching of children, particularly small children. As far as I understand it as a non-expert, the seminal creative figures in the field – Rousseau, Pestalozzi, Froebel, Dewey and Montessori – promote what is often called 'progressive education'. In his paper, 'Teaching and learning psychotherapy' (Evans, 1992), Michael Evans describes this tradition as supporting 'the notion that the capacity to learn is inherent and that the function of education is to promote personal autonomy and creative capacities, and to enable knowledge to be regarded as a means of discovery'. He quotes Dewey:

> To the growth of the child all studies are subservient; they are instruments valued as they serve the needs of growth. Personality, character, is more than subject matter. Not knowledge but self realisation is the goal. Moreover, subject matter never can be got into the child from without. Learning is active. It involves reaching out of the mind. It involves organic assimilation starting from within. The only significant method is the method of the mind as it reaches out and assimilates.

In contrast to this philosophy, Evans describes the traditional conventions of higher education.

> In Higher Education the prevailing method consists of the lecture or demonstration, closely followed by the seminar and the tutorial. At postgraduate level the tutorial takes precedence over the seminar and the lecture, and the student is expected to work more independently but is often isolated from other students because of his specialisation. These practices are characterised by an unquestioned common sense hierarchy, in which lecturers teach and students learn.
>
> The common assumption behind this system is that education consists of the transmission of culture by teachers which is received by pupils. At a later stage these facts and ideas are reproduced and it is assumed that learning has taken place. (Students frequently sell their books after their exams as if to demonstrate that their qualification proves that they have learned the contents.) The lecture theatre and even to some extent the seminar room are organised to express this hierarchy and the teachers exert their control and mastery through the system of devising aims and objectives, setting the syllabus, producing lecture lists, essay titles, marking systems, assessment criteria and examinations.

In the fields of education, philosophy and psychotherapy it has, in recent years, been suggested that the best way of reaching the truth is by conversation.[1] A conversation – a good conversation – is open-ended; there is no leader, no voice that is necessarily dominating, no truth other than the nearest approximation to it that will be arrived at by a group of people sufficiently relaxed and free from fear and constraint to say what they really think; and the due respect appropriate to those with much to contribute will not be allowed to inhibit the creative ideas of those whose knowledge of the matter under discussion is less at the moment; there are no prizes and no rewards other than enjoyment, play, curiosity and, if luck holds, some achievement.

Where, at the present time, does the teaching of psychotherapy stand in relation to the differing ideas on education? In some ways it stands clearly in the progressive tradition: the pupil gets more individual attention, by means of personal therapy and supervision than perhaps in any other occupation. Moreover, this attention is centred on his or her uniqueness and the limitations that stand in the way of fruitful living; even in supervision, the student's individual responses (the counter-transference) gains increasing emphasis. Also, as in progressive education, the focus is on activity: the student learns by doing: he or she sees clients.

In other ways, however, the progressive tendency is less in evidence and follows the conventions of traditional higher education: the transmission of culture by teachers which is received by pupils; teachers devise and organise a system of learning which students follow: there are assessment criteria and some kind of examination.

To my mind this system is as inappropriate to the teaching of adults as of children, and particularly inappropriate to the teaching of psychotherapy, a subject that depends far more on ordinary capacities of living (which teachers share with students and all members of the human race) than, for example, a much more technical undertaking like electronic engineering.

It was this line of thought that led some of us in Cambridge to set up a teaching scheme in psychotherapy, one in which the students' own drive to learn would constitute the energy by which the teaching scheme functioned and developed.[2] It was central to our thinking that students should be left as far as possible to learn and develop in their own unique way and their own time, and expect to be able to turn to each other for help in learning. There were to be no fixed conditions or rules.

It is now clear to us that we were pursuing an aim which, however justifiable as a valid method, could not be maintained in the modern world. There is now a widespread belief that training set-ups should be regulated by a central body in order that the public be protected from morally irresponsible and ignorant practitioners, that such a central body could effectively bring this happy state about, and that it could do so without stifling the expression of individuality in individuals and training organisations. This is a view which, I believe, involves a misunderstanding of the nature of good therapy, and which fails to recognise the gross distortions to creative work which such standardisations will bring. Nevertheless, in order to give our students a better chance of succeeding to achieve the necessary status to do the work they wanted to do, we elected to follow the trend. However, within this limitation, we have tried to keep to our original aim as far as possible. There is no formal hierarchy. What students do is decided amongst themselves, and there is no compulsion for individual students to follow any course of action with which they disagree. Nevertheless, certain expectations have developed which, although few, have a force comparable to rules, e.g. that candidates should be prepared to have individual therapy and supervision for a substantial – though unspecified – period.

In practice, what does this regime amount to? The students meet weekly to discuss psychotherapy; sometimes they invite one of the trained members to join them either as a participant in the discussion, or to lead a seminar, or give a talk; each month the whole group meets to discuss psychotherapy, sometimes inviting an outside speaker.

The students arrange their own programme, usually planning meetings for a few months ahead, and from time to time inviting one or two therapists to help them with their planning. It is understood that therapists are willing to meet any student to discuss a particular problem or advise on any matter, but this kind of help is, in fact, seldom asked for. Small study groups are arranged from time to time on an *ad hoc* basis. One of the problems is that, as therapists are not paid for the help they give, students are understandably reluctant to ask them to give their time. Occasionally the students have made a private arrangement with a therapist to provide a weekly series of seminars over a period of time, but this is not the norm. The group functions, to some extent, as a network. This has been formalised by an arrangement of pairing lasting six months each, by means of which members meet each other informally to discuss psychotherapy or anything else they like, and to give each other mutual support. It is hard to overestimate the value which students find in this arrangement.

I don't present this account as an ideal way of doing things, nor am I attempting to describe a group in which all is harmony and we are on our way to heaven. It has, like any group, its own particular awfulness. But it is a different way of doing things, and it appears to be able to grow therapists who show no obvious signs of being less competent or professionally dedicated than other training in the field.

One of the difficulties of giving a description of a teaching scheme is that we are easily drawn towards specifying the organisation and the practical arrangements, and leaving out of account the philosophy which informs the arrangements. The result is rather like that which follows from describing, in a mechanical way, the practicalities of psychotherapy – the setting, the cost, the frequency and so on – without saying what it is all about and what it feels like to be doing it. Yet what really matters in what we do as a teaching group is to keep in mind the principles and aims which brought us together and to observe, for example, whether we do manage to have conversations of the kind I have mentioned, and what appear to be the advantages and disadvantages of so doing. It is, I think, because it is so difficult to describe nuances of experience that most descriptions of training focus on the practical arrangements in the same way that much of psychotherapy focuses on the technique and simply assumes, for example, that the precise quality of what is called 'the therapeutic alliance' can simply be taken for granted and not explored.

The reasons which make it difficult to maintain the ideals of a training of this kind, and which have revealed themselves in our own group, seem to fall into three categories. (In what follows I am giving my own views; these are not necessarily those of others in the group).

1. *Practical.* As the group grows in size, it grows in complexity. In order to facilitate communication, avoid muddle and save time, more organisation and division of labour became necessary. This is at a cost of flexibility and intimacy. For example, we now have business meetings with pre-arranged agendas and minutes which are basically no different from those in most organisations, and out of these meetings come fixed procedures. To put the matter another way, it becomes more difficult to rely on the kind of goodwill and personal understanding of each other that make for congenial family life, and therefore procedures are established.

2. *The pull of normality.* Any organisation which departs radically from the normal way of doing things is under constant pressure from the outer world to get back into step, and it does seem to be the case that the creative edge of most organisations gradually succumbs to this pressure. The pressure towards normalisation comes not only from outside but is in the individual members. Habit, as William James has so eloquently taught us, is a powerful force. And those of us who have worked in organisations in which the traditional hierarchies and

procedures flourish tend to fall back on these methods when trying to solve problems. Moreover, members who are new to The Outfit often find it difficult to believe that the flexibility which it promotes is really there. For example, students from time to time ask if a certain line of behaviour is 'permitted' rather than saying 'Do you think this would be a good thing to do?'

3. *Emotional.* A set-up that is not based on rules and in which structures are at a minimum requires its members – particularly those who are students – to tolerate a considerable level of uncertainty. Security has to be based on the member's own self-motivation and on personal trust in other members, and less on a fixed framework and procedure. The insecurity shows itself, I believe, in attempts to establish hierarchies which are not formalised, and in attempts to control the activities of others and to discourage idiosyncrasies. For this reason, the original idea that each student should be allowed as far as possible to learn in his or her own particular way is hard to maintain. It is, of course, quite realistic for the views of the more experienced therapists to be given due weight, but I believe that that is a different matter from the degree of control which can easily be exerted by the elders – or indeed, by the organisation as a whole.

There is one particular area which proves to be a persistent problem: that of assessment and graduation. Appropriate, wise and unbiased feedback from others is a vital element in learning. However, the word 'assessment' usually carries connotations of an examination in which the degree of overall competence of the student is the matter in question. In other words, help with creativity can easily become muddled with judgement of capacity. Thus, a student may not be clear as to whether he or she is writing an essay for their personal development or in order to satisfy the expectations or demands of others. To the degree that a student feels watched and judged by an organisation that is concerned with fitness to practice, he or she will be insecure and less able to think boldly and creatively. Moreover, the time and energy absorbed by a preoccupation with assessment (which is part of the spirit of the age – we see it in schools for example) could more effectively be used to help students in other ways.

Although there are undoubted merits in having a means by which practitioners can be identified as having been well-trained, these are not as unambiguously useful as might be supposed. The stamp of authority given by a qualification is, sadly, no guarantee that the practitioner is a good therapist, or a good therapist for a particular patient, and the apparent guarantee can inhibit the potential patient from finding an intuitive answer to the question 'Is this the right person to help me?'. The criteria which one should use in estimating whether someone is capable of practising good therapy are elusive, for psychotherapy is, I believe, more akin to an art than a science, and are probably best served by intimate experience of the student and our best instinctive judgement, rather than, say, the writing of a paper or a quantitative measure of training achieved. There is no satisfactory answer to this problem at present. But I believe that a shift from measures such as assessment, monitoring and examination to the provision of a culture in which individual style, exploration and self-responsibility are given as much rein as possible provides our best chance of growing effective psychotherapists. The pressures towards conventionality have been enormously increased since we opted to join the United Kingdom Council for Psychotherapy. Because the UKCP was set up to monitor psychotherapy, regulations have become the centre of its philosophical approach. It exists in order to measure and to breed conformity, an outlook which is antithetical to the aims that I outline above. This is not the place to discuss in detail the ways in which The Outfit have felt obliged to restrict its creative activities in order to be acceptable. Although the UKCP has tried to take account of our unique aims, the fundamental difference in philosophy has been too great to bridge without loss of our driving force and spirit. It really does seem difficult for the Committee to understand that we have seriously considered the implications of giving such responsibility to the students and that this measure has proved rewarding over many years.

I have been talking about the principles and organisation of teaching rather than the content of what is taught. I don't feel that I've much to say on this subject. What we teach will vary according to our theoretical and ideological predilections, but I imagine that most therapists would give a lot of weight to Freud's ideas on resistance, transference and the influence of childhood experience. However, in view of what I've been saying about psychotherapy, e.g. that I see it as more akin to an art than a science, it follows that I'm bound to advocate a focus on the actual practice of psychotherapy and the nitty-gritty of what occurs in the therapist's room. How do we teach this?

A student at art college has the opportunity of seeing the work of the great artists in front of them, although not the actual process of its creation.

But the work of Freud and other pioneers is not there to be seen. We don't really know very well what it was like to be with them in therapy. The best the teacher can do (and this is perhaps most easily done in personal supervision) is to share as openly as possible his or her experiences in therapy without covering up (as is so often done when we write papers) the failings, uncertainties and the spontaneous ways of behaving which do not appear to be based on sound methodical ideas. I think, too, that the content of students' discussion groups and seminars could perhaps be more focused than they often are on the actual experience of being with patients.

In the matter of the content of our teaching, the UKCP has, to my mind, had a notably restricting influence. Because, on joining, we were obliged to place ourselves in one of the theoretical boxes available, we decided on the 'psychoanalytic'. The consequence is that because of a pressure to conform to the requirements of the section, we have, since joining, become narrowly analytical. The students confine themselves primarily to analytic books and formulae and, it seems to me, are afraid of being thought wild, unrigorous, irresponsible, naive or unscientific if they depart from the rigid expectations of being '*psychoanalytic* psychotherapists'. It is ironic that, as Rosemary Randall has tellingly observed (1995: 98), followers of Freud should forget his own cautionary advice, i.e. that 'The extraordinarily diversity of the psychical constellations concerned the plasticity of all mental processes and the wealth of determining factors oppose any mechanisation of the technique' (1913: 123).

One of the problems of learning psychotherapy is that much of the subject is written in jargon. This is difficult for a beginner to grasp and can be quite intimidating. The student can easily feel the awe which a small child feels in the presence of adults who command fluent speech and use words which to them are obscure. Personally I believe that psychotherapy is best communicated in *any* circumstances by the use of ordinary language insofar as this is possible, and that to do so in teaching eases the path of the student. No other medium of expression has the richness, or the resonance to convey the nuances of human intercourse. Of course, simply in order to be able to follow a discussion involving jargon it is desirable at some point that the student should become familiar with the language used (e.g. good object, bad object etc.), but this should not, I believe, be the accepted path to understanding therapy.

For a similar reason, learning about psychotherapy should involve wide-ranging discussion of cultural issues – of family, society, morality, etc. – which, if omitted, would leave us too far from the actual world in which we live.

If we are to find a way out of this mess, it will require something more than an alteration in organisation. We need to recognise the limits of our knowledge, the poverty of technique, the sterility of excessive control, the uniqueness of each and every therapeutic encounter and the fact that the human spirit stretches beyond the confines of experimental science.

References

Evans, M. (1992) 'Psychotherapy and educational theory', paper read to the Cambridge Society for Psychotherapy.

Freud, S. (1913) *On Beginning the Treatment*, Standard Edition, Vol. 12, London: Hogarth Press.

Lomas, P. (1990) 'On setting up a psychotherapy training scheme', *Free Associations*, 20: 139–49.

Randall, R. (1995) 'Does psychotherapy need NVQs?', *British Journal of Psychotherapy*, 12 (1): 98–102.

Endnotes

1. The Socratic dialogues precede this approach by two millennia, but Socrates was in his subtle way a very dominating teacher, and perhaps not a good model in this context.

2. I wrote about the early days of this endeavour in 'On setting up a psychotherapy training scheme' (Lomas, 1990).

Therapy in New Paradigm Perspective: The Phenomenon of Georg Groddeck IV.3

Richard House

> The answer to human life is not to be found within the limits of human life.
>
> (C.G. Jung, quoted in Lorimer, 1990: 220)

Introduction: modernity, spirit and the 'profession'

> I cannot send a prospectus of my small clinic .... There is no prospectus. My charges are adjusted to the means of my patients .... I have not forgotten during my life as a doctor that man's true profession is to become a human being.
>
> (Groddeck [1930] at age 64, quoted in Schacht, 1977: 1)

In Chapter 8 of his book *Whole in One*, David Lorimer (1990) writes incisively about what he calls 'the eclipse of the spiritual world-view' that has been under way since the seventeenth century, and which has been paralleled by the inexorable rise of the scientific materialist world-view. Barrett (1987) has also bemoaned the loss of the soul in modernist discourse, and how this loss seriously compromises our ability to form an adequate philosophical understanding of 'mind'.

Before Descartes, the phenomena of nature were typically accounted for teleologically with reference to their purpose, and not merely their physical or mechanical causes (Lorimer, 1990: 227, 255): 'nature was explained as animated, alive, having not yet succumbed to the deadening influence of mechanical philosophy' (p. 228). The seventeenth century heralded an ontological shift from a concern with connections within the whole to a preoccupation with the mechanisms of separate parts: the metaphor of the organism was replaced by that of the clock, knowledge of the workings of which can best be discovered by taking it apart (ibid.: 230). Accompanying this shift in world-view was a radically different definition of truth – an objectivist 'correspondence' theory which assumes that the scientific method gives us reliable access to an accurately describable world that exists independently of our perception of it – and which, crucially, is also unaffected by our perception of it. This Galilean scientific world-view purports to explain all phenomena as 'by-products of matter and physical forces'; and any kind of dualism of soul or body is disdainfully scorned as 'unscientific' and mystical (ibid.: 246, 248).

As will become clear in what follows, recent developments in the fields of physics (e.g. Bohm, 1980 and Clarke, 1996) and biology (e.g. Sheldrake, 1981 and Goodwin, 1994, 1997) are beginning to cohere into a so-called New Paradigm world-view (Woodhouse, 1996) which is challenging quite fundamentally the old-paradigm consensus of objectivist positive science. Yet the fear aroused by, and the resistance to, revolutionary ideas can be considerable – sometimes uncontainable (Clarke, 1997): William James commented that, 'in admitting a new body of experience, we instinctively seek to disturb as little as possible the pre-existing stock of ideas' (quoted in leaflet for the SMN conference cited at Clarke, 1997). The questions raised by the explicitly spiritual New Paradigm (NP) world-view are quite central to the philosophy of psychotherapy and counselling as healing practices. Put differently, whether or not one subscribes to a NP world-view will profoundly influence one's approach to therapeutic practice, one's philosophy of the person, and how one conceives of the therapeutic change process – not to mention, of course, one's attitude towards professionalisation and its associated ideologies and practical consequences.

Within the therapy field, the so-called 'transpersonal' approach (Rowan, 1993) tends to be partitioned off and neatly categorised as just one of many alternative therapeutic approaches – with little recognition of the fact that the experience of working transpersonally, with spirit or soul, can't just be picked up and used or not as the mood or fashion takes one, but rather, necessitates a fundamentally different world-view which is philosophically incompatible with alternative approaches that are rooted in the old-paradigm philosophy of Galilean science. The view, as Rowan for example has argued (1992: 165), that the whole field of therapy can somehow be treated as one unified 'profession', in which the differences between distinct approaches are less pronounced than are the commonalities that unify them, ignores the fundamental ideological incompatibilities in world-view between different approaches. At least some of these incompatibilities will be the focus of much of what follows.

Jutta Gassner (personal communication) has referred to her own counselling work not as a profession, nor even as a career or a vocation, but as a *calling*. This terminology is crucial: the term 'calling' immediately conveys a transpersonal or spiritual dimension which, from this perspective, *is an indissoluble aspect of therapeutic work* – and is one which so easily becomes submerged or lost under the deadening practices of credentialisation and career-mindedness. Of course, many (spiritual) healers do not, as a matter of principle, charge a commercial fee for their healing work; and one can see how practitioners working within a transpersonal NP world-view can experience the commercialisation and commodification of the therapy world as alienating and quite incongruous with their value system. On this view, the whole edifice of institutional professionalisation, preoccupied as it is with status, the 'power-over' dynamics of hierarchy, career development, personal and professional security, registration and accreditation-mindedness, is firmly rooted within an old-paradigm materialist philosophy which privileges conscious, rational knowledge, causal-linear ways of reasoning and knowing, measurement and controllability, guarantees of allegedly measurable competencies, and all the other leitmotivs of the modernist scientistic world-view.

If we accept Jung's view that we cannot hope to discover the meaning of life from within the limitations of conscious, rational human experience, then it follows that *human-made structures* of institutional professionalisation cannot begin, from within the modernist paradigm, to touch or help to throw light upon that which really matters in the realms of human potential. As Krishnamurti resoundingly stated, 'Truth cannot be organised; nor should any organisation be formed to lead or coerce people along any particular path .... If you [organise a belief], it becomes dead, crystallised' (Talks, 1929 and 1974, quoted in House, 1997: 31).

Georg Groddeck – the unaccreditable 'wild analyst'

> We know or seek to know what we can get by learning. Groddeck sees and knows without making this detour.
>
> (Georg Simmel, quoted in Schacht, 1977: 8)

The 'phenomenon' of Georg Groddeck (1866–1934; I use the term advisedly), the brilliant physician-cum-healer-cum-analyst and contemporary of Freud, provides us with an extremely revealing vehicle for considering just how – if at all – spiritual perspectives might subsist within a licensed field of therapy. By common consent Groddeck had quite remarkable success with a whole range of often chronically ill patients who had been abandoned as beyond cure and hope by the medical establishment of his day (quoted in Groddeck, 1951: 5–6).

Groddeck had a very strong sense of the ineffable level of human experience: he stressed the impossibility of putting words to our most essential experiences, and he went as far as to say that it is with language that the falsification of truth begins (Schacht, 1977: 22). (There are echoes here of Wittgenstein's 'prison-house' of language.) Groddeck coined the term 'the It' (which we might call 'life force', spirit or soul) which, he believed, had to be harnessed if the patient was to be healed. (In fact, Groddeck himself used the word 'soul' when writing about the It, thus: 'it would be desirable if people showed more interest … in the manifestation of the It, the mute and yet so insistent entreaties of their innermost soul which strives desperately to get a hearing ….' ibid.: 24–5.)

For Groddeck (1977: 212), the It 'means nothing else but the whole of all the life forces that make up an individual from the moment of his conception'. Elsewhere he wrote, 'I liked the indefiniteness about [the term "It"] …. My It … suggests that only a fool would try to understand it. There is nothing there to understand' (letter, 1930, quoted in Schacht, 1977: 11). Elsewhere, he wrote: 'The sum total of an individual human being, physical, mental, and spiritual … I conceive of as a self unknown and for ever unknowable' (Groddeck, 1951: 73); and a bit later, 'It is absurd to suppose that one can ever understand life ….' (p. 84); 'Life does not let itself be analysed, one can only speculate about life' (quoted in Grossman and Grossman, 1965: 158).

For Groddeck:

> *any* sort of treatment, scientific or old wives' poultice, may turn out to be right for the patient, since the outcome of medical or other treatment is not determined by the means prescribed but by what the patient's It likes to make of the prescription
>
> (1951: 78–9, original emphasis)

Elsewhere, he wrote that 'every method is right and … I myself use any method that works, no matter what name or technique it may follow' (quoted in Schacht, 1977: 20). (In passing it is notable that, in the light of

Groddeck's ontology, therapeutic 'eclecticism' is perhaps by no means the dirty word that it currently seems to be in some circles.) Groddeck was also refreshingly undogmatic and non-programmatic about the healing or therapeutic change process: 'efforts at making repressed material conscious may often have a therapeutic effect, *yet as often such results do not occur* and conversely there are many cures without any attempt at treating unconscious or repressed material' (ibid., emphasis added).

This line of argument shines a highly revealing light on the controversial issue of practitioner competency and therapeutic outcome. The ideology of credentialisation and registration is substantially founded on the assumption that the *therapy practitioner* is the 'active ingredient' in successful therapeutic outcome. If this were shown not to be the case, however, then what is perhaps the principal argument favouring practitioner licensing would be decisively undermined. In fact, the important recent paper by Bohart and Tallman (1996) on 'the active client' cites copious research evidence to show that *the locus of therapeutic change always lies with the client*, and that 'Ultimately all therapy is self-help' (ibid.: 7). And prefiguring by nearly 70 years the Bohart–Tallman paper, Groddeck wrote in 1928 that 'the essential contribution to a patient's recovery is not [the practitioner's] effort but the patient's will to get better' (1977: 217). The Bohart-Tallman paper confirms previous findings of Russell (1981), who, after another comprehensive literature review, concluded, *inter alia*, that untrained or minimally trained paraprofessionals achieved, if anything, better results with therapy clients than trained professionals (Mowbray, 1995: 118; see also my Chapter II.2, this volume).

Now all this would have come as no surprise to Georg Groddeck, for he advocated an ontology which makes complete sense of these counter-intuitive and, until fairly recently, quite mystifying findings. Here is Groddeck: '[The It] takes something from the environment to cause recovery when it wants to manifest itself in a state of health. It treats itself .... *There is no right or wrong treatment.* This and this alone explains the reasons why most illnesses cure themselves without a doctor, *why many people recover more readily when treated by an old shepherd or clairvoyant than by a university professor*' (quoted in Schacht, 1977: 20, emphases added).

In the light of Groddeck's 'transpersonal' therapeutic ontology (to be outlined later), then, it makes complete sense that, as research evidence has repeatedly shown, all forms of counselling and psychotherapy seem to yield very similar success rates (Russell, 1981; Bohart and Tallman,

1996). For Groddeck, 'having found that all roads lead to Rome I do not consider it vastly important which road one takes, so long as one is willing to go slowly and is not too eager for wealth or recognition' (Groddeck, 1951: 85). Groddeck's genius therefore cuts a swathe through the whole efficacy debate, threatening to undermine and make largely redundant a large corpus of research on efficacy in the therapy literature – showing it to be founded on the naively false premise that it is the nature of the particular approach or technique(s) used by the practitioner, or the practitioner's expertise or discrete level of competence, that determines therapeutic outcome.

As soon as we accept this Groddeckian view of healing and change, our attention quite naturally shifts to what might be the blocks to self-healing that the client's It is creating, rather than embarking upon the wild goose-chase of 'scientifically' specifying which treatment modalities are most efficacious when 'applied to' the client. In passing, too, we may note that the latter approach is firmly rooted in old-paradigm thinking, preoccupied as it is with control, instrumental reasoning, the objectification of a relational process which is indissolubly intersubjective (Crossley, 1996), and so on.

It should be clear from the foregoing that Groddeck explicitly shunned any pretensions to expertise or privileging of technique in his healing work (cf. Mair's Chapter II.1, this volume), and it is little wonder, then, that Groddeck's belief in the physician's relative unimportance was truly galling to his professional colleagues (Grossman and Grossman, 1965: 76). Groddeck wrote that 'My task is not to teach, it is not to help, to give or take responsibility, the doctor's profession is only concerned with the moment, the doctor has to be, not to act … the more the doctor *is* instead of *does*, the easier it will be for the patient to use him' (quoted in Schacht, 1977: 2, original emphasis). Thus, Groddeck preferred to see the doctor as a servant rather than as a therapist (Schacht, 1977: 20). In his 1934 obituary for Groddeck, Keyserling wrote, 'He [Groddeck] took the view that the doctor really knows nothing, and of himself can do nothing …, for *his very presence* can provoke to action the patient's own powers of healing' (Groddeck, 1951: 12, emphasis added). Groddeck's radical view that there is no valid ontological differentiation between health and illness also prefigured the arguments expressed some 70 years later by Ian Parker et al. in their important book *Deconstructing Psychopathology* (1995): for Groddeck, '*Illness is a sign of life*, and even the most celebrated scholar knows nothing about the causes of its origins and as little about the causes of its disappearance' (quoted in Schacht, 1977: 10, emphasis added). One is reminded of J. Krishnamurti's steadfast refusal to accept the 'expert authority' that people repeatedly tried to foist upon him.

Groddeck also challenged the then prevalent reductionistic view that the human body is nothing but a machine assembled from many parts (ibid.: 18): he explicitly treated 'the whole organism irrespective of symptoms' (p. 19), and he quite specifically eschewed *technical* medical-model forms of treatment, for 'up till now every step forward in technique has been paid for in increasing blindness to human life' (Groddeck, 1951: 205–6). For Groddeck, what was crucial in successful healing wasn't technique, but 'that place of utter sincerity and selflessness where to be human is enough' (Collins, quoted in ibid.: 29).

Groddeck was concerned with the role of unconscious forces in organic disease as early as 1888, well before Freud's started to formulate his own psychoanalytic theories (ibid.: 26); and although Groddeck was enthusiastically embraced by Freud and admitted into the fold of psychoanalysis (despite having received no formal analytic training), his concept of the unconscious 'It' was far more extensive than Freud's. In reading Groddeck's biography (Grossman and Grossman, 1965), the running tension between Freud's own scientific-materialist world-view and the more spiritual-mystical world-view of Groddeck is continually erupting to the surface in their often intimate correspondence (much of which appears in Groddeck, 1977). Writing in June 1925, for example, Freud wrote to Groddeck, 'I do not, of course, recognise my civilised, bourgeois, *demystified* Id in your It' (quoted in Schacht, 1977: 14, emphasis added); and elsewhere, in 1922 Freud wrote to Groddeck, '... I do not share your Panpsychism, *which amounts almost to mysticism*, but rather admit my agnosticism much earlier; ... I believe you too-early despised reason and science' (quoted in Grossman and Grossman, 1965: 123–4, emphasis added); and Freud is said to have remarked that 'It mythology carries me nowhere' (ibid.: 129). Again, in 1917 'Freud stubbornly repeated that the Unconscious was sufficient and that Groddeck was seeking to involve unwarranted philosophical assumptions' (ibid.: 87).

Yet despite their differences, according to Schacht, 'Freud's genius was able to understand and tolerate the very different genius of Groddeck' (1977: 27). Indeed, it may well be that in Groddeck, Freud unconsciously saw and embraced the spiritual part of *himself* that he was systematically denying and disowning in order to render the evolving 'science' of psychoanalysis scientifically respectable in the materialist, deterministic

Zeitgeist of his day. Such a view is certainly consistent with the fact that, despite Groddeck's notable lack of psychoanalytic qualifications and training (Ernest Jones was at the time complaining about untrained people, termed 'wild analysts', setting themselves up as teachers of psychoanalysis! – Grossman and Grossman, 1965: 62), and despite his unpopularity with many other analysts (Ernest Jones dismissed Groddeck as 'an amusing oddity'! – ibid.: 93), Freud had a great deal of time and affection for Groddeck, and corresponded with him over many years (see Groddeck, 1977).

Despite his apparently strong desire for Freud's approval, Groddeck did not yield on his view of the 'It', which at times has the feel of the mystic, or of a Buddhist initiate, or even of a Krishnamurti: 'There is no such thing as an I, it is a lie, a misrepresentation to say: I think, I live' (quoted in Schacht, 1977: 11); 'The It cannot be analysed whether it is Freud's Id or mine which share a common name' (p. 15); 'I maintain the position that everything human is dependent on this infinitely mysterious entity and I also persist in maintaining that nobody can fathom the depths of it' (ibid.). Furthermore:

> *The It exists before the formation of the brain*, the brain is an instrument of the It ... [the It takes care] that the brain deludes us into believing all sorts of strange notions which are peculiar to man, such as the belief in an I.
>
> (Ibid.: 16, emphasis added)

And elsewhere, and again echoing the mystics of the ages,

> the ego is something ... in essence illusory, something existing only in our imagination. It comprehends only a very small part of man.... [N]one of us lives in accordance with our knowledge, for we are all under the spell of the ego idea .... We all fancy we must have a core at the centre, something that is not merely a shell ... we do not realise, cannot realise, that we have in fact no kernel.
>
> (Ibid.: 26)

(Note Groddeck's statement that 'the brain is an instrument of the It'; this is a classically anti-materialist, NP conception of 'mind' which reverses the conventional materialist view that subjective experience is supervenient upon the physical activity of the brain, rather than the other way around [cf. Steiner, 1917]. This is a particularly 'hot' debate within consciousness studies, the philosophy of mind and so-called 'neuro-psychoanalysis' at the present time.)

In the light of these views, it followed quite naturally and organically that Groddeck's views on thinking and ego were also radical, and ontologically far removed from the natural-scientific mentality of his day. Again, we see interesting parallels with the spiritual philosopher J. Krishnamurti: thus, in a transpersonal vision that closely echoes the teachings of Krishnamurti, Groddeck referred to 'the tyranny of conscious thought' (Groddeck, 1951: 103), with the thinking ego having 'left us without a faith in anything greater than ourselves'. Indeed, he goes on to say that the thinking ego 'is in large measure responsible for the troubles which are threatening our very existence today' (ibid.: 106; cf. Hall, 1993) – prophetic words indeed, written as they were some 70 years ago .... And in a statement that again echoes a Krishnamurti teaching, that to try is nearly always paradoxically to bring about the opposite of one's intention, Groddeck wrote: 'the more [man] struggles after exactitudes in charting the world outside himself, the more deeply does he sink into his bondage to the ego' (1951: 105). And for Groddeck, '[The I] forces us to see everything, particularly our Self, in distortion ....' (in Schacht, 1977: 25). There could hardly be a stronger indictment than this of the deluded world-view of one-sidedly positivistic science which posits, and actually demands, the so-called detached 'objectivity' of the autonomous observing 'I' of the scientist.

In our ego-bound and control-oriented Baconian way, furthermore, we delude ourselves in believing that we are masters of nature and of ourselves – a view which is 'assuredly false', but which it is necessary in our everyday lives to assume to be true (Groddeck, 1951: 77). Tied up with such a perception is our highly mechanistic conception of the nature of causality itself. For Groddeck we can never know exact causes of illness or of cures. Grossman and Grossman describe Groddeck's view thus: 'A given virus *causes* a given disease, they say .... What, then, causes the virus to become active so that one falls ill? Physicians ... fall back on the phrase "lowered resistance", which illuminates nothing and merely describes what has happened' (Grossman and Grossman, 1965: 85, original emphasis). Groddeck again: 'because we live we are bound to believe that ... there are such things as causes and effects ..., whereas we really know nothing about the connection between one event and another' (1951: 77). There are echoes here too of Jill Hall's *The Reluctant Adult*, in which she writes, 'the time has come to go beyond causal thinking .... When we come to try to understand the psyche causal thinking is not only inadequate but is even positively dangerous' (Hall, 1993: 2, 7; cf. Chapter I.6, this volume).

The essential quality of man is, according to Groddeck, 'his overestimation of himself' (1951: 78) – perhaps as a deep and primitive defence against a phantasised terror of impotent victimhood or annihilation (Hall, 1993). In his *Peer Gynt* essay, Groddeck implores us to 'be a thou, a thou to thyself .... Stop being an "I".... Make yourself a part of the great whole, the universe' (Schacht, 1977: 25). And relatedly (and no doubt unwittingly), Groddeck parallels the radical progressive educational philosophy of J. Krishnamurti when he argues that the child is much nearer to self-knowledge than the adult, and that developing ego consciousness actually constitutes a *barrier* to self-knowledge; so it's not surprising, therefore, that 'children are the best teachers' (ibid.). Yet at this stage in the evolution of human consciousness the developed ego is most reluctant even to countenance the view that 'everything important happens outside our knowledge and control' (1951: 78).

In a prophetic admiring reference to the Goethean scientific method, Groddeck prefigured the very recent New Paradigm revival in Goethean science by almost a century (Bortoft, 1996; Naydler, 1996; Scientific and Medical Network, 1997). Like Goethe, Groddeck was fascinated by the perceptual process, believing that the eyes were the most commonly used organ for expressing emotional difficulties (Grossman and Grossman, 1965: 97). He identified two ways of seeing: the outward–inward seeing of normal vision and the inside-outwards way of the dreamer or visionary (Schacht, 1977: 19). Old-paradigm positivist ontologies are preoccupied with the former, typically assuming a naive mechanistic '*correspondence* theory of truth', such that the act of seeing is assumed accurately to capture an objective reality assumed to exist quite independently of the observer's perception. New Paradigm perspectives, in contrast, honour the inside-outwards way of seeing – amounting to a '*congruence* or *participatory* theory of truth' (Heron, 1996: 163–9; Skolimowski, 1994: 309–26), in which the observer and the observed are not asssumed to be completely independent of one another (Krishnamurti, 1970: 79–82; 1973), and in which the observer participates in and actively *creates* the reality she is apprehending.

The foregoing discussion, and not least the consideration of NP philosophy, points to a wider question regarding what it is precisely that contributes to effective practitionership in the therapy field. Following the tenor of the current discussion, my strong hunch is that whatever those qualities are, they are possibly *in principle* beyond the ambit of rationalist discourse – and are hardly measurable or accreditable according to the old-paradigm cannons of measurability and verbal-rational articulation. By all accounts Groddeck 'was able ... to touch some key to the forces of life ... The real essence of Groddeck's treatment was his silent presence' (V.M.E. Collins, quoted in Groddeck, 1951: 9, 12). So perhaps at least some of the 'active healing ingredients' were presence, faith and love (cf. Shohet's Chapter I.4, this volume). Groddeck prefigures Karl Menninger's views, expressed many years later (Menninger, 1963, Chapter 15), on the role of faith and the other so-called 'intangibles' of treatment: 'where it [faith] is lacking the doctor can be of little use, whatever resources may be at his disposal' (Groddeck, 1951: 266; cf. Frank, 1978). (There are also clear and interesting parallels here with the theory of the placebo and so-called 'non-specific' factors in healing and change – see Jospe, 1978; Shepherd and Sartorius, 1989; Scientific and Medical Network, 1996; Ekeland, 1997.)

With regard to love Groddeck had this to say: 'Without the arrow of Eros no wound can heal, no operation succeed' (1951: 189). I have written extensively elsewhere on the role of love in therapeutic change (House, 1996); and in general, it seems that Groddeck was offering an early kind of what Lawlis (1996) has recently called 'transpersonal medicine' – the essence of which is seen by Lawlis to be love.

In sum, and according to Morris Robb (quoted in Groddeck, 1951: 15) – and accreditors and registrators please note – 'it is impossible to schematise such a [therapeutic] process, and *to talk of training anyone else to achieve its results is absurd, yet some approximation to a character of this sort is the only basis on which psycho-therapeutic power can be built*' (emphasis added). Perhaps it was in this spirit that Groddeck wrote that 'Psychoanalysis cannot be taught, for the simple reason that it is innate in all of us, that it is a human ability like seeing or hearing' (quoted in Schacht, 1977: 23 – echoes of the late Peter Lomas here). According to Collins, Groddeck's ideas 'were indeed so strange and unexpected: so contrary to the crass materialism of his own generation, that it may be years before his contribution to medical science is fully understood (Groddeck, 1951: 28). Sadly, perhaps little has changed in the 50 or so years since this was written – although recent moves towards a NP world-view, referred to elsewhere in this chapter (and also in Heron's Chapter IV.4, this volume), do hold out at least some hope for the realisation of Groddeck's inspired vision.

In many ways Groddeck was a New Paradigm thinker *par excellence*, decades ahead of his time: echoing Goethe, he writes of 'a union with Infinite nature, a being at one with the creative universe, a surrender and dissolution of the barriers of personality so that the part, the ego, becomes merged with the whole' (ibid.: 49). For Groddeck, the mentality of 'objective' science was just another expression of fantasy that has no right to the pre-eminence that its proponents claim for it: 'the unconscious forces at work in human behaviour are too obscure – and by their very nature will probably always remain so – to be confined in strictly scientific terminology' (ibid.: 40).

Throughout his writings Groddeck made it clear that he completely rejected false dualities between mind and body, and that for him there was no ontological distinction between organic and mental illness: thus, in his very first letter to Freud he writes, 'the distinction between body and mind is only verbal and not essential, that body and mind are one unit ....' (quoted in Schacht, 1977: 9). It comes as no surprise, then, that Groddeck should write that 'I almost never depend solely on the psychotherapeutic method in its widest sense, though I always use it' (ibid.: 20).

In a paper published in 1925, and referring to Freud, Groddeck wrote:

> For him there is just as little division between body and soul as there is for me and every human being. But *for the purposes of his profession as a specialist in mental illness he named these things in different ways, more appropriate for his purposes*, and confined himself apparently to the fields of neurosis and psychosis.
>
> (Quoted in Schacht, 1997: 14, emphasis added)

From his holistic ontology Groddeck could not but challenge the rationale for the existence of Freud's profession, psychoanalysis, which artificially splits the mental from the physical, creating a misguided and distorting fetish of 'the mental' in the process. The kind of emerging NP philosophy, of which Groddeck's world-view is an early harbinger, would certainly agree wholeheartedly with Groddeck's assessment – i.e. that if holistic NP philosophy is anything like right, then there is no rationale whatsoever for the existence of a specialised profession of *psycho*-therapy; and any attempt to so construct one is merely perpetuating an outmoded reductionist, deterministic world-view which can only now do harm rather than good if its ideology continues to be perpetuated – certainly in the realm of human relationship.

Conclusion: the professionalisation of spirit?

> When the scientists focused more of their attention on [the] irregularities [in nature] they formulated the theory of relativity and quantum physics, and things never looked the same again. Something of the sort is needed in the field of psychotherapy.
>
> (Kotowicz, 1993: 151)

That Groddeck was a mystical-spiritual practitioner, with a transpersonal ontology that thoroughgoingly challenged the prevailing modernist world-view of Baconian positivist science, cannot be doubted:

> I have searched for a way leading into my untrodden, the pathless. I knew that I was moving close to the borders of mysticism, if not already standing in the very thick of it .... I do not see the borders between things, only their running into one another ... *Systematic heads need for their value people of my kind.*
>
> (quoted in Grossman and Grossman, 1965: 69, 114–15, emphasis added)

And William Inman wrote of Groddeck as possessing 'the reverence of a mystic for the forces which carry man along the path of life' (ibid.: 155).

From a New Paradigm, spiritual perspective, surely the very energy of professionalisation, along with its associated ideologies and practices, is fundamentally antithetical to the kinds of NP spiritual values which are now gaining increasing ground, as the inadequacies of the old world-view become increasingly obvious. One area in which this trend is particularly important is in the field of therapeutic ontology and its relevance to therapeutic practice. In drawing upon the work and philosophy of Georg Groddeck, I have argued that the kinds of qualities that are really decisive in therapy work are crucially beyond rationalist discourse and scientific specification and measurement. And any professionalising ideology that pretends otherwise is not only fundamentally barking up the wrong tree, but – far worse that this – it threatens to do untold (and untellable) damage to those very ineffable processes that are so foundational to creative and effective practitionership.

Certainly, in today's climate the maverick genius of Georg Groddeck (who, to quote Georg Simmel, cured so many 'incurables' – Grossman and Grossman, 1965: 166) would surely never have been registered or accredited: he consistently refused to follow conventional orthodoxies just for the sake of it, and was a free thinker who was seemingly relatively unconditioned by the modernist cultural milieu in which he lived. He 'owed his training to no-one but himself', 'hat[ed] anything that savour[ed] of official action', and despised 'those worn-out medical dogmas, which, with professional egotism, made the physician instead of the patient the centre of the medical picture' (ibid.: 167). And Groddeck would no doubt have shared J. Krishnamurti's deep scepticism about the value of organisations and institutions (quoted earlier) – not least because of the way in which they usurp the intrinsic authority of the individual.

The psychoanalyst Joyce McDougall has recently written that 'It would be presumptuous to imagine that it is our theories that bring about psychic change and symptomatic cure .... *Is not our leading perversion ... the belief that we hold the key to the truth?*' (1995: 236, 234, original emphasis). I believe that the long-overdue injection of such modesty and honesty into the therapeutic realm is crucial for the healthy development of the therapy field – and I hope that the foregoing discussion gives at least some clues as to the directions that such healthy developments might take. Certainly, it will come as no surprise to the reader that in my view, the *spirit of professionalisation*, with its commercialisation, commodification and all the other accompanying leitmotivs of the institutional professionalisation process, makes the *professionalisation of spirit* a highly inappropriate and potentially damaging move, antithetical as it is to the core foundational values that underlie and inform transpersonal ontologies and practices.

As Juliana Brown and Richard Mowbray write so poignantly, 'Where there is a genuine need for structures, we should develop structures that foster our values rather than betray them' (quoted in Mowbray, 1995: 225).

References

Barrett, W. (1987) *Death of the Soul: From Descartes to the Computer,* Oxford: Oxford University Press. (Original work published 1986)

Bohart, A. C. and Tallman, K. (1996) 'The active client: therapy as self-help', *Journal of Humanistic Psychology,* 36 (3): 7–30; reprinted in Y. Bates and R. House (eds) (2003) *Ethically Challenged Professions: Enabling Innovation and Diversity in Psychotherapy and Counselling*, Ross-on-Wye: PCCS Books, pp. 258–74.

Bohm, D. (1980) *Wholeness and the Implicate Order*, London: Routledge & Kegan Paul.

Bortoft, H. (1996) *The Wholeness of Nature: Goethe's Way of Science,* Edinburgh: Floris Books.

Clarke, C. J. S. (1996) *Reality through the Looking-glass: Science and Awareness in the Postmodern World,* Edinburgh: Floris Books.

Clarke, C .J. S. (1997) 'Superstition or liberation: heretical ideas and the physical sciences', paper presented at the Scientific and Medical Network Conference, 'Science, Heresy and the Challenge of Revolutionary Ideas', London, May.

Crossley, N. (1996) *Intersubjectivity: The Fabric of Social Becoming,* London: Sage.

Ekeland, T.-J. (1997) 'The healing context and efficacy in psychotherapy: psychotherapy and the placebo phenomenon', *International Journal of Psychotherapy,* 2 (1): 77–87.

Frank, J .D. (ed.) (1978) *Psychotherapy and the Human Predicament: A Psychosocial Approach,* New York: Schocken Books.

Goodwin, B. C. (1994) *How the Leopard Changed Its Spots: The Evolution of Complexity,* London: Weidenfeld and Nicolson.

Goodwin, B. C. (1997) 'Challenges to Darwinian orthodoxy', paper presented at the Scientific and Medical Network Conference, 'Science, Heresy and the Challenge of Revolutionary Ideas', London, May.

Groddeck, G. (1951) *The World of Man,* London: Vision.

Groddeck, G. (1977) *The Meaning of Illness: Selected Psychoanalytic Writings,* London: Hogarth Press.

Grossman, C. K. and Grossman, S. (1965) *The Wild Analyst: The Life and Work of Georg Groddeck,* London: Barrie and Rockliff.

Hall, J. (1993) *The Reluctant Adult: An Exploration of Choice,* Bridport: Prism Press.

Heron, J. (1996) *Co-operative Inquiry: Research Into the Human Condition,* London: Sage.

House, R. (1996) 'Love, intimacy and therapeutic change', *Self and Society,* 24 (1): 21–6.

House, R. (1997) 'From professionalisation towards a post-therapy era', *Self and Society,* 25 (2): 31–5.

Jospe, K. (1978) *The Placebo Effect in Healing,* Lexington, MA: Lexington Books.

Kotowicz, Z. (1993) 'Tradition, violence and psychotherapy', in L. Spurling (ed.), *From the Words of My Mouth: Tradition in Psychotherapy,* London: Routledge.

Krishnamurti, J. (1970) *The Krishnamurti Reader,* Harmondsworth: Penguin Arkana.

Krishnamurti, J. (1973) 'Can the fragmented mind be whole?', 1st Public Talk, Brockwood Park, Hampshire, 1/9/73 (audio cassette).

Lawlis, G. F. (1996) *Transpersonal Medicine,* Boston: Shambhala.

Lorimer, D. (1990) *Whole in One: The Near-Death Experience and the Ethics of*

Interconnectedness, Harmondsworth : Penguin Arkana.
McDougall, J. (1995) *The Many Faces of Eros: A Psychoanalytic Exploration of Human Sexuality*, London: Free Association Books.
Menninger, K. (1963) *The Vital Balance: The Life Process in Mental Health and Illness*, New York: Viking Press.
Mowbray, R. (1995) *The Case Against Psychotherapy Registration: A Conservation Issue for the Human Potential Movement*, London: Trans Marginal Press.
Naydler, J. (ed.) (1996) *Goethe on Science*, Edinburgh: Floris Books.
Parker, I., Georgaca, E., Harper, D., McLaughlin, T. and Stowell-Smith, M. (1995) *Deconstructing Psychopathology*, London: Sage.
Rowan, J. (1992) 'Response' (to K. Mair, 'The myth of therapist expertise'), in W. Dryden and C. Feltham (eds), *Psychotherapy and Its Discontents*, Buckingham: Open University Press, pp. 160–6.
Rowan, J. (1993) *The Transpersonal – Psychotherapy and Counselling*, London: Routledge.
Russell, R. (1981) *Report on Effective Psychotherapy: Legislative Testimony*, New York: R. P. Latin Associates.
Schacht, L. (1977) 'Introduction', in G. Groddeck, *The Meaning of Illness: Selected Psychoanalytic Writings,* London: Hogarth Press, pp. 1–30.
Scientific and Medical Network (1996) Conference on 'The Placebo Response: Biology and Belief', University of Westminster, London, 9–10 November.
Scientific and Medical Network (1997) Conference on 'Perception, Intentionality and Science', Regent's College, London, 5–6 July.
Sheldrake, R. (1981) *A New Science of Life*, London: Blond and Briggs.
Shepherd, M. and Sartorius, N. (eds) (1989) *Non-Specific Aspects of Treatment*, Toronto: Hans Huber Publishers.
Skolimowski, H. (1994) *The Participatory Mind: A New Theory of Knowledge and the Universe*, London: Penguin Arkana.
Steiner, R. (1917) 'Anthroposophy and psychology', lecture given in Zurich, 5 November; in R. Steiner, *Anthroposophy has Something to Add to Modern Sciences*, Beechmont, Australia: Completion Press, 2004, pp. 15–43.
Woodhouse, M. B. (1996) *Paradigm Wars: Worldview for a New Age*, Berkeley, CA: Frog Ltd.

A Self-Generating Practitioner Community IV.4

John Heron

Part 1

Starting with ends

What constitutes a healthy practitioner community? I start my answer with the notion of intrinsic value, of what is good as an end in itself. What states of affairs, for human beings, are worthwhile simply by virtue of what they are, not as a means to anything else? Such states are the ultimate ends of action, the final human rationale for individual behaviour. Each person's intrinsic values are the non-negotiable ground on which they stand up to be counted.

Statements of intrinsic value are, on my view, autonomous; they rest on their own epistemological ground, not to be justified by theological assertion or statements of fact. If well-founded, they are also subjective-objective, relative-universal in their formulations. On the one hand, they are relative to the person and to the cultural context out of which they have emerged. On the other hand, they have reference to the needs and interests of our common humanity within shared features of the human condition. No statement about what is good in itself is ever final, because of its contextual relativity, but every such statement that is thoughtfully put together claims general relevance.

What I present here is my account of intrinsic values. It is certainly not a prescription for other practitioners, who will evolve their own account. But if there are other practitioners whose own autonomous values significantly overlap or resonate with mine, then we constitute a viable network of value. We can commence a fruitful dialogue about the nature of a healthy practitioner community. This chapter is my contribution to that dialogue.

Practitioners within the Independent Therapists Network in the UK would seem to have values that relate to mine, from what I have heard, and from what I have read (Totton, 1995). I am not a member of this network since I live in Italy and work internationally. But there is clearly a strong basis for co-operation.

An account of intrinsic values

The state of affairs I take to be desirable as an end in itself is *human flourishing* in individual and social life. I conceive this flourishing as a process of social participation in which there is a mutually enabling balance between autonomy, co-operation and hierarchy; and which is interdependent with the flourishing of the planetary ecosystem.

- By autonomy I mean a state of being in which each person can in liberty determine and fulfil their own true needs and interests. I do not here mean the autonomy of the isolated and dissociated Cartesian ego, but the autonomy of the person in a deeply participative relationship with being and other beings (Heron, 1992, 1996).
- By co-operation I mean mutual aid and support between autonomous persons, including negotiation, participative decision-making and conflict resolution.
- By hierarchy I mean a state of being in which a person appropriately takes temporary responsibility for doing things to or for other persons for the sake of their future autonomy and co-operation. This is part of parenthood, education and many professions.

What is valuable as a universal means to this comprehensive end is participative decision-making, which enables people to be involved in the making of decisions, in every social context, which affect their flourishing in any way, and through which people speak on behalf of the wider ecosystem of which they are part.

This is a dynamic account of intrinsic values: to do with the politics of choice and action. Autonomy is about deciding for oneself, co-operation about deciding with others, and hierarchy about deciding for others. And this order seems to be paramount. Only persons who know what their own preferences are can negotiate and co-operate effectively in conjoint decisions. People who do not really know where they stand on an issue have no proper ground for co-operation, and can only huddle together in the middle of a fudge.

Even more critically, a person who does not know how to be autonomous and co-operative cannot make effective decisions for other people to empower their future autonomy and co-operation. Leaders who are not inwardly free can only lead people into sustained submission and subpersonhood. So hierarchy has human value when:

- It is manifested by a person well-grounded in their own autonomy and co-operation, both rooted in a deeply participative relationship with being and other beings.
- It is exercised to empower the emergence of autonomy and co-operation in others.
- It is reduced as that emergence occurs.
- It is abandoned when that emergence has occurred; otherwise it is disvaluable and oppressive of human emergence.

Nikolas Berdyaev (1937) affirms human personhood as the creative process of divine spirit, manifesting as the self-determining subjectivity of persons engaged in the realisation of value and achieved in true community (*sobornost*). This gives a theological account of human autonomy and co-operation. But whether theologised or not, the above account of what is intrinsically valuable stands firm, in my view. And it subsumes, within the notion of autonomy as the freely chosen fulfilment of human needs and interests, many other states of being of intrinsic value.

Part 2

The challenge of hierarchy

The challenge of human development on this planet could be construed as the challenge of learning how to manifest hierarchy – deciding for others – in an appropriate and flexible way that honours the flowering of autonomy and co-operation. It is the great challenge of parenthood, itself the primary form of helping, in which deciding for and on behalf of young children is shaped from the outset by a concern for that future flowering, and is progressively reduced over the years as that flowering occurs. The parent is between the Scylla and Charybdis of too little hierarchy, or undercontrol, and too much hierarchy or overcontrol.

A few years ago I was involved in making a TV programme for the BBC on parents and teenagers, which had the unfortunate, but telling, title of 'Living with the Enemy'. In the research for it, it became painfully clear how many parents in the UK are stuck in a compulsive attitude towards their teenagers of overcontrol. It was also clear how counterproductive and useless this attitude is. A teenager cannot learn how to live and emerge as a young adult by being told how to live, but only by the practice of making their own choices, by being supported to be responsible in increasing measure for their own lives.

The parents repeatedly justified their useless overcontrol on the grounds that they were seeking to protect their teenage sons and daughters from the snares and pitfalls of the adult world. But over and again this inappropriate seeking-to-protect merely generated sullen resistance or overt rebellion. And since modern societies have no appropriate rites of passage to initiate teenagers into the real challenges of adult autonomy and co-operation, teenagers today have to make a leap into adulthood simply by virtue of the turn of the years and the external structure and demands of the social system. To meet these demands they learn to exercise a modicum of an apparent autonomy and co-operation, but it is not grounded in a real emotional and volitional inner entry into adulthood.

Political acting out

The political Scylla and Charybdis within family dynamics of too little or too much hierarchy is echoed in all other forms of human association between the family and the state, and beyond that within federations of states and the total international community of states. Democratic institutions seek to find the balance by making the temporary hierarchical control of their officers periodically subject to the autonomous voting rights of their members.

However, the adults who hold office are ex-teenagers who missed a real entry passage into adulthood. Hence they tend to act out in office two left-overs from the unresolved tension of their teenage years. These are the interacting poles of internalised parental overcontrol and adolescent resistance and resentment. The first is acted out as a tendency toward centralised overcontrol, often justified by an assumed need to protect some group or other from an assumed danger; the second as a regular relapse into factional fighting and compulsive resistance, at the expense of exercising any real personal autonomy and social co-operation.

We see both these tendencies at work in our parliamentary democracy in the UK. We also see them at work in many supposedly representative institutions, especially those seeking to court the approval and imprimatur of the government of the day. Thus the United Kingdom Council for Psychotherapy 'continues to work to achieve statutory regulation of the profession' and justifies this work, and the Council's existence, on the grounds of 'adequately protecting the public' (Tantam and Zeal, 1996).

The public, of course, cannot be protected by the statutory regulation of any profession. Such regulation just lulls some people into an uncritical dependence on legalised dogmatism. The public can only be educated to be self-protecting, by learning to claim its right:

- To have satisfactory evidence from practitioners about their credentials and competence.
- To know what constitutes such evidence.
- To be fully informed by practitioners.
- To participate in whatever decisions practitioners make.

The public has never needed the legalised professionalisation of a few experts. What it has always needed, and still needs, is the widespread and competent laicisation of itself, so that it becomes empowered to relate effectively to practitioners of any kind, whether legalised or not.

So here within the UKCP the first tendency is at work: a strong compulsion to overcontrol the profession, to regulate it centrally, justified by a specious concern to protect the public. Needless to say, significant numbers of the public will inevitably and healthily discount and ignore all this, just as they have ignored conventional medicine's attempts in the past to protect them from alternative medicine. And the second tendency is at work too, for the UKCP has already been riven by factional splits and infighting between psychoanalytic diehards who want to maintain a patriarchal hegemony over mere psychotherapists, and other groups who resist this (Young, 1996).

Part 3

Finding a model

It surely behoves adult practitioners within the helping professions to step outside this dynamic, which looks very much like adolescent insecurity and mayhem sententiously masquerading as social responsibility. Counsellors and psychotherapists need to find a model for institutional forms and processes which are free of centralised overcontrol and compulsive factionalism, and which have the sort of empowering hierarchy which serves the flourishing of autonomy and co-operation among its members. It seems fairly clear that if professional helpers are incapable of practising these values in their own working lives, they are in no place to empower their clients to do so.

I believe there is a basic model of community process which has relevance here. It is that of a self-generating culture. Within its broad aegis there are two sub-models which have particular relevance for a community of practitioners: self and peer review, and co-operative inquiry. I will first sketch out the self-generating culture idea in general, then look at how the idea could apply within a practitioner network, including the use of self and peer review and of co-operative inquiry.

A self-generating culture

A self-generating culture, which I have discussed elsewhere (Heron, 1993), is a vision of a community whose members are in a continuous process of co-operative learning and development, and whose forms are consciously adopted, periodically reviewed and altered in the light of experience, reflection and deeper vision. Its participants continually recreate these forms through cycles of collaborative inquiry in living.

In its most comprehensive, society-wide version, it includes many strands: forms of association; forms of decision-making and political participation; forms of economic organisation; forms of supervision and quality control; revisioning a wide range of social roles; forms of ecological management; forms of habitation; forms of education and personal development for all ages; forms of research; forms of intimacy and parenting; forms of conflict resolution; forms of recreation; forms of aesthetic expression and celebration; forms of transpersonal association and ritual.

What all this entails is individual and co-operative commitment to experiential learning and inquiry through living. Each person in the everyday process of his or her personal and professional life is adopting an informal experiential inquiry cycle, what Torbert calls action inquiry. For Torbert (1991) this means extended consciousness-in-action, widening attention to encompass your vision of goals, your strategies to achieve them, your current actions and their outcomes, and what is going on in the world around. It also means noticing and amending, either through action or internal revision or both, incongruities between these components of your lived inquiry.

Such action inquiry will have its idiosyncratic private strands, its shared and face-to-face strands with people at home and at work, and its more collective strands within organisations and the wider culture. It will involve phases of intentional, aware living; with time out for phases of collaborative reflection, review and goal setting. The totality of all this, applied within each of the several strands of social life, is what I call a self-generating culture. The concept of the learning organisation points in this direction (Garratt, 1987), as does a wide range of recent work on community building (Gozdz, 1995).

Torbert, working within the field of management training, presents a similar notion. For him, personal action inquiry 'aims at creating communities of inquiry within communities of social practice'. It exhibits 'transforming power' which

> operates through peer cultures, liberating structures, and timely actions. Cultures are truly peer-like, structures are liberating, and actions are timely, if they simultaneously promote widening inquiry about what is the appropriate mission, strategy, and practice for the given person or organization or nation, while accomplishing established objectives in an increasingly efficient, effective and self-legitimizing manner.
> (Torbert, 1991: 100)

A 'liberating structure' within an organisation is one in which there is a sense of shared purpose among its members, an increasing self-direction amongst them, and a commitment to generate quality work by them. It is a structure which simultaneously cultivates amongst its members both quality improvement in their work on the one hand, and action inquiry and personal development on the other. 'If liberating structures succeed organizational members will increasingly take executive responsibility, will increasingly treat one another as peers, and will increasingly create their own liberating structures' (Torbert, 1991: 100). In short, they manifest the values of autonomy, co-operation and empowering hierarchy.

For Torbert, the leader who exercises transforming power to bring a liberating structure into being essentially invites mutuality and participation in power. This is similar to my notion of empowering hierarchy which serves the flourishing of autonomy and co-operation. Thus, any practitioner exercising this kind of empowering hierarchy will take initiatives for and on behalf of other interested practitioners, and will invite them to participate in a professional community in which the values of autonomy and co-operation are paramount.

Part 4

A self-generating practitioner community

A healthy practitioner community is one, then, that is self-managed in the spirit of a self-generating culture, a liberating social structure. Such a self-generating community of practitioners includes a selection of strands from the society-wide version. It particularly attends to three clusters. In characterising these I am, again, not making prescriptions, but putting forward my own contribution to a dialogue with other practitioners with similar sorts of values. I have had experience, in one context or another, of all the different forms I describe below.

The first cluster deals with basic social structure and process.

- *Forms of association*
  - Local face-to-face self and peer review groups of practitioners within a loose federation.
  - A federation characterised by a commitment of all participating groups to the values of autonomy and co-operation within each group and between groups.
  - Elected federation officers exercising the kind of empowering hierarchy that enhances autonomy and co-operation within and between local groups.

- *Forms of decision-making and political participation*
  - A form of co-operative decision-making within a group in which each person has a voice which is heard, in which authentic differences are affirmed, and in which there is a commitment to a creatively negotiated outcome. The same applies to federal decision-making between groups.
  - Decisions about basic policy and practice, to do with the main activities of practitioners in association with other practitioners, are made heterogeneously and idiosyncratically within each group.
  - Dialogue, exchange and conference among local groups are further to enlarge and extend the autonomy and co-operation within each of them, not to achieve homogeneity, standardisation and conformity between them.

The second cluster attends to the main activities of the practitioner community.

- *Forms of supervision and quality control*
  In all these forms, the role of the peers is to enable each individual rigorously to deepen the integrity of her or his self-appraisal.
  - Varieties of peer supervision with regard to professional practice, using self and peer feedback, assessment and review. Feedback is informative, assessment is evaluative, and review is revisionary. I describe several different kinds of peer supervision in *Group Facilitation: Theories and Models for Practice* (Heron, 1993).
  - More formal peer review audit, in which: the main components of the job are identified and revised; the criteria of professional competence with respect to these components are identified and revised; the practitioners do on-the-job self (and where possible peer) assessment of their competence, applying these criteria and keeping records of the assessments; the practitioners meet periodically in an audit group to present these on-the-job findings and to process them by self and peer assessment. A full description of this sort of peer review audit is given in the same book (Heron, 1993).

- *Forms of research*
  - Varieties of participative research, in which research is done with people, not on them or about them. Co-operative inquiry, which I practise and about which I have written, breaks down the distinction between researcher and subject. All those involved are co-researchers, doing the thinking that designs, manages and draws conclusions from the research. They are also co-subjects, engaged in the experience and action which are the focus of the inquiry. They move cyclically several times between reflecting and planning as co-researchers, and action and experience as co-subjects. And they use a variety of validity procedures to secure the process against uncritical subjectivity, consensus collusion and other hazards of the method (Reason, 1988; Heron, 1996).
  - Co-operative inquiry can be applied to all forms of peer supervision or peer review audit, and of continuing professional education, raising them up into systematic research into professional practice.

It can also be used by practitioner–client pairs and groups, and by client-only groups, to explore relevant concerns and interests. Its strength is that it is a form of research that fully honours personal autonomy and group collaboration.

- *Forms of continuing education and development*
  - Practitioners need to attend to their own ongoing professional education and personal development, through the whole range of adult education and growth strategies: conferences, seminars, peer teaching and learning, literature and Internet searches, training workshops, co-counselling, individual sessions, ongoing experiential groups, and so on.

And the third cluster deals with supportive processes.

- *Forms of conflict resolution*
  - Psychotherapists are notorious for incompetence in committee and bizarre forms of factionalism and infighting (Young, 1996). A healthy practitioner community could address this propensity by working out and agreeing, within each local group, forms of dispute and conflict resolution. These forms need to separate out authentic and honourable differences that are to be properly acknowledged and accommodated, from misunderstanding, misrepresentation, manipulation, and unaware projection of unprocessed distress.

- *Forms of ceremony and ritual*
  - A practitioner community, as a systemic whole, has an ethos which transcends any purely linguistic description of its values, norms and beliefs. This ethos of a body of practice can be felt. It can be grasped imaginally and intuitively. It can be invoked through metaphor and indicated by symbolic presentations. Above all, it can be honoured corporately by the use of creatively devised ceremony and ritual.

This kind of self-generating practitioner community is grounded in relatively small peer groups in which the basic processes of self and peer review, and co-operative inquiry, can proceed effectively. With its basic values of autonomy, co-operation and empowering hierarchy, such a community affirms the principle that, in the last analysis, all authority about practice rests with each practitioner's well-informed discriminating judgement, a precious metal refined within the crucible of rigorous peer process.

Part 5

Ending with starts

I began this chapter with some axiology, a consideration of value, in particular with the idea of what is intrinsically worthwhile, an end in itself. I'll conclude it with some ontology, thoughts about the nature of reality, in particular with the idea of innovative reality, the reality of new starts. Revisionary thinking across a wide array of disciplines from physics and biology, through medicine to social science and consciousness research, is articulating a new-paradigm world-view. This differs in fundamental respects from the old-paradigm positivist account – inherited from Descartes, Newton and others – of reality as an objective physical world, independent of the human mind, which we can all set about studying as if it had nothing to do with us. There are various overlapping ways of characterising the new world-view, and here is my account of three of them:

- Reality is transactional, relational, to do with dynamic interconnectedness.
- Reality is subjective-objective, a transaction between the human mind and the cosmically given, in which persons participate in what there is without separation from it, and in the process shape it perceptually and conceptually (Skolimowski, 1994; Heron, 1996).
- This reality, co-created by the mind and the given cosmos which it conjoins, is in process of emergent evolution, which is unpredictable and innovative, generating new starts.

One wing of the new paradigm is the science of complexity, or complexity theory, which seeks to give a comprehensive account of the emergence of creativity and innovation in the dynamics of complex systems in nature and culture. It is a recent development which claims wide relevance, from the weather and ecosystems to elaborate human societies (Lewin, 1993; Goodwin, 1994). Reason and Goodwin (1997), in an interesting paper on complexity theory and co-operative inquiry, take six principles of complexity theory and use them as metaphors for what goes on in a co-operative inquiry. These principles can also be used as metaphors for what happens in the kind of self-generating practitioner community (SGPC) which I have outlined above. In saying that this is what happens, I am extrapolating from my experience, in diverse contexts, of the different forms I have included within my account of an SGPC.

- Complex systems have variegated, multiple patterns of interconnections between diverse components. The interconnections are not simple and uniform. This is a precondition of the emergence of unpredictable novelty.

  The SGPC form of association, with its loose federation of local groups, has a rich diversity of ways in which autonomy and co-operation interact both within and between the local groups.

- In complex systems, novelty arises by the repetition of cycles of a regular pattern of activity, in which both convergent and divergent processes interact.

  Within an SGPC, the use of both peer supervision and of co-operative inquiry involves repeated cycles of activity within which there will be innumerable varied patterns, both concurrent and serial, of converging on the same and diverging over the different. Thus, everyone explores the same issue, but each a different aspect of it; or everyone explores a different issue, but each the same dimension of it; and so on.

- The order that emerges in a complex system cannot be predicted from the nature of the interconnected entities that comprise it. It can only be discovered by going through the cyclic processes that constitute it. The order within an SGPC consists of the values, criteria, beliefs and procedures related to the professional practice of its members. These cannot be derived by some process of abstraction from the views of individual members. They can only be discovered by their emergence through the cyclic processes of self and peer review within local groups, and as between local groups.

- The novel order that emerges in a complex system is holistic. It results from the interactions among constitutive parts of the system. It is not determined by the properties of a privileged set of parts, by preordained instructions coded in them. It is the dynamic interconnectedness of the whole that has the potential for emergent novelty.

An SGPC does not have a central privileged committee that shapes policy and which controls the organisation of the profession. It is the dynamic relations within and between its loosely federated local groups that gives rise to its innovative order.

- Complex systems are characterised by variable and transient fluctuations between chaos and order, which at a certain point may lead over into the emergence of complex and novel organisation. The fluctuations may also go the other way, and involve a transition from some degree of initial organisation to chaos.

  The organisation of an SGPC fluctuates between chaos and order. The members of an SGPC live and work within this fluctuation awarely as part of the challenge of being co-creators within emergent innovative evolution.

- A complex system is most adaptive, flexible and innovative when it is at the edge of chaos where large fluctuations between chaos and order occur, since it is here where novel order emerges.

  An SGPC is continuously involved, through autonomous self and peer review groups, in a deeply grounded revisionary exploration of its members' professional practice. They put all at risk by moving away from the security of established and authoritative definitions of practice, and by moving towards self and peer definitions, attending rigorously to their own experience. They may flounder at times in the rough seas of uncertainty, confusion and chaos, before spacious new continents arise from the depths.

There is, of course, nothing sacrosanct about complexity theory, itself part of the emergent process it seeks to describe. But for those of us who have worked with autonomy and co-operation within peer groups of various kinds, there is an interesting isomorphic resonance at work. And the kind of SGPC I have derived from a consideration of intrinsically worthwhile ends of action – as well as, it must be said, from a great deal of practice – is consonant with the new paradigm world-view that affirms a participative reality of emergent starts.

By contrast, it seems that the over-control of professional practice by centralised bureaucracy, evident in much current psychotherapy professionalisation, is very much an expression of the old-paradigm world-view. Positivist science regards the whole as the mechanical sum of its parts. Specialist experts divide a domain into its simple parts which can then be intellectually and technically managed to gain control over the whole. This breeds a rigid and restricted view of what constitutes reality, since it has no way of honouring the creative emergence of novelty.

If a group of senior and specialist practitioners analyse the whole field of psychotherapy and counselling into its component parts – the numerous schools and modes of practice – and then use this analysis to devise a way of managing and controlling and organising the whole, there can only be one result: a rigid and restricted view of human helping, with no way of honouring creative helping at the forward edge of evolutionary emergence.

References

Berdyaev, N. (1937) *The Destiny of Man*, London: Bles.

Garratt, R. (1987) *The Learning Organization*, London: Fontana.

Goodwin, B. (1994) *How the Leopard Changed its Spots: The Evolution of Complexity*, London: Weidenfeld and Nicolson.

Gozdz, K. (ed.) (1995) *Community Building: Renewing Spirit and Learning,* San Francisco: New Leaders Press, Sterling and Stone.

Heron, J. (1992) *Feeling and Personhood: Psychology in Another Key,* London: Sage.

Heron, J. (1993) *Group Facilitation: Theories and Models for Practice,* London: Kogan Page.

Heron, J. (1996) *Co-operative Inquiry: Research into the Human Condition,* London: Sage.

Lewin, R. (1993) *Complexity: Life on the Edge of Chaos*, London: Phoenix.

Reason, P. (ed.) (1988) *Human Inquiry in Action,* London: Sage.

Reason, P. and Goodwin, B. (1997) *Complexity Theory and Co-operative Inquiry*, Centre for Action Research in Professional Practice, University of Bath and Schumacher College.

Skolimowski, H. (1994) *The Participatory Mind*, London: Arkana.

Tantam, D. and Zeal. P. (1996) Circular letter to the three analytically oriented sections, London: UK Council for Psychotherapy.

Torbert, W. (1991) *The Power of Balance: Transforming Self, Society and Scientific Inquiry*, Newbury Park, CA: Sage.

Totton, N. (1995) 'The Independent Therapists Network', *Self and Society*, 23 (3): 31–3.

Young, R. M. (1996) 'The psychodynamics of psychoanalytic organisations', online paper, http://human-nature.com/culture/ppo1.html.

Part V
Pluralism and Self-Regulation in Practice

Practitioner Development through Self-Direction: The South West London College Counselling Courses V.1

Val Blomfield

> No (one) can reveal to you aught but that which already lies half asleep in the dawning of your knowledge.
> (*The Prophet* by Kahlil Gibran)

Twenty years' experience of counselling education may make me no more of an expert than those colonials who spent twenty years in India and mistakenly thought they knew the country. However, I have explored this counselling country in different vehicles and over difficult terrain, and I now present my particular, subjective journey.

My association with the radical counselling courses which started at South West London College (SWLC) began in 1976 as a student. Later, I spent ten years on the courses as a tutor. More recently, I have worked as external examiner on other counselling courses and have supervised individuals and groups on diploma courses which have been awarded, or are applying for, accreditation.

SWLC Courses had a programme devised each year by the students on that course. Assessment was by a portfolio of work whose contents were negotiated within the student group and assessed by self and peer assessment. Tutors acted as a support and as a resource but did not assess. Workshop topics were suggested by students, and might be facilitated by tutors or students, or a combination of the two. External examiners validated the process and the general standards of the course.

There was always a battle in the large group between what I saw as 'Task' and 'Process' people. Task people wanted to get on with it. They got frustrated with group dynamics and wanted to concentrate on learning the appropriate skills. Process people wanted to pay attention to feelings in the group, to make sure difficulties were brought out into the open, to let strategies for devising the programme emerge.

As in most conflicts, both sides were expressing one whole. Each had vital qualities to contribute. Yet they were always at loggerheads. It seems to me that in recent years, the Task people have won the educational battle. There has been an educational backlash which concentrates on outcomes, at the expense of more subtle qualities, valued by Process people, such as intuitive understanding of another person, patience, unpretentiousness, and trust in the other's potential for wisdom. Qualities which counsellors need for the 'I–Thou' communication at the heart of relationships. These attributes come from an openness to self-learning which is hard to convey in a course with primarily functional aims.

Even when courses value personal growth, the demands of the accreditation process put the emphasis on academic achievement in a way which can lead to a high drop-out rate for students who are not from a conventional white, middle-class background. This is worrying because, as a person-centred counsellor, I want to move towards inclusion rather than exclusion. The academic perspective is one useful aspect of learning, but in my experience as tutor and supervisor, it can re-inforce feelings of stupidity in people who have not fared well in the school system. I myself was one of these people.

SWLC courses placed emphasis on the fact that we all have our own unique contribution to offer to the community, as in the counselling model – it would be ludicrous for counsellors to value clients only for their academic achievements. SWLC attempted to encourage individuality, while also promoting communal responsibility – to celebrate our differences and also to see them as indispensable parts of the whole.

My experience as a student

I was a secondary school teacher when I heard about the South West London College Counselling Courses. I was feeling trapped. The system seemed to be imparting information from the notes of the teacher to the pens of the students without passing through the minds or hearts of either.

As a student, SWLC was a revelation to me. I kept waiting to feel the 'iron fist' hitting me with hidden rules and restrictions, but instead found that the 'velvet glove' had reality, leading me by the hand, helping me look for my own answers.

The self-directing nature of the course was developed in the mid-1970s by Brigid Proctor, influenced by John Heron's Human Potential Resources Project at Guildford, and by Gaie Houston and Tom Osborn from the self-directing Diploma in Applied Behavioural Science at the then Polytechnic of North London. When I joined the course, Brigid and Gaie were the tutors together with Pat Milner, whose ideas have been influential in the person-centred movement. It was not a diploma course at the time. There was a heated group discussion about the possible effects of a diploma on the course. Would it make us too keen to get the qualification and forget about the qualities of inner learning? Would an academic assessment destroy the fluid and creative nature of the course?

These concerns now seem far from today's emphasis on standards and accountability. But in them we were detecting the move towards professionalisation. What we were questioning was whether a diploma would mean that the outcome of the course would determine its content, rather than this being open to negotiation based on our learning needs. I appreciated the arguments about values, and I knew I needed a recognised proof of my competence so that I might get a job in counselling and escape the classroom grind.

The group consensus was to go for the diploma. We invited an ILEA inspector to meet us, so that, together with the tutors, we were instrumental in making ours the first diploma year of the course.

In those heady days of the late 1970s we were very well-funded. Course fees were low and free individual supervision was included. We only had to name a model we wished to learn about and a top figure from this field would be engaged for a six-week workshop. These were the days of ILEA, of experimentation, of creativity.

We were all inventing the course together

I had a degree in Education, and I had loved academic study, but this course showed me a very different way of learning. As a secondary school 'failure', leaving school at 15 with no qualifications, I had thrived on interest and encouragement from tutors in my life as an adult student. To feel I could be trusted to define my own educational goals and standards by tutors I respected was a surprise, a delight, and a challenge. Sometimes, it's true, I yearned to be told what to do, to be given marked essays, to place myself in a hierarchy with the other students. To have my image of myself defined by others.

But I felt alive and excited. I adopted the course philosophy with gusto. I was never forced to read a book or produce an essay, although when I asked about essays I was told it was fine for me to submit them and the tutors would give me feedback if I did.

I learned through my experience

I learned that education could be fun. I remember a Gestalt workshop where we role-played being our five-year-old selves on our first day at school. Several of the men, usually very respectable professionals, behaved in a way which got quite out of hand. In their 'boy' roles they threw everybody's shoes out of the first-floor window, actually breaking a pane of glass. The community had a meeting about this to decide what should be done, and I recall being in a delegation to appease the manager of the site so that we should not be evicted. This is an extreme example, but it also shows the communal feeling of responsibility for the actions of individuals.

I had always seen myself as a writer, but had never written unless directed to do so. Now, poetry poured out of me like lava from a volcano. I once wrote 14 poems on the tube home, each about a student on the course. This ability has never deserted me, and I am now a performance poet and a playwright as well as a counsellor.

I learned not to impose limits on my life, that I had a right to happiness and personal fulfilment, that there is always more to learn. I learned that life is very serious and you can always get a good laugh out of it.

Through triad work and group discussion I learned the Person-Centred Approach. I began to recognise my intolerance of people who were defensive and not open, as I believed I was. In a course which questions conventional attitudes, those with traditional opinions can find themselves isolated and feel misunderstood. Traditional power structures were turned on their heads.

The Person-Centred Approach became my grounding, my 'counselling backbone'. It was new to me; it contradicted my previous psychodynamic model. I also became a bit of a zealot of non-directiveness. We were the 'non-directive mafia', fighting the Freudian baddies for the rights of clients. We shared anecdotes about analysts who knitted, slept or wrote shopping-lists behind the recumbent backs of patients on couches.

As the first diploma year, we had to devise our own assessment system. In fact, each course in later years devised their own system. I recall finding it daunting – we had to get down to the bones of what counselling values are, and try to work out how to assess skills and what makes them good enough, bearing in mind the welfare of future clients. We set up Portfolio Groups – of up to five people, giving each other support and feedback on our written work and on counselling skills.

When it came to portfolio time, I got into the normal state of total resistant terror. I used Gestalt to help me, and wrote a piece called 'Gestalt

Voices' which began, 'I feel my knot of fear …', and in this way got it all out of my system until I began to think clearly. I included these murky thoughts in the portfolio as well as lots of my new-found poetry. And I also produced three essays on TA, Gestalt and the Person-Centred Approach, which the external examiners asked to use as teaching aids on other courses.

I did this after at last embarking on extensive reading and then deciding that I would talk about what each of these models meant to me. It seemed more in keeping with course philosophy than 'sitting at the feet' of Berne, Perls or Rogers and merely regurgitating their words. The fact that I would be writing about my experience of these models freed me from the despairing 'I know nothing' syndrome. Because I did know about my experiences, successful or otherwise. And I could describe them if I meditated on that which 'lies half asleep in the dawning of (my) knowledge'.

Drawing out that 'half asleep knowledge' is the kernel of the person-centred way of teaching and the kernel of the counselling process itself. I appreciated having to write a portfolio. Because of my fear of not being good enough, I produced a portfolio which surpassed my expectations.

The course ended with a residential assessment weekend. Several students were referred. One repeated the final year. Does this mean we were astringent enough as self and peer assessors? Who were the people who did not pass? Was it easier to confront vulnerable students than those with more personal power on the course? Can tutors handle the process any better than peers? Can you devise a purely objective assessment procedure when counselling skills depend so much on sensitivity and self-awareness? How can you measure such things except subjectively, in which case how can you not be biased in your assessment?

I know that the assessment weekend was a peak experience for me, and the next day I went for an interview as a school counsellor in a boys' comprehensive and, in the heat of achievement, did remarkably well and so got the first job in my life which I actually enjoyed.

My experience as a tutor on SWLC counselling courses

Three years after qualifying I was appointed as tutor during a self-directed interview. This was an experiment in which we, as twelve applicants, had to devise a method of being interviewed for five vacancies. This was hard, as interviews are by nature competitive and do not lend themselves well to co-operation. The experiment was not repeated in that form.

The residential planning weekend

As the courses developed, core structures were added, such as a counselling skills module, a video to be self and peer assessed at the end of each year, and access was given to current students to look at past students' programmes and portfolios. It was always a question as to whether to constantly get students to 'invent the wheel', or if we gave too much information, would we inhibit them from inventing new, unique structures.

During the early years, the programme was entirely open to student planning. Each year started with a residential planning weekend where the main object was to enable each student to make a learning contract and to plan the first term.

Each student year-group would develop a very individual group personality. These early stages were like a birth, and the skilfulness with which the delivery was handled determined the ensuing healthy (or otherwise) character of the group as it developed over its three years of life. The staff team needed to be balanced between being able to nurture to create safety, and having the ability to energise in order to encourage and motivate students to risk planning their programme creatively.

There was a staff/student ratio of 1:12. Student groups varied in size from 35 to 50. One year on the residential weekend, students were divided into two groups of 35. Was it a mistake to invite both groups to the same residential venue? Students began to get suspicious about why they had been put into a particular group. Meetings were held. I remember 20 groups of three or four dispersed over the sun-dappled lawns in intense discussion.

Thinking about it now, I try to recall our role as staff that weekend. Did we challenge students about issues of boundary testing, rebellion against parental figures, power struggles? And would that have been a manipulative ploy if we had? As a staff group we came from diverse backgrounds, from psychodynamic, person-centred, family systems, gestalt. But we were all, in our way, committed to self-direction. We answered practical questions, and let the group throw up its natural leaders who suggested structures to aid discussion and decision-making. At length, the group decided that they would join into one large community. We as staff joined into a six-strong staff group with a community group of 70 students. It felt like a risk, but this group was so successful that the staff decided to repeat the experiment, making the next intake also comprise 70 students. However, this time the group found it hard to gel.

The missing factor was student choice. How important it is for each of us to feel listened to and heard, our wishes acted upon. What a stimulus for self-motivated learning this is.

And it is not as simple as that. Students and staff had chosen to join this course knowing its central philosophy of self-direction. This commitment provided the opportunity for an underlying element of goodwill which usually got us through the sticky moments. Students came on this course expecting to be self-directing, sometimes fearing this, but also on the look-out as I had been, for the iron fist of hidden rules.

Staff set up structures to enable students to work out their learning contracts and course programme. This might all go according to plan, or it might be changed by issues which arose from the community. This is because our Task was to produce a course design, but the Process was to give students a taste of self-direction and to help them see how they functioned in a community group.

In fact, detailed plans made on the weekend were often scrapped by students on the first week of term, and a new design formulated. As if the supposed task was secondary to the community and individual learning. As if the experience of negotiating, challenging, experiencing fear, anger, discomfort and joy was where the real learning lay.

I noticed that devising this new programme was often very quick, very clear and co-operative. Once the underlying issues had been faced and dealt with, carrying out the task became a simple matter.

Course self-design

The Life Map

On the planning weekend, staff would provide group experiences to help focus on individual learning needs. One such was a Life Map. After drawing a map of key life experiences, students were asked to list resources they brought to the course – for example, looking after young children at home, or running a small business, entail management skills and patience. The map could also cover the future, and ask the questions:

- Where do you see your life going?
- What does this mean about what you want to learn?
- What topics might you want included as a participant in a workshop?

- What might you want to teach
    - in an ongoing workshop?
    - a one-off community workshop?
    - on your own?
    - with fellow students?
    - with staff?
    - with a mixed staff/student group?

These issues would be aired with partners, in groups of three and four and more, and in the big group. Over the first few weeks of the course, this map would be used to write the individual learning contract. This would be the basis of assessment for the portfolio of work to be assessed at the end of the course.

Chinese Procession
After a short meditation on what sort of workshop might best meet an individual's learning needs, each student would write their preference on a large sheet of paper. For example, someone might write 'Person-Centred' on a sheet, another might write 'Disabilities'. Each would hold up their sheet and parade around the room, looking at others' sheets to find similarities, talking to students or staff they hoped might facilitate, and ending up with several viable groups.

There were various issues which might make the choosing of workshops difficult. Firstly, there was the issue of whether tutors would declare their specialisation. The thinking went like this: If I declare my specialisation, students will be attracted through their anxiety to choose this rather than devise a workshop more suited to their needs, say on cultural diversity or how differing theories of counselling hang together. They may also hold back from offering workshops of their own or supporting other students to offer workshops.

Then there was the individualistic trap. In the offer of self-direction is the hidden promise that, at last, we can all get what we want and not have to bother about anyone else. So if only one person wanted a workshop on work with adolescents and nobody else did, that person could hold up the proceedings in great disappointment that her/his needs were not being met. Negotiation could assist – they could join a similar group, engage in private study in workshop time, make a bid at the next planning session. But the underlying cause might be a feeling of betrayal – 'The course said it would meet my needs!' I remember finding this confusing. Because we were rejecting martyred selflessness, would we just be totally selfish and inconsiderate? I now think of the words of Rabbi Hillel, written in the sixth century:

> If I am not for myself, then who is for me?
> And if I am only for myself, then what am I?
> And if not now, when?

In the age of self-assertion, the first line is a revelatory contradiction to childhood oppression, but without the second line, community and society collapse.

The programme

Two aspects of the course which had to be decided were, firstly, the structure of the day, and, secondly, the content of the programme. We met on one day a week for five hours.

There was often a similarity in programmes over different years. A community group for one hour at the beginning and a support group at the end for an hour was usual. This could vary. Sometimes a time for free study might be built in. Or one-off student workshops might take place. The differences were important. It was the fact of choice which created energy, excitement and motivation.

During the day there would be one or two workshops. Later, there was an obligatory workshop on counselling skills. Students would then chose workshops, usually based on a particular model. Sometimes, in the first year, there might be 'taster' workshops which introduced different models, to enable students to make choices about more in-depth study. Nowadays, the move is towards a one-model course (cf. Feltham's Chapter II.4, this volume), which is understandable. But, when counsellors have practised for some time they do tend to become more eclectic. Students from SWLC often went on to study a model in more depth after leaving the course, but they also had a fairly sophisticated background knowledge of various counselling techniques. I went on to train in Psychosynthesis, as it seemed to me to pull diverse strands of counselling together within a framework that included spirituality.

Decision-making

So in this oasis of negotiation, how were community decisions made? How can you make decisions if you have no strategy for doing so? A straightforward majority vote meant that a minority of people would be overruled. One system which worked well was to take a 'straw poll' and then to ask those who'd 'lost' to give their views. The majority would then adapt the decision to allow for these reservations.

Another system involved going to different parts of the room according to your opinion and conducting a discussion between each section.

A 'fish-bowl' might be suggested, in which four or five protagonists sat in an inner circle for a public discussion with empty cushions for members of the larger community to temporarily join in with comments, before returning to their seats. The staff group might sit in the middle to muse on what they were experiencing and thinking about the process, while students could comment from the empty cushions.

Sometimes we would stop the discussion and go round the group, with each person sharing their current feelings to see what might be getting in the way.

If discussions became contentious it is likely that this was caused by underlying issues of power and competition. As in my interview for the job, to endorse another's idea could feel like giving up power. Decisions about assessment procedures provoked much anxiety and regression, and if that was acted out but not directly expressed then we would sit in the group for hours feeling stale and stuck – the worse it got, the harder it was to move.

The role of the tutors – sharing leadership

As tutors, we were invested with a lot of power by students. If we made any suggestion, it tended to be immediately taken up, as opposed to the arguing which went on about the ideas of fellow students.

I stayed on the courses for ten years, because they were continually surprising, enlivening and challenging. Each year had a different personality and would draw from me my own new resources and learning. In spite of this, the role of the tutor could at times be confusing. Because of the students' eagerness to adopt our ideas, I often held back on my own spontaneous leadership in order to leave space for them to take power. But the tutors also acted as models of group behaviour, so was I modelling passivity – or presenting a blank screen and encouraging transference? When students chose which tutor-led workshops to attend, I felt some pressure to sell my wares to the populace. It was hard not to feel competitive with other tutors.

I suspected that students could sense these things, unconsciously – or perhaps it was obvious. When there are uneasy issues which do not feel safe enough to confront, they prevent clear group decisions being made.

Although we wanted to celebrate difference, counselling in this country has tended to be a well-meaning white, middle-class profession. In later years I came to realise that it is not enough to expect all groups to fit into the expectations of this 'mainstream'. Black people, for example, who felt subtly excluded, could protest – to the confusion of the 'well-intentioned' whites. Since then, in Re-evaluation Co-counselling, I have realised the value of working on esteeming our own identities and working on our own feeling of being oppressed. It is from this hurt place inside us that we hurt and oppress and exclude others.

When difficult issues were being faced in the community, staff teams could be a useful source of support for tutors. When we worked well together as staff, it could feel like being allowed to play with your best friends all day long. Sometimes, especially when there were questions of cutting back on staffing, or issues of inequality, our fears could exacerbate rivalries between us. As a staff group, we were also trying to evolve as a co-operative team. Outside pressures affected us in the same way that cutbacks and 'the market' act against co-operative learning today, and can lead to rigidity and insistence on rules and standards at the expense of personal growth – a theme which recurs throughout this book.

Self and peer assessment

The method by which assessment is made in any educational setting determines the content and learning environment of the course of study being assessed. The SWLC courses were putting forward a model of counselling education which mirrored the humanistic counselling process. In this model, counselling is a way of helping clients to come to their own wise decisions, based on a concept of inner wisdom and inner resources which we as counsellors respect and encourage.

Counsellors do not evaluate their clients, but encourage clients themselves to evaluate their own lives and choose courses of action. If tutors had been responsible for the final evaluation, this knowledge would be present throughout the course, and the power-sharing dynamic of negotiation and course ownership by students would have been undermined.

In 1985, an action group on assessment was set up, chaired by a tutor, Liz Noyes, with student members Joy Davies, Heather Longhurst, and Gillian Thurlby. This group set out information about the experience of previous course years in the area of assessment. It was available to later courses to use as a starting-point for devising their own assessment procedures.

There were advantages of having a system devised and assessed by students. Firstly, it led to an intense level of debate about the first principles of counselling; to discussions on equal opportunities and how they were affected by counselling methods and approaches. The desire to enable fellow students to gain a diploma was weighed against the need to ensure the safety of future clients.

Underlying this, it faced students with taking responsibility for their community, and taking time and effort to act ethically and with care to enable the learning of others, and in so doing extend and deepen their own learning.

It was also important to recognise the anxieties brought up around assessment and how this could get in the way of clear group decision-making. How it could lead to avoidance and prevarication and endless argument. To recognise that in co-operative learning, we have to own our feelings of competition and rivalry, and fear and contempt of others, repeatedly discharge them and find ways of choosing to act in a way that furthers the best interests of ourselves and our community.

Did the system produce competent counsellors?

What are the attributes of a competent counsellor?

The Shorter Oxford English Dictionary defines 'competence' as: 'Suitable, fit, proper .... Answering the requirements of the case'. I like this definition because it implies that to be competent is to be flexible and responsive to the needs of differing clients. Each client will have had a different experience of early infant care. So there will be variations in the sort of counselling relationship which each client needs to feel safe enough to build trust. Clients from groups which have been oppressed in this society may want to know where a counsellor stands on issues of racism or homophobia, and know they have permission to challenge the counsellor if they do experience assumptions or prejudices. Counsellors need to have developed sensitivity, empathy and the courage to take appropriate risks.

Another 'requirement' is that counsellors are able to accept and emotionally 'hold' clients, especially when they are distressed, so that they do not feel abandoned to their feelings of shame, despair or rage. This means that counsellors will have needed to face their own uncomfortable feelings, and recognise how hard it is to develop a sense of compassion towards one's own vulnerability.

The most important safeguard for competence is the ability to reflect honestly on one's practice, to face mistakes and difficulties, to see where one has done well, to accept where there is need for growth and change in oneself – to learn from supervision and to develop an 'internal supervisor'. I have one who sits on my shoulder, noticing what's going on between me and my client; within me; making links, lightly noticing where I might have blocked a client's progress; checking out what might have made me do that; acting on that information.

Richard House (1996), in his article 'Professional vs. vocational training in practitioner development', writes about the capacity 'for intimacy and relating' which lies at the core of counselling. Behind this needs to be a sturdy framework of applied knowledge and skills. Theoretical models of counselling can fire our enthusiasm, help us make sense of what we are doing, enrich our intelligent understanding of ourselves and our world, and provide a structure to inform our thinking which enables us to feel safer and more boundaried. But remember – each model was originated by a person having insights and intuitions based on his or her own preferred personal style. Their formation was often produced in rebellion against previous originators for whom they were disciples. Freud engendered many new theories in rebellion against his own – Jung, Perl, Rogers – I could go on. The model is not a religious tract. It is only useful to counsellors in practice if they can apply it to the benefit of their clients. Competent counsellors, in my experience, become more integrative with time in the field. This stems from their ability to learn and grow in their practice. So I would want a requirement that there is an ability to integrate new knowledge.

How did we assess and measure such attributes?

Firstly, a community group would get together to devise a Community Contract for assessment. They would brainstorm a list of counsellor competencies to be assessed. Time boundaries were givens because of end of term dates, leaving time for appeals and the necessity of giving the external assessors a firm date. But the method chosen for demonstration of competency was left to individuals. It might include poetry, artwork, flow-diagrams, or be entirely on tape. The aim was to include those for whom academic expression was not their prime ability, even though they might be excellent counsellors.

The action group mentioned previously defined three core aspects of assessment:

- *Monitoring* – Checking what is going on and reflecting on it, with a view to developing practice over time.
- *Evaluating* – Asking how good the work is. What are the good points? What could be better? By what values do I evaluate?
- *Assessment* – Deciding in the light of evaluation if a good-enough level has been reached.

Expectation of content would usually include a personal philosophy, knowledge of theories of counselling, evidence of counselling skills, evidence of self-evaluation and assessment, evidence of peer evaluation and assessment.

In later years on the course, audio and video tapes of counselling sessions would be included in which the ability to accurately and honestly reflect on the session was more important than the display of skills shown. Each year's community group devised their own system of assessment. There were often groups monitoring and evaluating each aspect of portfolio work, written work, counselling skills, and personal growth in support groups. Assessment was usually in groups of three – possibly random, sometimes chosen or a mixture of the two. Tutors did not assess, but acted as facilitators of groups or as consultants.

I think the most difficult area was the definition of criteria for assessment. How good is good enough? Does one's knowledge of a person outside of their presentation of their portfolio influence one's evaluation of them as a counsellor? Should it do so – is it appropriate or might it reflect your own prejudices about how well you get on with them? These questions would be just as relevant for tutors assessing students as for students peer-assessing their fellows.

Did the system produce competent counsellors?

The aim of the system was to mirror the counselling process. My own success or otherwise with clients depends a lot on the client's willingness to engage, work on their obstacles and resistances, motivation to confront painful feelings and ability to act on their new understanding. In SWLC, the same would apply to students. So some students would thrive in the creative, sometimes threatening, sometimes outrageously boring environment. People like myself, who had previously felt stupid and incompetent in previous educational settings, could really use the opportunity to learn and grow, and develop skills and potential in counselling and in their lives. The lessened boundaries and lack of firm direction could at times feel difficult and confusing. There was a major emphasis on the need for personal growth on the course. It was students who found this area difficult who might flounder.

How can I answer this question? Past students on the course have gone on to be leaders in the counselling field, to be honest and ethical counsellors, to be influential in the field of education and management, to undertake further training. There was an emphasis on congruence, on ethical behaviour, on difficult though honest debate. There was engendered a belief in community, and in the importance of giving mutual support even while struggling to understand the dynamics of the large group and confronting one's feelings within it. The whole evaluation and assessment process rested on being able to give relevant feedback, and one of the main criteria of assessment was in the ability to receive, digest and learn from such feedback.

The main criticism of the course from past students and staff I have contacted has been around the area of theoretical knowledge. The emphasis on the course was certainly on personal development, especially in regard to the capacity for intimacy and relating, and community negotiated learning. The workshops were experiential, with varying amounts of didactic teaching, depending on the style of the tutor. If you were a student who was well motivated to learn, there was a wide range of reading and expertise to learn from. But there was no coercion, and the theoretical aspect was not perhaps given its due weight. There could also have been more emphasis on counselling skills training.

I do feel that students received an education. They learned to be open to new knowledge, to be committed to their own personal and professional ongoing development, and their sense of community showed that it is necessary and acceptable to care for other people and thus to care for the well-being of their clients. SWLC was the beginning of their journey to being competent counsellors.

Messages for counselling education today

What is important is that we need to take into account the philosophical and social effects of the procedures we adopt. At SWLC, the sheer challenge was that we actually attempted on a daily basis to provide a course which would go against our hierarchical and often oppressive society.

Counselling education today has largely changed its emphasis. We wondered all those years ago whether adopting a diploma would change our values and aspirations. We were concerned that the gaining of a qualification would become an end in itself. Hierarchical learning can mean that power shifts from the students to the accrediting body who set the programme for the tutors, who in turn decide the programme for their students.

I always noticed a battle between those who favoured Task and those who favoured Process. It was hard to agree on a middle way. Today it seems materialism has won. There is an emphasis on theory and skills, overshadowing process values such as personal growth, the capacity for intimacy and relating, and particularly the search for inner wisdom and creative potential, which is what makes the counselling relationship work successfully for clients.

In SWLC students were allowed to learn at their own pace. On the whole, the community worked in a very responsible way. The feeling of being trusted and given the power to choose ways and topics of learning led to a vibrant, exuberant and expressive course – often the highlight of people's week, and a turning point in their lives. I would like to see more courses having the courage to trust students to have more input into their learning, creatively discovering their potential.

Knowledge and skills are obviously vital in counsellor training. This needs to be balanced by emphasis on personal development and choice. My worry is that there is too much content, too many academic demands, too many hoops to jump through and not enough positive feedback and support. The course becomes an endurance test, and students learn to be martyrs who do not take enough care of their own well-being and happiness – a well-known ailment of the counselling profession!

SWLC was a course where I and many others felt alive and fulfilled. I hope its influence will live on to make ethics and love a factor in counsellor education and in society.

Acknowledgements

I would like to thank the following past students and tutors of the course for their feedback and help in writing this chapter: Madelyn Brewer, Sheila Broderick, Claudio Calvi, Veronica Denby, Joy Davies, Isha Mckenzie-Mavinga, Martin Jelfs, Grazina Kowzun, Wendy Laird, Richard Lovegrove, Pat Milner, Brigid Proctor, Leisl Silverstone, Janet Stott, Gail Taylor and particularly Penny Travers.

References

House, R. (1996) 'Professional vs. vocational training in practitioner development' (mimeo).

Osborn, T. (ed.) (n.d.) *South West London College Counselling Courses – Student Manual.*

Three Experiences of Self and Peer Assessment V.2

Michael Eales, Catherine Hayes, Michael McMillan & Jill Brooks

1. Developing Self-determination: The Institute for the Development of Human Potential (IDHP)

Michael Eales

Assessment and accreditation have become a focus point for the growth movement in the 1990s. For the past 21 years the IDHP has been using and developing self and peer assessment and accreditation, both in its selection of course facilitators, and in the ongoing and final assessment and accreditation of participants on its postgraduate diploma in Humanistic Psychology and Facilitation. I would like to outline some of the background and some of the learning we have gained from this approach.

My first experience of self and peer assessment and accreditation was as a participant on an IDHP Diploma course at the University of Surrey in 1982–4. It sounded from its description that it might be easy, although the facilitators warned otherwise. In practice it turned out to be an extremely rigorous process, and much harder than any written exam I had ever sat. Imagine having to assess yourself, both your strengths and weaknesses with depth and honesty, and then to have that 'rattled and shaken' by peers, and then to be given in-depth and honest feedback – I came out of the experience knowing more about who I really was, and feeling confident about my abilities.

In 1987 I decided with my working partner, Anouk Graav, to apply to the IDHP to co-facilitate the very same diploma at the University of Surrey. The selection procedure again used self and peer assessment. Firstly, the course outline and our individual self-assessments were prepared with a support person, then these were rattled and shaken by a representative of the IDHP committee. There was then a final self and peer assessment process with the whole committee. It was extremely challenging to feel that I was a peer amongst the great and the good of the facilitation world. Again the end result was that I felt empowered and supported, and well prepared for the task ahead, as the feedback drew so much from the collective experience of the peer group.

At the end of the diploma course, whose aim it is to move towards a peer learning community, Anouk and I took part in the final self and peer assessment, looking at both our roles as primary facilitators, and at our own development through the course.

It seemed to me to be yet another layer of self-challenge to self-assess my role as a facilitator and get honest and thoughtful feedback from participants on a personal basis – no hiding behind a post-course questionnaire.

I have since co-facilitated two more diploma courses, have participated in the selection of other IDHP facilitators, and have introduced self and peer assessment in countless other environments over the last 14 years. I still believe in its rigour, and feel I can stand behind the work of those I have had the privilege to peer assess and accredit.

From the outset, one of the main objectives of the IDHP was empowerment, defining an 'educated' or 'professional person' as:

> ... an awarely self-determining person, in the sense of being able to set objectives, to formulate standards of excellence for the work that realises those objectives, to assess work done in the light of those standards, and to be able to modify the objectives, the standards or the work programme in the light of experience and action; and all this in discussion and consultation with other relevant persons.
>
> (Heron, 1982: 15)

This is, for me, the benchmark definition of professionalism – where the person has ownership of maintaining their own professional practice, rather than giving the role to a quasi-parental professional body who will watch for misdemeanours. It also defines professionalism as an ongoing process, rather than a once-and-for-all gateway.

The founders of the IDHP believed that if this were a valid definition of professional practice, then the educational process in most institutions of higher or professional education did not prepare students to acquire such self-determining competence, as staff unilaterally determined student learning objectives, student work programmes and assessment criteria, and then unilaterally did the assessment of students' work. This developmental stalemate still persists. In fact, many so-called new developments seem to be taking a backward step as traditional models of professionalism are reintroduced.

There seems to be a classic anomaly where professions acknowledge the ideological case for its members acquiring self-determining and co-operative skills but the education system from which the professions emerge is highly authoritarian. The aim of such education is often to further (or create) an established tradition. This can inhibit creativity and inventiveness – the very qualities that were the foundations of the 'tradition' in the first place:

> For talk of inventiveness is empty unless the individual is brought up in a tradition which enables him to see and find a way round a problem when it arises. Some situations are called problematic because they cannot be dealt with by an established tradition .... Individual inventiveness can only emerge against a background of a public tradition which has provided both the milieu for problems and the procedures for tackling them.
>
> (Peters, 1966: 57)

Self and peer assessment and accreditation was therefore seen by the IDHP as a cornerstone of a professional education process that directly addresses this anomaly, and also as a method of assessment which elicits the maximum learning from experience, i.e. focusing on the process as a basis of product; developing self-criticism; developing the skills of giving and receiving honest and direct constructive feedback; developing the ability to set realistic goals; and understanding the interpersonal and group dynamics involved in such a process.

Self and peer assessment

The self and peer assessment process is carried out in a group, or sub-sets of a group, with each person having a set time for uninterrupted self-assessment, and then receiving an equal time for feedback. It is vital that the self and peer components have equal time. This gives equal validity to, and encourages, self-audit rather than giving it second place to outside feedback – which would perpetuate the notion that the outside authority always knows best, and the resulting dependency culture which that creates.

Assessment is based on criteria selected by the participants prior to the self and peer assessment process, and reflects the scope of the assessment and the time available. The criteria could be:

- a fixed set of criteria applicable to the whole group;
- key criteria applicable to all, with options to be chosen by individuals;
- a free choice by individuals.

Where participants choose their own criteria, then that choice is also up for assessment (e.g. too easy, too hard, irrelevant). Participants are encouraged to balance negative and positive in their self-assessment. The peer assessment is also based on the criteria selected. A clear distinction is made between the criteria for assessment and the 'whole person'. This is not an occasion for unsolicited or generalised criticism of another group member, or for dumping previously undealt-with feelings.

The peer assessment may include clarifying and/or drawing out questions. Constructive negative feedback (which could include 'devil's advocate' feedback) and positive feedback must be of equal time, and the positive must always come last. This is to contradict a common tendency to hear positive as a sweetener to the negative, 'I like you ... but ...', or for the negative to cancel out the positive.

A subsequent review of the whole process could focus on contribution rates in the feedback process, the quality and balance of feedback, and such things as gender issues and competitiveness. The assessment therefore becomes a part of a learning process, where assessment skills can be honed.

The final accreditation is through a formalised process of written self-accreditation, which is then reviewed and revised in the light of peer feedback. It is important that participants receive feedback from all group members. This feedback may be focused through an elected 'rattle and shake' person, to support individuals in drawing up the final self-accreditation. The self-accreditation is honed until a consensus, or agreed majority, can stand by it.

From this outline model various adaptations are possible, but the basic principles are central to current IDHP practice.

Learning from the process

Certain issues have clearly emerged from my experience of using the model. The demands of the self and peer assessment process connect with the ongoing process of the training group, or professional supervision group.

If it is a training group, then the facilitators have to be clear about the aims and objectives of the course as a whole and of individual strands. There also needs to be clarity about standards, and facilitators need to be prepared to model, train and confront on these issues throughout the course.

The facilitators need to support participants in defining their individual learning needs, and relate these to their development throughout the whole course. In this respect the facilitators are not simply 'peers', they have responsibilities which they are paid to carry out.

The facilitators need to trust in participants' ability to become self-determining, and be prepared to work on their own issues of letting go of being inappropriately hierarchical as the course progresses. They also need to help foster a self-accepting atmosphere, and be willing to work with the feelings generated by the process. The interpersonal skills of the group are needed here. Personal and interpersonal skills development needs to begin early in the course, and in activities not directly related to assessment. It is important for the facilitators to model giving clear and direct feedback, both negative and positive.

Facilitators need to maintain an ongoing commitment to their own development – i.e. having encouraged participants to set and monitor their own learning, they need to be open themselves to feedback and change. If it is a professional supervision group, then unfinished business has to be worked through regularly so as not to contaminate the process. Issues that may affect the group as a whole, e.g. competitiveness, fears about how others see their competence, and other issues endemic to professional life, need to be addressed. Individuals need to define their own developmental needs and to commit themselves to openness.

I personally have a lot of experience of both self and peer assessment and traditional assessment as a lecturer in Higher Education (where I have introduced new forms of assessment where I can). I have no doubt that self and peer assessment is more challenging to the facilitator than traditional forms. The facilitator needs to be clear about when the role of hierarchy is appropriate, knowing when to support and challenge, or when to disclose, share or confront as a peer. The traditional hiding place of the unchallengeable authority has gone. I am sure that the continuity of the process is also rigorous for course participants, and means that the final accreditation can at last become a celebration of the whole process, rather than a disembodied, disempowering ritual which can do no other that assert the power of the unilateral authority.

2. The Diploma in Counselling at the University of East Anglia

Catherine Hayes & Michael McMillan

Introduction

We trained together on the Postgraduate Diploma in Person-Centred Counselling at the University of East Anglia in 1995–6. This is a rigorous full-time training, and trainees are required to meet external criteria in order to satisfy suitable standards determined by the university examination board. Throughout the course, trainees mainly learn within group situations which include training sessions, supervision groups, lectures, personal development groups and community groups. The community group is considered by many to be the most effective learning environment. In addition to the study of counselling theory, the course structure also involves input on, and the exploration of, the spiritual dimension. Clients are seen throughout the training, and tape transcripts and case studies are drawn from this work.

In the final term each trainee considers their understanding and achievements of the year, reflecting on the qualities they have developed, as well as aspects of self which they feel need further attention. With these considerations in mind, the trainees formulate questions to ask each other and their trainers about how they are experienced by them. The trainees have their own feelings and observations that are also essentially trustworthy. The result of this process is an 8,000-word self-appraisal statement. At the end of this statement the trainee chooses whether or not to award themselves the diploma, being able to defer the award until a later date if this seems appropriate.

We have chosen to present our experiences of the self and peer assessment process separately. We offer our experiences in this way because it is in keeping with the process itself: our different styles, thoughts, feelings and reflections illustrate exactly why the process is such a stimulating and rich interaction.

Catherine Hayes

> A person-centred approach is based on the premise that the human being is basically a trustworthy organism, capable of evaluating the outer and inner situation, understanding herself in its context, making constructive choices as to the next steps in life, and acting on those choices.
>
> (Rogers, 1978: 15)

The process of self-assessment presents an extraordinary opportunity at the end of an incredibly challenging and intensive training. I could begin to synthesise the many strands that I had been discovering throughout the year. Being given the freedom to structure this final piece of work in a way that truly represented my journey was a perfect conclusion to a unique experience.

I decided the nature of the questions I wished to ask my trainers, my supervisor and my peer group. I had a clear idea of the questions I wished to ask my tutors and supervisor, having been used to a termly tutorial and weekly supervision. When it came to my peer group, the questions were not so clear. The sense of vulnerability heightened as various recollections of events during the course lurked in foggy corners, and the unpredictable quality of personal development issues hung in my mind as I pondered over what I would risk asking. Then there was the open-ended question: 'Is there anything else anyone would wish to add that has not been addressed?' Even the most brave would quake at that moment. The beauty of the process was in recollection that we all fundamentally cared for each person in the group. We each knew where we were in our own process. It was clear there would be no nasty shocks during feedback, but self-saboteurs lurk and edge in to make heart-stopping moments an inevitable part of the self-assessment.

This was clearly a delicate time. Situations had evolved in the community around boundaries and secrecy. This had caused some frustration and discomfort. The inevitable ending of the course allowed us to hold the community together in a way that was constructive and supportive. This process of reflection and evaluation enabled perspective to develop and deepen. We were each other's midwives, and within that there was an awareness that issues could be resolved beyond the ending of the course.

Each one of us had access to another 17 reflections of our self to comment on their experiences of us as counsellors in training. Very little could be avoided or overlooked. I chose to question my supervision group. As people talked, trains of thought would go through the group and trigger off other responses which addressed a different aspect, and so it continued very much in the manner of the dance which experiencing the core conditions had become.

I cannot think of anything I have ever experienced in my life that could possibly compare to the process of giving and receiving this feedback. There was a sense of a communion of souls. Here was a group who had together contacted deep joy, fear, pain and grief: people with whom I had explored the most devastating truths about myself and confronted fundamental aspects of my being. Now came the moment when I had to listen and bear what was said. It was such an intimate experience ... shared between ten people. Perhaps that is the unique quality of the process? How rare it is that we are able to be alongside a group for so many hours over a period of ten months, exploring the most intimate aspects of being, then finally, ask them how they experienced you? It is, to coin a phrase, mind blowing.

I recently read my self-appraisal statement and listened to the recordings I made of the responses to the questions I asked. I have been able to recognise where I was then and where I am now. Interestingly enough for me, where I am now enables me to hear the responses with more clarity than perhaps I had at the time. During the process of self-assessment so much is happening: it is the critical moment of birth. A profound sense of loss has been building over the weeks as this process represents the ending of being together. Hanging in the air is the decision as to whether 'I am ready for this diploma'. The empowerment of the self, the validation of the self, gradually edging its way into the senses and nudging into consciousness, aching for acceptance whilst necessarily aware of the continuity of being in process as an essential element of continual growth.

What I have listened to has informed me about the nature of being in transition. During that particular time, one is caught in a moment where the self is attempting to integrate its various aspects which, during the process of training, may well have been thrown up into the air. Listening to positive confirming statements about myself created a mixture of feelings. The overwhelming one then and now is humbleness. Allowing the nurturing, positive feelings that we as counsellors are hoping our clients may find in themselves, to now take a firm hold inside, must be a part of the training that cannot be guaranteed but truly hoped for: a deepening.

For us all to be around each other and experiencing each other in this way created an environment that encourages the bubbling up to the surface of feelings and attitudes that, if brought into focus, can be taken on board at the time, or at a later date. What strikes me as dependable is the overriding sense in the self of where you are within this process.

My self-appraisal statement focused on client work. By drawing on the rich resources I found in my clients, I could truly demonstrate the theory, evaluate myself as a person-centred counsellor who had grown throughout the year, and accept the diploma. Fifteen trainees reached the same conclusion for themselves. Two trainees postponed accepting the diploma.

Michael McMillan

I have come to realise that the self and peer assessment process was invaluable in my reaching a fairly accurate understanding of myself, both as a person and as a professional at that point in time (i.e. the end of the diploma course). I feel that this understanding was facilitated in three different, yet interrelated, ways: one, the feedback I received confirmed what I had already believed about myself and therefore consolidated that belief; two, the feedback added a new perspective on aspects of myself of which I had already been aware, thus presenting me with nuances of meaning about myself and my behaviour which I had not previously considered; and three, the feedback highlighted elements which were simply not in my awareness at that time. Let me discuss these in a little more detail.

The most important issue for me, the one which reoccurred throughout my personal and professional development on the course, was that of my self-expression. My initial lack of expression was a struggle for me personally, but was also inhibiting me as a counsellor as the *communication* of the core conditions of empathy, congruence and acceptance is a necessity for an effective person-centred therapist. By the end of the course, and after much personal exploration and experimentation with new ways of being, I felt that I had made huge strides toward expressing more spontaneously, and with more depth, what I was experiencing. This was confirmed by peoples' comments: one person said that the most significant change she had experienced about me was that I was now so expressive; another likened this change to 'a flowering' and felt that the actual quality of my voice had changed, now having more depth and timbre: a physical manifestation of the change which had occurred. Responses such as these by fellow students consolidated my beliefs about how I had changed, and verified that the change was as real for others as it was for me.

Such verification was, of course, not only useful in consideration of what I felt to be 'positive' aspects of myself and my development, but also confirmed my thinking in respect of qualities which I had identified as 'negative'. For example, at least two people commented directly on what they had perceived as my struggle to express my feelings towards another where this expression might cause difficulty or be upsetting for the person concerned. This was certainly something of which I was aware: communicating my thoughts and feelings when there was a risk of causing pain was something I found very difficult, despite acknowledging that sometimes this communication may be very important for both parties concerned. Receiving feedback from others in relation to this enabled me to clarify that whilst I had made some progress in resolving this issue, it was undoubtedly an aspect of myself which warranted a great deal more consideration and exploration.

Some of the feedback I received went further than offering confirmation that my beliefs about myself were true, in that others' perceptions added implications which had not previously occurred to me (the second way in which the peer assessment process was useful). This was highlighted by one trainee in particular, who made an observation about the commitment I showed to my fellow students and to the whole learning experience of the course. He commented on how powerful this had been for him, as he had experienced my enthusiasm as a positive energy and suspected that there may be similar implications for the way that clients experienced me. The key issue here is that I was aware of my own enthusiasm and what that meant for me, but I had not really considered what effect that might have on the people around me, or on those with whom I was engaged in a professional relationship.

Finally, some feedback touched upon aspects of myself which I had simply not identified or, at best, was only very dimly aware of. The most important example of this for me came from a fellow trainee who had been on the receiving end of my refusal to accede to her requests regarding practical issues which, though seemingly straightforward, were nevertheless very emotive and significant for her. She commented that normally she would have experienced this type of incident as a very powerful rejection. But because she had consistently experienced me as a loving and valuing person, she could free herself from this sense of rejection as she was able to allow me to value myself and my boundaries because she knew that I *also* valued her: the two were not mutually exclusive.

This observation is particularly important because it directly concerns my difficulty around communicating feelings and thoughts that I suspect may be painful for another person to hear (as mentioned earlier). What my fellow student had highlighted was that it is precisely because I am loving and valuing that I can also communicate what may be upsetting/painful for another to receive. This does not give me permission to go around trouncing everybody's feelings with whom I come into contact! But what it does suggest is that another person is capable of receiving my love *as well* as my anger, or any other aspect of myself which might have a 'negative' effect if expressed. This is an insight which I would not have arrived at on my own, and has implications for my personal relationships as well as for my work with clients.

Conclusion

The self and peer assessment process that we experienced at the end of our training held enormous value for us both. It has become increasingly clear, especially through writing these contributions, that its value still has potency for us in our lives today. We therefore conclude that this process of peer feedback, which seems a very effective way of monitoring each counsellor's 'health' within their practice, is one to be nurtured and encouraged beyond the initial training period.

3. Assessment Tension on a University-Based Counselling Training Course

Jill Brooks

Ten years ago, I started a part-time, three-year, University Certificate of Counselling. On completion, I became an 'apprentice' tutor for the same course (three years), then continued co-tutoring over the past four years. Although what I'm going to say in this contribution may sound critical of a particular course, in fact my disquiet is far more with the general question of the culture-wide environment in which university-based courses like my own are increasingly having to operate. In that sense, what I will have to say about my own course could, I'm sure, be applied in broad terms to university-based training courses up and down the country.

Assessment, since my initial course, has developed in a way that I experience as being externally driven. The increasing pressure to standardise qualifications in counselling and to meet the need of the funders for greater numbers of students completing assessed courses has taken its toll of the more liberal nature of adult education. The spirit of enquiry, which laid the foundations for my becoming an autonomous learner and reflective practitioner, has been superseded by an obsession with complex registration and assessment procedures. As a counsellor, how do I prove I am not harmful to my clients? As a tutor, how can I guarantee that the students on the courses I run are accountable and practising ethically? It is not enough to instil the need to strive towards personal 'integrity, impartiality and respect for the individual in their work' (AHPP, 1996: 29), but so-called professional safeguards of qualification and long experience are now required. The very word 'assessment', with its academic connotations, has replaced evaluation or appraisal, as if people's beings can be quantified, their behaviour monitored and competence conveyed in terms of prescribed learning outcomes. Criteria are set, whether student or tutor devised, as if the messy business of self and other discovery is a linear process, and students' development (as people who can relate with care and delicacy to others) reduced to skills that can be ticked off or marked on a list.

My argument is not so much that there is no need for raising awareness of skills, that there is no progressive development in acquiring these skills and that there is no need to track that development in the learning individual, but that the emphasis should be on the real nature of learning, especially when we are the subjects. To break down whole people into parts must not be more important than experiencing ourselves as whole people first, with all the difficulties and confusions that abound within and without – 'this fear of jumble and the terrors of exchange', as Adam Phillips (1994: 80) so eloquently puts it. And to do this, we need a safe place to develop, to cultivate our respect for persons, including ourselves and for intellectual, emotional openness. I agree with Ellen Noonan (1995: 382) when she writes that the process of producing intellectual and emotional autonomy 'cannot flourish if we have to keep stopping to ask how we are doing, checking that we are on track, pinching the unripe fruit'.

Student experience

When considering the self and peer assessment elements on my initial course, I realised that these would not be separated into conveniently distinct areas of development, but rather lay at the heart of the learning process and the person-centred and psychodynamic philosophy of counselling that the course embraced. From the beginning we were being shown how to use our experience of ourselves and others to build our knowledge of human relating which is at the core of counselling. Our natural desire for knowledge related to living was deepened and broadened, as we were provided with the skills to acquire and communicate that knowledge. Attention to our own and others' processes, acceptance of how we are, free from judgement yet grounded in our lived reality and awareness of the multitude of communications from which we select and project particular messages, some conscious some not, were actively promoted, and formed a consistent framework for our learning in contracted groupwork, skills development and theory presentation over the three years.

Self-assessment was not formalised into a list of specific criteria, such as, 'Where am I now?' 'Where am I going?' 'How do I get there?' – the sort of skills-based assessment that seems to be so in favour at the moment. Peer assessment was not formally introduced as a process different from any other interaction with learning others. Rather, our development as counsellors was equated with our development as persons. A clear framework (an enquiry group with a specific contract) was given which encouraged honest, accepting, attentive feedback. Our evaluations of ourselves and others were being constantly challenged. Prejudices, beliefs and opinions needed revising and often abandoning. Intense feelings, pleasant and unpleasant, were elicited, and could be enquired into and learned about at a pace dictated by the individuals in the group. Those with anxieties about their worth and the judgements of others were on an equal footing with those feeling confident about themselves. We all had to struggle with the demands of relationships, the stresses of being in the dark, of not knowing, and the strains of strong feelings, of love and frustration, persecutory fears and the poignancy of sharing. We were not in the business of assessment, but we were in the business of relating, of risking – and being enhanced by – intimacy.

Our termly written assignment also explicitly encouraged us to explore our own judgements with reference to our experience of the theoretical material, groupwork, counselling practice and the processes of learning itself. Originality was consistently sought after – we were expected to develop our own voice, our own model of counselling which would have a relationship to others we experienced but would also emerge from our personal experience of the world. Most of us became adept at self and other appraisal and the evaluation of our own learning.

At times, the clarity might have been helped by having the purpose more articulated, and I came to appreciate at first hand the need for clear, open and ample opportunities for communication in order to question, understand and negotiate the learning process. This was most clear when, in the second year, an attempt to introduce a mark was made which we could arrive at ourselves in conjunction with our peers, and a final discussion with the tutor should there be a discrepancy. This seemed anomalous and rather ridiculous as there were no previously agreed criteria, but we were told that a mark was needed for forwarding to the University to comply with their system of assessment. Coming from an academic background, I found no difficulty in accepting that my written work could be assessed for content and style (as indeed dissertations were), but to try and pin down my 'standard of learning' to a mark out of 100, without a framework except my own idiosyncratic response to the course provision and understanding of my own 'worth', was a spurious activity in the extreme. I was challenging to the course leader about this, and an explanation was given which revealed the essential conflicts between the University academic ethos (albeit in the guise of liberal studies) which based its notion of competence on essay skills and top-down tutors-as-expert-assessors judgements, and the course ethos, which was person-centred and psychodynamic. As a student I was encouraged and enabled to question and tease out, then take responsibility for, my own response to these difficulties, but these were intimations of a fundamental and as yet irresolvable tension.

'Apprentice' tutor

I became a tutor mainly on the strength of my psychology degree. I had also just trained as an early years teacher. Although not formally identified as such, I consider that these three years were probationary, during which my development was 'monitored' and my inexperience absorbed and tolerated by my two more experienced colleagues, one of whom was the Director of Studies and as such my 'line manager'. I attended several training days with tutors from parallel courses and, in the second year, a funded one-year supervision course.

Over this time, I left the fielding of questions by students regarding assessment issues to my more experienced colleagues whilst fulfilling a relatively narrow tutor assessment role: giving my written response to students' essays, thus managing to avoid the inherent difficulty of quantifying for the Board students' progress and ability in relating.

Co-tutoring

I was invited to continue tutoring (with a different co-tutor) for the next four years, now that the structure had been changed to a two-year Foundation Course followed by a two-year Psychodynamic Certificate Course. Self and peer assessment had become a very live issue. During an increasing number of tutor training days, along with increased opportunities for tutors to share, reflect and evaluate their methods and the content of their teaching and more two-way communication with the external examiner, internal moderator and administrator, our chief focus was devising a Personal Statement of Learning (PSL) for students to self and peer assess. There was external pressure to replace the students' written self-evaluation of their own learning and development, completed each term, with a standardised and quantifiable form.

This was partly to fulfil the requirements of assessment to carry a credit rating within the national, Credit Accumulation and Transfer Scheme (CATS) to which the Certificate courses now belonged, a service to students, apparently, for the purposes of mobility between Higher Education institutions. Tutors and the Board were also mindful of changes in BAC requirements and the movement to establish NVQs in Advice, Guidance and Counselling, all part of a more general move towards greater standardisation in what to expect of counsellors. Discussions and changes were shared with students and trialling of the PSL began, all within an atmosphere of tacking on an extra externally derived requirement. So instead of an assessment/evaluative climate which relied upon an ongoing dialogue with students about the way their development manifested in their experience of the course, 'evidence' of 'learning outcomes' was now required. Students were asked to 'rate' themselves and their peers in two areas: increased awareness of basic counselling skills, and increasing ability to recognise and use psychodynamic skills.

We seemed to be a long way from the counselling room. How did this reflect good practice in counselling? Were we wanting to develop a reductionist skills-based, criteria-driven notion of the counselling relationship? The Board was pushing through changes to provide information for outside moderators, examiners and accreditors, not to give valuable feedback for the developing student (which was already in place). The PSLs had been introduced after the beginning of courses and had not had the chance to become integrated. Resistance from tutors such as myself, who had only a hazy idea of the implications and had serious doubts as to its usefulness, were glossed over. I had difficulty in justifying to students the need for prescribed documentation (rather than articulation for themselves) which included quantification of the essentially unquantifiable.

This all had a subtle effect on the cohesiveness and power base within the course. Anxieties, intrusive and irrelevant to the empowering philosophy of counselling, began to surface. Some students felt inhibited and intimidated by a system which awarded marks (even when they themselves were giving the mark). Giving marks was generally perceived as deadening, extracting the immediacy of the live process of dialogue and working out. I felt it undermined the autonomy of students to select the areas of development they felt the most need to focus upon, and that unnegotiated assessment would become paralleled in the counselling relationship. The subtle and deep development of empowering others was being replaced by the need to please the power-holders. In addition, the pace of the change meant there was seldom long enough to tackle the many ambiguities of interpretation that were present.

As a tutor, the challenge of how to devise means by which students could retain the development of their own sense of autonomy (power-with), within the confines of an hierarchical (power-over) institution and the more overarching pressures of accreditation and registration, has become a most urgent concern. John Button (1997: 4) recognises that 'the problems faced by many clients have to do with arbitrary externally imposed power-structures which reduce them to powerlessness and inertia'. Students too are facing these difficulties, as well as tutors. I feel strongly the need to maintain opportunities for real, clear, openly debated and available choices for all involved. This lived experience of autonomy is not an easy option. It lacks certainty but celebrates an essentially optimistic passion for authentic living in all people.

Combined references

Association of Humanistic Psychology Practitioners (1996) 'Code of Ethical Principles', in *Membership Directory,* London: AHPP.

Button, J. (1997) 'Safety in numbers: creating safe space in groupwork', *Self & Society*, 25 (2): 4–11.

Heron, J. (1982) *Assessment,* London: British Postgraduate Medical Federation.

Noonan, E. (1995) 'The ends of education', *Psychodynamic Counselling*, 1 (3): 377–90.

Peters, R. S. (1966) *Ethics and Education*, London: George Allen and Unwin.

Phillips, A. (1994) 'Depression', in *On Flirtation,* London: Faber and Faber.

Rogers, C. R. (1978) *On Personal Power*, London: Constable.

The Independent Practitioners Network: A New Model of Accountability V.3

Nick Totton

The Independent Practitioners Network is a response – or at least, began as a response – to the pressure for compulsory registration of psychotherapists and counsellors: from practitioners who, as Denis Postle has put it, preferred therapy to remain an *occupation* rather than becoming a *profession*. In other words, they take the position that nothing is broken, so nothing needs fixing: that all the sound and fury of the registration/professionalisation process is at best unnecessary, and at worst destructive of what already exists.

This position deserves and needs support, and I want to describe here how the Network, as well as providing this support, has taken on many further positive and creative aspects, becoming an initiative for a new model of accountability and a new way for practitioners to organise and relate to each other.

Origins

Over the last few years, many people in the therapy and counselling world, along with other practitioners who use relationship in their work, have become deeply unhappy about the process of regulation and control which has developed under the banner of 'registration'. Out of this unhappiness came, in late 1994, a proposal for 'an alternative model of accountability and validation ... which actually makes use of what we know as therapists about human interaction'. Em Edmondson and myself invited people to attend a conference which would set up a network composed of *groups* of therapists – rather than either individuals or training organisations – involved in mutual self and peer assessment and accreditation: a network where

> there will be no distinction of more or less qualified or 'registered' members, since we recognise that therapeutic ability is not based on

> hours of training or numbers of essays written. Nor will we be scrutinising each other's qualifications. In other words the structure will be horizontal and multi-centred rather than vertical/pyramidal.

The aim, as outlined in the leaflet advertising the event, was 'to provide intending clients with a context of basic security within which they can make their own decisions about which practitioner is valuable for them'. The Network would 'not attempt to define terms like "therapy", or to distinguish between different styles of work, since we see a richly pluralistic and multi-skilled ecology as the ideal'. Above all, the Network would not be run by a 'trainers' club' in the same way as the UKCP: accreditation would be mutual and horizontal, rather than trickling down from the top to the bottom.

Some 60 people attended this meeting, and most of them agreed to set up a Network along these lines. There was strong emotion involved – many people spoke of feeling that they had found a home, a place where they belonged. Two and a half years later, and after several more large gatherings, about 400 people have expressed interest and over 200 people are actively involved in forming potential member groups.[1] Some of these are long-established groups of practitioners – for instance the Open Centre and AMAP in London, Six of One in Norwich, the Derby Counselling and Therapy Centre; some are groups that are newly forming around the Network, and often finding the peer assessment and supervision function of the groups extremely valuable in its own right. As of May 1997, four groups have fulfilled the criteria to become members, and at least another half dozen are close to this point.

Principles

The best way to communicate the approach of the Network is probably to reproduce here the first part of its Interim Constitution.

1. The Network exists to further and support among its members good practice which is open about its aims and underlying principles.
2. The Network also seeks to provide people looking for help with a context of basic security within which to make their own decisions about which practitioner and which form of work is appropriate for

them, in the confidence that Network members are able to provide and sustain a suitable environment for the work they offer.

3. To the above ends, member groups recognise that practitioners must take responsibility for ensuring that they are able adequately to fulfil their role. Member groups are committed to supporting this responsibility through continuous self and peer assessment, monitoring, and challenge.
4. Member groups know and stand by the work of the individuals who comprise them. Each group takes responsibility for resolving any problems that emerge in the practice of its members, including any complaints made by clients; and is prepared for this process to be monitored by other member groups, and ultimately for its membership of the network to stand or fall by how it carries out this commitment. Similarly, each group takes responsibility for helping to resolve any problems that emerge in the practice of its peer groups.
5. The Network has no commitment to any specific model of therapy, therapeutic training, or the therapeutic relationship. It specifically favours diversity and ecological complexity.
6. The Network seeks to develop a culture of openness, mutuality, support and challenge within and between its member groups, so as to ensure good and empowering practice.

Structure

The constitution establishes that the unit of membership is a group of at least five, and usually no more than ten, members who stand by each other's work, vouch for each other's good practice, and sort out any problems that arise. Each member group must in turn be linked with at least two other such groups in a similar relationship of mutual validation and responsibility.

This means in effect that each practitioner's integrity is bound up with that of their colleagues – a minimum of 14 other people in their own group and the two link groups. If that practitioner is found to be acting unacceptably, then those 14 other people will have to account for their failure to prevent the problem; if they cannot satisfy their own link groups, then they will no longer be members of IPN – not through a formal 'expulsion' process, but simply because if those groups withdraw their links, their membership will automatically lapse. The structure attempts to model itself on ordinary responsible relating.

This relationship of support and responsibility extends outward, through inter-group links, to the whole of the Network. The safeguard for clients is that if grievances arise, they can take them to any of these 14 or more people – or indeed to anyone in the Network; and that if the group to which their practitioner belongs doesn't resolve the issue to the satisfaction of its link groups, those links will be withdrawn and the whole group will lapse from membership. (As a balancing factor against trivial disputes, the group withdrawing its link would itself no longer be a full member, and would have to find a link elsewhere to restore its own status. The structure encourages groups to ensure themselves of each other's integrity, but not to argue over details.)

The Network's structure is thus what the Network stands for: mutual openness, support and challenge at every level. There is no one shared code of practice; but each member group must publish its guidelines (and the names of its members) to the whole Network. Similarly, there is no shared position on therapeutic methods, theory or training: the Network supports diversity and plurality, and recognises that there are many ways of becoming an effective practitioner. Participation in the Network is open to anyone, 'with the presumption that at least some of their activities could be taken for psychotherapy, counselling, growth work or facilitation'.

The central goal of the Network is given in the constitution as 'furthering and supporting good practice'. The question of what 'good practice' *is*, however, does not have a single answer; but openness about our practice allows a wide and ongoing debate, including criticism and challenge. The Network's whole ethos is that there is no centre to give authoritative judgement; individuals must take responsibility for their own definition of what good practice means, and share this definition publicly.

The current situation

The Network unambiguously *exists*, and thrives. Its sound construction needs a lengthy exploratory period in which we really get to know each other, each other's practice, and what membership of the network actually means. Accordingly, at this moment (August 1997) the Network has just three x 2 full member groups: that is, three x 2 groups who have gone through the process of:

a. *Formation* – each individual satisfying themselves that they are willing to stand by the other individuals' work.[2]

b. *Linking* – finding two other groups who are satisfied with the integrity and validity of the processes included under (a), and with the ongoing monitoring process; and for whom the same is also true in reverse – that is, the first group is also happy about the second group's processes and procedures.

c. *Satisfying the other requirements of full membership* – i.e. a group needs to have at least five people in it; a statement of ethics; a name, and a contact address.

We know that there are at least 32 groups working towards this position – as well as many individuals seeking to form groups; and we hope soon to be able to 'go public' as a resource for members of the public who are looking for accountable and responsible therapists.

Accountability

Personally, I am happy to acknowledge that the accreditation debate has brought home to many of us that there is a real need for therapists and other practitioners to be accountable for their actions. There may be, as I have said, nothing broke and in need of fixing; but there is an appearance, and to some extent a reality, of a lack of open communication between clients and practitioners about the problems that arise between them. Until a few years ago, many of us were in a deep trance around this issue; and I feel grateful to those who organised UKCP and BAC for waking us up. However, I and others in IPN profoundly disagree with the way in which these organisations have tried to create accountability.

There are two main issues here: how can potential clients establish whether they would be in safe hands with a particular practitioner? And how can a practitioner be held accountable for her or his work – and those who have underwritten the practitioner be held responsible for their judgement?

With both of these questions, we believe that the Independent Practitioners Network has come up with a better solution than other organisations. Rather than relying on qualifications and hours of training, we use precisely the qualities at the heart of our own practice – ongoing face-to-face relationship, authenticity, honesty, and personal responsibility. The members of an IPN peer group know each other's work in a real sense – they have to, because they are staking their own reputation on it. They have spent hours in peer supervision, perhaps in a formal self and peer assessment procedure, perhaps even exchanging or watching therapy sessions. In whatever way each group chooses, they have worked through to a real confidence in each other.

And this confidence, this 'standing by' each other, arises not only from support in the simple sense, but also from confrontation and challenge. If a problem arises between practitioner and client, then the peer group should be both able and committed to seeking resolution: not through a fixed and formal procedure, but in a way which is tailored to the specific situation, and to the specific outcomes sought by both the client and the practitioner. (This stress on desired outcome seems likely to be very fruitful as a way of moving from the 'trial' model to one of conflict resolution.) If the peer group cannot cope alone, then it has two link groups to call on, and they in turn can call on others as needed for either 'fresh eyes' or specific skills and resources. We believe that our approach will be both more flexible than those of other organisations, and more profound in the questions it seeks to answer: not just 'Has someone done wrong?', but 'What has gone wrong here, and why – what conscious and unconscious issues are being acted out, and how has the whole situation failed to contain them?'

Looking forwards

It has become clear over the last two and a half years that the underlying principles stated above lead to a structure based not on representative democracy, but *on autonomous self-responsible action*, and on *pluralistic consensus*. This means that the ideal outcome of decision-making is to find a way forward which allows *everyone's* goals and methods to be pursued *in parallel*, rather than to install one option over the others. This may sound (and may be) cumbersome, but it is part of what seems to us an important and exciting adventure in moving away from pyramidal hierarchies of authority into new territory of self-responsibility and multi-centred networks. If our work is about empowerment, as many of us would agree, then our organisational structures should surely also be empowering.

In particular, we find ourselves trying to build a network that can stand up to the critical voices, both external and internal, which tend to dominate discussion of accreditation: the voices which tell many of us 'You're no good,' and pressure us to bow to the assumed authority of others. Internal messages of this kind strengthen the actual political oppression of the pro-regulation campaign. Through working to disarm these internal critics, we have moved from a somewhat defensive approach towards one which, fully acknowledging the need for accountability, places it within a positive context of learning and support.

For the Network to work successfully requires a high degree of commitment, response-ability and awakeness from those who are part of it. It won't work as a union card, an automatic safety-net on which we can rely unthinkingly. This is how the traditional top-down system works, or doesn't work; and undoubtedly some people prefer not to have to be responsible. (This may turn out to represent a limit on the Network's appeal.) In a whole number of ways, we need to put energy into the Network's functioning: not only administering the structure, but the circulation of information of every kind, and finding out about each other's practice.

IPN intends to be exemplary in our field. We are offering a jewel beyond price: a network of practitioners who feel good enough about themselves and their work that they are prepared to share it openly with others; who feel good enough about each other's work that they are prepared to share responsibility for it. With the Network, through confronting the structures of transference and projection which seem so often unexamined in our institutions, we have a chance at seeding a new culture of therapy and counselling.

In fact, what is starting to emerge is a sense of the Network as part of a wider social movement towards the restructuring of institutions of all kinds on a pluralistic and non-hierarchical basis. However, we don't want to lose sight of its central function of providing support. Support for *clients*, through a model of accountability which delivers what it promises; and support for practitioners, through peer supervision and feedback in an occupation which tends so strongly towards isolation.

Endnotes

1. It's not easy to gather accurate information on the Network and its members: like every living organism, it grows in unexpected and unregimented ways! However, as groups reach 'full member' status, an accurate list will develop.

2. The concept of 'standing by each other's work' has become a fruitful and complex question, constantly subject to further discussion.

Self and Peer Assessment: A Personal Story V.4

Juliet Lamont & Annie Spencer

Self and peer assessment is an extremely good model for people who are training to become, or are working as, psychotherapists. It is a process that mirrors what we hope to achieve with our clients. It models and reminds us of good practice. If our aim is to empower our clients to see themselves in their wholeness and make decisions based on their self-knowing, then self and peer assessment is an appropriate process for us to go through ourselves, for it has these same aims at heart. We believe that it would be hard for these principles to be applied in sessions by therapists who have trained in a hierarchical organisation. A structure in which power is exercised from the top is less able to engender trust in the therapist's ability to know their own skills and develop their authenticity.

Our intention in this piece is to describe our own experiences of self and peer assessment and to give an outline of the model we used, its history, how it was useful to us, and how it might be problematic or need adapting with a different or less experienced group.

We have both been involved with self and peer assessment as a practice for many years through our association with the Institute for the Development of Human Potential (IDHP),[1] which has been developing this model over the past 20 years. As founder members of the Independent Practitioners Network (IPN), we needed to set up our own IPN group, and to find a basis for standing by each other's work. So we naturally looked to self and peer assessment as our model. After adapting it, we find that it is working well.

When we were setting up our IPN group it became clear that we wanted to limit our membership to experienced psychotherapists, and later members were invited to join on that basis. The actual composition of the group represents a great diversity of experience. Although we are all humanistic, our training and preference range from psychodynamic, co-counselling, gestalt and psychosynthesis, to Reichian/shamanic. Far from being a source of confusion, this diversity has enriched and expanded our understanding of therapeutic approaches. Because we were not always familiar with one another's style we had to confront our doubts about appropriate practice. This meant that we really had to learn about one another's techniques and find a way of experiencing each group member's integrity and skills.

We had some hairy times now and again. One of us would gulp at hearing a detail of the other's practice. Have I been mistaken? Can I really stand by this person: 'You answer the doorbell during a session?' 'You are seeing an ex-client's brother?' Also there were moments of excitement: 'You dare to ... how exciting! Could I incorporate such an idea into my practice?' We discovered how hard it is to make general rules as each particular situation was unravelled in all its detail.

The model of self and peer assessment that we developed in our group was intended to be rigorous and yet not too stressful. It grew out of a long period of discussion, and was a modification of the IDHP model. We were at pains to ensure that the structure we finally worked with would honour the principle of supporting and challenging each other, while also meeting the needs of this particular group.

Self and peer assessment is a mutual activity. The practitioner and her peers work together to produce an assessment that they can all agree upon. We chose to base it on a written statement followed by verbal feedback. A key part of the aim is to explore how close a 'fit' there is between the practitioner's self-description and the other group members' experience of her, both as a person and in relation to the supervision they have shared. We are looking to bring to awareness areas that may have been overlooked: blind spots, lack of self-care, anything that might get in the way of good practice. We might also draw attention to a tendency on the part of the practitioner to underplay her strengths. The aim is to help her produce as clear and accurate a picture as possible, keeping in mind the important point that the assessment always belongs to the practitioner.

It is an interesting and democratic alternative to other methods currently in use. It is an opening-up process rather than a limiting one. It empowers the practitioner, who shares in the setting of the conditions, and writes the report on which the assessment is based. The content of the assessment is generated by the practitioner rather than the parameters being set from the outside.

We decided to start with a practice statement.

> ***Annie:*** I found this tremendously exciting. To give myself time to sit down and write about my practice, my philosophies, my ethics. We

were careful, with the first drafts, to give no guidelines and to give ourselves a deadline so that nobody should read anyone else's work before they had completed their first piece. We wanted to give ourselves absolute freedom to formulate our ideas and make choices about what we felt was important without influence. I found it a creative and empowering experience. I was also surprised at how much relief I felt as I ordered and clarified my ideas and discovered that I could address these issues, and I did have coherent thoughts on them.

At this stage we started to look at each other's writing and to notice our differences: how some people had put in a curriculum vitae, some had spent more time on philosophical issues, some were more pragmatic. This was a time when we could see the range and diversity of our approaches and thus honour our individuality. After this we spent some sessions considering the whole issue of assessment, and brainstormed, considered and finally drew up a list of guidelines for ourselves around issues that we thought it would be appropriate for each of us to cover. This is what we came up with:

Self-reflection including motivation, curriculum vitae and relevant history, own therapy; supervision, peer support, weaknesses and strengths; who we can and can't work with, gender, race, class, ethics, power; beginnings and endings, practice management, self-care.

Juliet: We were definitely in the creative soup at this time. The group had several times reached the point of embarking, only to realise we weren't ready. First we needed to give more consideration to the form: how much time for presentation, feedback and other details. How did it need to be different from the IDHP model which some of us had worked with, but some hadn't? Later, the group took in three new members. We had to meet several times over a period of some months and give time to supervision before we all knew each other well enough.

Finally we got started and here is the outline we came up with:

Two group members agree to go first and circulate their written pieces among their peers in the group. They read it and formulate their own opinions without communicating with one another. So when we meet for our first discussion, each person is unaffected by the others' views.

We start the assessment by giving the practitioner ten minutes to talk about her work and this is followed by an hour for clarifying questions and general discussion. If we are all happy with the presentation, then we declare that we're prepared to stand by this person's work.

If we fail to agree or we come across problems that we can't resolve at this point, we then adjourn until a later meeting. This gives the practitioner time to amend her statement in view of comments received. It also gives her peers an opportunity to communicate with her and one another before coming together for a second attempt to come to agreement. At this point it may be appropriate for the practitioners to choose a member of the group as a support person or ally. This person can then contact, support, lovingly confront and generally be a resource for the practitioner. We have decided that if one member gets stuck on an issue that doesn't trouble the rest of us, we will also look for signs of projection, or whether there are unresolved interpersonal issues. We have also agreed that no more than one group member can be absent on the day for an assessment to be valid.

How did we find this?

Annie: The second piece proved less fun to write. I was nervous about including everything that I 'should'. I had started to compare my written pieces to those of others, not just the content but also the style and presentation, even though I knew that such matters should carry little weight. After all, I was being assessed neither for my writing nor my presentation skills, but on how I operated as a psychotherapist. I was reminded of the growing emphasis on academic qualifications and written work in current training. Neither of these skills are central to what is primarily an oral profession.

I also remembered how important it had been for me to grope my way fairly blindly as a new therapist (all the while within the protection of weekly supervision). The skills that I have found most useful over the years have been my developing intuition (an umbrella term for a collection of skills) and what I call 'seeing emotions around a person'. Had I had a more traditional training, my ways of experiencing others would have been in danger of remaining buried under a collection of other people's theories assimilated by a fairly formidable intellect. At the time, I thought I was recovering a feminine way of experiencing the world. Now I might further describe it as 'right-brain activity'.

> ***Juliet:*** When it came to my turn, I felt full of anticipation. Giving feedback, and hearing my peers expand and elucidate their self and peer assessments, had been a great relief. This wasn't so alarming. It felt as though the preparation had brought me to a place where I felt relatively clear. I could give an account of myself which felt true to me, to the extent that I can have insight into my process. It is also overwhelmingly important that I feel, with this group, that they have insight into me and are willing to challenge me. I have to be prepared to expose myself, and I can only do that where I can trust, so all the time we've spent struggling, learning, running forwards and holding back has been essential to bring us to this stage of preparedness.

We found that it took a long time to establish a trusting relationship between group members. The route we took was laborious, as many of us were unfamiliar with one another's work and we were scattered geographically between Bristol, Bath, Chiswick and Norwich. It would clearly be easier or at least quicker, for an established peer supervision group to put themselves through this process.

It is clear that this way of proceeding is open to accusations of collusion. This problem is addressed by the commitment to stand by one another's work. The fact that we are taking responsibility for accrediting[2] this colleague to practise means that we share at least moral liability in the event of a public complaint. Everyone involved in the process will clearly need to be convinced of the reliability of the others. They will therefore be at pains to be rigorous: self-protection can transform the most friendly co-supervisee into a formidable challenger.

We see this as a healthy system which is designed to support the autonomy of the practitioner. If there is doubt or disagreement, the assessors have to take the time to understand the detail of the practitioner's case. They cannot override her arbitrarily. If they are unable to accept her self-assessment as it stands, the system allows for one or more 'caveats' to be added. For example, these might limit her client group; they might ask for further training in particular areas to be completed within a time limit; they might ask for increased supervision.

Our disquiet about the move towards psychotherapy becoming a post-graduate profession is based on the knowledge that gaining academic qualifications requires skills that are often not relevant to the practice of psychotherapy. Neither of us feels that our academic qualifications contribute to our ability to 'be with' another human being or give us insight into individual process. It would be more useful for every practitioner to have some individual psychotherapy and experiential learning of process prior to formal training, than to have an academic degree. When considering applicants, other qualifications could be given equal weight to academic ones. For example life experience – as in rearing children – career experience and travel, spiritual discipline etc. The focus needs to be on the trainee's ability to show her awareness of her own learning thus far, rather than on their skill at absorbing theories.

Our own early experiences of being assessed had been unsatisfactory and left us feeling cynical about the university system and the status of qualifications.

> ***Juliet:*** My experience of gaining a first degree as a mature student encouraged me to believe in my intellectual abilities. Beyond that, it offered me nothing that I can identify as contributing to my skills. I discovered early on that I was part of a system that had to be manipulated in order for me to come out with a reasonable degree. I learned how to write a competent essay, how to develop topics that were part of the curriculum, how to be curious only to the extent that it was useful. On the whole, my abilities were assessed by people who hardly knew me, and the experience of taking finals left me determined that I would never submit myself to such a system again. I felt the weight of the external examiner behind me.

> ***Annie:*** On gaining an Oxford degree, I was surprised to discover how people who had previously paid little attention to my opinions now deferred to me. So by the time I came to train as a psychotherapist I was fairly disillusioned with paper qualifications, which seemed to me to encourage hypocrisy.

Self-assessment (in the model we have used) requires a substantial written piece, describing the work of the practitioner in all its aspects. It requires great depth of self-reflection. You can't be clever with intellectual arguments or apposite quotations, or hide behind theories or philosophies. While philosophies are important, the bulk of the work really does focus on our own practice, the methods we have developed and examples drawn from client work.

We do feel the need as individual psychotherapists to have a relationship both with our colleagues and with the wider world. The support and fellowship of belonging to a professional group is certainly welcome and necessary. It is important, however, that the group you join broadly shares your beliefs and aims. As the UKCP system started to gain ground, many of us realised our own need to form a group that would represent our values, one that could be a support and protection to therapist and client alike.

Juliet: I want to belong to an organisation that I respect and that respects me, and I want that organisation to have sufficient gravitas so that I can name it as my professional body.

Annie: And I want it to support me so that I don't become isolated, excluded and marginalised. I hope that my self-assessment will lead to accreditation through a system that is inclusive rather than exclusive. It is a way for me to get out into the world and be recognised on my own terms.

We struggled with all these issues in the early months as we worked our way to a point where we were ready to go through the process of self and peer assessment. So what was it like for us both?

Annie: I was surprised at how relieved I felt. I approached it with some familiar paranoia. They're going to find me out at last. Something that I have been doing by myself, building up by myself without a clear (or accredited) training, can't be good enough. When I centred myself, I became aware of a much stronger reaction – a feeling of confidence. I know what I'm doing. I have worked for 15 years without a complaint and with a lot of positive feedback from both my clients and my peers. I realised that I do feel solid. Even if some people questioned my work, we would sort it out. They were not going to fail me as a therapist.

I remembered the self and peer assessments I had been through in the past, and realised that I found each one an empowering experience. I have grown in my ability to stand by my own judgement. I have been supported in my statements, and through this support and the challenges have learned to know myself. So I realised that in fact I was looking forward to this process. Also, I knew that my assessors would honour my statement, and that it would be the basis for the final outcome, however much it might be altered along the way. This allowed me to be self-revealing and vulnerable. Again, it was a relief to be honest and to describe what I saw as my weaknesses, to admit to my fears as well as describe all the areas in which I felt confident.

And my expectations were well-founded. I did feel met. I felt held by the scrutiny of my peers, who worked hard to explore my statement and to root out blind spots. What I did not expect was the relief I felt when it was over. For the first time in my career I had held my work open to scrutiny by experienced people whom I trusted. I felt safe and as if I were now part of a group, rather than sitting out there on my own. I had revealed my inadequacies and fears; they had questioned some statements and still they decided to stand by me.

Juliet: There was a lot of joking at first. I remember noticing the humour and realising it was helping me to deal with my anxiety. As soon as I got started I felt fine. I knew the questions were aimed at clarifying, not at trying to catch me out. It was all right to say that I was not sure, or that I needed to stay aware of something or give it further thought. Sometimes I could hear myself getting clearer as I spoke, discovering something about my ability or my ideas in the moment of communicating.

When it was over I was cheerful and relieved, then, briefly, I was filled with anxiety. The fear that I had been sitting on before the event had a brief rampage through my body, then it dissipated. My strongest feeling afterwards was of being treated respectfully by these people who were prepared to stand by my practice, who believe that I act in good faith, that I am good enough.

After the event we realised how well this model suited us as a group of experienced psychotherapists. The process we went through was one of evaluating our practice rather than testing our training. This raises the interesting question of whether a group of fledgling practitioners could follow this process meaningfully. Relatively inexperienced therapists would need to bring in a facilitator to help them through the process and ensure that they really understood the pitfalls. This would in some ways be similar to an external examiner, except that the final assessment would still have been initiated and hammered out by the practitioner and her colleagues. The facilitator would bring an experienced eye to the proceedings. If they were to work with the rule of consensus, the facilitator's agreement would only be as important as that of any other individual. Alternatively, a facilitator could be brought in to observe and comment on the process but have no formal role or vote in the assessment.

If people form a new group – as we did – then a great deal of commitment and stamina is required before they are ready to do self and peer assessments. This process is very rewarding, and for us has resulted in a high level of engagement, strong affection, respect and humour.

There is a distinction to be made between the way in which this process serves the individual and the group. For the individual, the close scrutiny of their work helps them to cast light into areas which may be shadowy. To acknowledge the extent of their experience. To pull together the different strands of their work and make a coherent picture. More broadly, it supports the individual in terms of balance between work and the rest of life, to look at their self-protection and boundaries. It helps them to deepen their awareness of their strengths and weaknesses; to illuminate blind spots. They can be encouraged to explore areas for further development. By writing about their work they have the opportunity to clarify their own style and hold it up for others to see.

An important aspect of self and peer assessment is that it is ongoing, and the process lends itself to a regular repeat. It is organic and alive. It works well when a person is struggling to make a major change in her method, or has lost a sense of her style. This is an ongoing process that provides support throughout a working life.

For the group as a whole, self and peer assessment enables us to feel solid, bonds us. Group members are reassured of the capacity of the individual to do the work. The formality of the procedure is useful. It ensures rigorousness and equality, as everybody has to consent to be part of the same process. It is a ritual acceptance, a rite of passage.

We hope that by describing our own experience we have been able to communicate the value we put on the self and peer assessment process. As a group, we have tested this procedure to ensure that it is good enough to satisfy our requirements: that it demands and achieves transparency; that it ensures, to the best of our ability, holding of and respect for the client; and that it can be returned to and re-used as we change and develop as practitioners.

Endnotes

1. As is fitting for what is a quintessentially pluralistic and innovative peer psy organisation, the IDHP has gone through several incarnations over the past three decades, and at the time of writing is again in the process of reconstituting itself (eds, 2011).

2. We are using 'accredit' here as meaning 'vouch for'.

Stepping Off the 'Game Board': A New Practitioner's View of Accreditation

V.5

Marion Abernethy

I would like to begin by saying that there are still paths for a 'new worker' in this field, without necessarily going down the line of accreditation. Too many believe that accreditation, registration and the move towards professionalisation are simply the direction in which the train is going, and that if you do not jump on you'll be left behind. Had I not been involved with a group of therapists in Norfolk who continually affirmed that this was not necessarily the case, I am sure that I too may have panicked and jumped on that train. From where I stand now, though, I feel grateful that I was able (with encouragement) not to automatically buy into all the current fears. This gave me the freedom to reflect on the growing hysteria surrounding these concerns, which clearly indicated that a lot more was going on than simply 'improving standards' and 'protecting the client'. However, the sad state of affairs at present is that many potential new workers genuinely do not think they have an option, and are not aware that they are blindly consenting to a system of thought which can be seen by many as contrary to what the humanistic psychotherapies have stood for.

Let's dare to step off the consensus 'game board' – one where we still seem to be caught in thinking that authority is something that can be given to us from 'out there'. That behaving with integrity and excellence is something that can be proved by being on a registration list. Let's step beyond competing with each other and trying to justify our increasing need for outside validation.

My intention behind writing this is to encourage any potential new practitioners who may be reading to choose the training which you feel is the best one for you – accredited or not – but make sure it is YOU that is making the choice – not your fear.

I chose to be trained within an 'apprentice-type model' and one in which the focus was on experiential learning. I chose what I considered to be a most challenging and growthful way of learning. I wanted to be put on the line and to have to really look at and explore myself – my strengths and weaknesses. I wanted to train in an environment where I could dare to be honest, and where I was less likely to fall into the trap of trying to please my trainer or of concentrating more on my fears around passing or failing rather than the job in hand – to work on myself and to learn some skills. I hasten to add, the training I chose was not accredited.

I find the rush towards standardising trainings quite extraordinary in a field of human endeavour that, at its core, is surely about encouraging uniqueness, continuous growth and expansion, and exploring beyond the 'tried and tested'. Surely this is what the cutting edge of human exploration is all about. Whoever conceived of the idea that it *could* be standardised and controlled – and why have they forgotten that control is *always* about fear?

It seems to me vital for the profession as a whole, and for therapists and clients alike, that potential new practitioners in the field are not intimidated into thinking that their only option is to seek accreditation. We are conditioned to believe that accreditation and registration are the only methods that will ensure that standards are kept high. However, before potential trainees can even question this, the real fear that is instilled in them is that if they are not accredited, they will have no chance of succeeding in their chosen profession. I know of a number of people who have chosen accredited trainings over and above non-accredited courses not because they felt the accredited one offered a better training (and in a few instances they felt the exact reverse to be true) but because the accredited training appeared to offer a more secure and lucrative path ahead for them.

To my mind, the whole rush toward accreditation, registration and professionalisation tempts our worst and not our best sides to come to the fore. It encourages competitiveness, status-seeking, and the elevation of ourselves above those who we claim we want to help. Insurance and trainers' fees zoom, and many of us go along with it, because we feel too intimidated and self-doubting to do anything else. When one is continually fed the line that the move toward accreditation and registration is the only responsible way to ensure standards of excellence, it is easy to automatically take this on board as a 'truth' (in spite of there being a great deal of research showing that the opposite may in fact be the case). However, it certainly makes for an apparently easier life to take on these views unquestioningly. Those wary of the notion of accreditation are not against rigorous, comprehensive and excellent trainings, and it is ridiculous to think we are not concerned about having high standards and good practice. The point simply is that we believe that the most fruitful and often the most challenging learning environment is one where passing or failing is not always at the back of one's mind; and it is simply a lie to suggest that accreditation and registration constitute the *only* responsible way to ensure good practice. The very fact that I *do not* have certificates from an accredited training course or belong to organisations that would assure people of my credibility does, if anything, mean that I take *even more* responsibility for my conduct and the way that I work with people. There is nothing to protect me or to close ranks around me if I *do* fall short.

I would like to clarify that I am not necessarily even against accredited trainings; what I am against, though, is the growing exclusivity and the increasing move towards outlawing those who may have undertaken a training which is equally rigorous but which chooses not to fit the increasingly standardised form of an *accredited* training. It is the *insistence* (and behind it, the assumed moral high ground) that there is *a* way, that to my mind is so dangerous. If to have had an accredited training and then to have to be on the register becomes the *only* way one is allowed to practice, then the whole field will have become seriously limited and impoverished. However, this can only happen if we allow it to. The more of us who refuse to be bamboozled into believing that it *is* the only way, and who dare to make a growth choice rather than a fear choice as to which training we undertake, the more it will enable a wide range of options to be held open for others as well. Many will still choose accredited courses and that is fine, but I am also convinced that a great many also would not. It does not have to be either/or.

I chose to train in 'Mind Clearing' (a psychotherapeutic process based on the Eastern understanding of clearing levels of the 'mind' combined with Western communication techniques) because having 'Mind Clearing' myself opened up a whole new world for me. A world where I no longer felt just influenced by that of others but began to really sense and then to experience my own autonomy. A world where I came to know that the limiting beliefs I had about myself were within my power to release. It was and continues to be a process of self-acceptance and empowerment that enables me, increasingly, to lessen my need to 'force' or 'resist' others, and be able to just 'be'.

When I chose the therapy I wanted, and then later the training that I wanted, worrying about whether my therapist or trainer were accredited was not the key issue. As a potential client, the key issue was: 'Do I trust this person? Do I feel the skills they are offering are what I want? Is the price reasonable? Did I come away, after an initial interview with them, with my intellect, intuition, emotions and body giving me the feedback that this was *the one to go for*!?' At the time, I had nothing against them also having a piece of paper (or, more often, a framed certificate suitably placed on their wall), and of course I wanted to know about their training, but not *just* their training; I also wanted to get a sense of who they were as a person and where they seemed to be 'coming from'.

Being an actress at the time I was well aware that having gone to the 'best' Drama School may well have taught one how to speak and move properly (and often did ensure that those who had, would get more auditions), but did not *necessarily* mean they had more talent, presence or compassion for the characters they played. We all know that in any walk of life the 'right' education or training certainly helps one to get on, but does not *necessarily* ensure that one is better equipped or more talented for the job.

Insistence on accreditation, registration and the move towards professionalisation is all supposedly being done to protect the client. Well, having been a client myself I feel offended and patronised to be told that I need someone else to tell me who I can and can't trust (cf. Mowbray's Chapter I.3, this volume). And then, even more ridiculous, to fob me off with the notion that an accredited certificate proves anything other than that the person has undergone that particular training – which may well be impressive and say a lot for them – but what if I still don't like them, or for some reason something about them worries me; am I wrong? It is one of the most disempowering things that I have ever heard of, to be force-fed the fallacy that the more 'respectable' one is or the more letters one has after one's name, the less likely one is to abuse one's position. This encourages me, as a client, to hand over even more of my power; and if an abuse then does occur I may well be even more damaged by it.

Just because I am seeking therapy does not mean that I have overnight lost all discerning powers and have to ally myself with 'big daddy' organisations that can tell 'poor little old me' who will and who will not be able to help me. It gives vulnerable clients a false sense of security. No therapist can *ever* be guaranteed, and clients lay themselves open to abuse if they are encouraged to believe that they can be. Surely the point of therapy is for the client to start trusting in *themselves* and their abilities to discern rather than putting all their trust into the therapist. In the name of protecting the public, the public are in fact patronised and infantilised into believing that 'governing bodies' and not *themselves* know who is to be trusted. This encourages a frightening and de-powering view of the world. No one is to be trusted unless someone else gives them the licence to be. And the covert message to the client is 'I'm not to be trusted unless someone above me (for example, my therapist!) gives me the OK'.

The same dynamic occurs when people are deciding which training they wish to undertake. We are encouraged to believe that anything other than an accredited training could be dangerous and certainly would not be a shrewd career move. However, I knew from my own experience as a client, what an incredibly valuable form of therapy 'Mind Clearing' was; and having over the years explored a wide variety of approaches within the humanistic field, felt that for me (especially since 'Mind Clearing' works within a spiritual framework) it was the most authentic path for me to take.

However, by choosing to train in a form of therapy that is not accredited, have I ducked out of the system because deep down I fear my own incompetence and fear being tested? This of course is something that I have to continually check in on and never get complacent about. However, I remember all too clearly how I relished being tested up until making the decision to change careers and train as a therapist. I did not doubt my ability to get through exams, gain a good degree and pass the appropriate tests – that was the easy part – it was the gnawing realisation that by achieving in that way and fitting the system I was even more undermined and lost than ever. Because it was not me who was being validated but my ability to appear confident, remember the appropriate information and the skill of being able to trot off other peoples' theories. I find this way of learning and achieving questionable, even in purely academic arenas, but for it to be encouraged within the field of therapy I find truly alarming. Learning about theories is, of course, important, but cannot be replaced by the *living* of them. And the danger of identifying psychotherapy as a 'profession' is that more and more status is increasingly given to theorising, and less and less given to the human relationship which cannot be experienced (however eloquently one writes about it in one's thesis) other than by living it.

Another aspect to consider is that if my focus is on getting the piece of paper, I am hardly going to delve into my shadow sides, explore my need for clients to need me etc. with the very people who are giving me a grade of 1 to 10 on everything I do. No, I am going to present myself as a 'first-class trainee'. This was a very real danger for me, being the daughter of two humanistic psychotherapists and having learned psychological concepts almost before I could talk; having started going to groups in my teens and then having been a professional actress for a number of years.

In my early twenties I participated in many therapy groups but so ashamed was I to have a problem with shame (not a problem that I felt the daughter of psychotherapists should have!) that I projected most successfully the persona of an integrated individual that was able to double bluff, i.e. talk about my shame and act it out etc., brilliantly camouflaging the depth of my unspeakable shame. I hasten to add that a number of the leaders encouraged me to pursue psychotherapy as a career as I was so exceptionally free with my emotions and so honest!! For me then to have undertaken an accredited training where the onus is on succeeding or failing, who are we kidding if we think someone like me, at that stage, would have dared to make themselves truly vulnerable in admitting their horror of failing? (though I would of course have admitted just enough so as to divert full knowledge of my problem); all the more would I want a piece of paper to prove my worth and assuage, at least for a little while, my fear and hollowness.

Had I not so utterly changed directions in my life, I think that I too may have wanted to enter into a 'respectable profession' where I was trained by experts to become an expert. Where I could distance myself from those I wanted to help – elevating my status and thereby gaining esteem, albeit false, *that* way. Where I could believe that more letters after my name proved that I was trustworthy. I would have been thrilled with the notion of having 'arrived' as a therapist once I had received my stamp of approval, and would have all too easily taken refuge behind my glittering image and been relieved to inwardly close the door on really delving into my shadow sides whilst outwardly still 'working on my growth' up to a point, and attending the appropriate number of weekend courses and supervision sessions.

It is ironic how we aim to create a safe and non-judgemental space for our clients but at the same time, those who need that almost more than anyone – those trainees who are soon to have the huge responsibility of creating that space for their clients – are denied it themselves. What client wants to share a weakness if they think they are being judged. What trainee would dream of being so stupid as to fully share their weaknesses honestly, when they know they are being judged. This is enough of a problem in non-accredited trainings as assessments are of course still being made, and therefore it is likely that trainees will to some extent still fall into 'presenting themselves'. This problem will always be there but my concern is that with the current trend it will begin to encroach more and more and ultimately will no longer be challenged, and may even go unnoticed. Trainers of course like to think (just as I would) that they are able to see through such machinations and may genuinely believe that standardising trainings helps this process. I take a different position, and hold that it is much easier to present what you know is being asked for if you are aware of set criteria, and if an increasing amount of the training is theory rather than experience based. I know this to be true because I have done it, and looking back now I can see that I did so with frightening ease.

Competitive and judgement pass/fail environments are counter-productive in a field where these very qualities are anathema to the process. The notion of rigorously standardised methods of assessment undermines the very thing we need to encourage – that individuals *are* equipped to sense another individual's authenticity and uniqueness. We are reaching a state of affairs where clients cannot trust therapists unless they are accredited, and the therapists cannot trust *themselves* unless they are accredited. But then, the assessors of those involved with the implementation of accreditation cannot trust themselves to *accredit* unless they are supervised, and then of course the supervisors need assessing etc. It is as if we are all passing the buck on to someone else, forgetting that the only way to create trusting environments is by first daring to trust ourselves; but no, the message is clear, it is not safe to do that. We need to set up organising bodies and tests and inspectors and rule books and multiple-choice questions and graphs plotting self-knowledge and techniques teaching the most caring (but absolutely not stepping over any boundaries) ways of holding a client's hand. The message is clear – stay within the system – fit in – don't dare to be your own person and trust your own instincts – we know what is best for you! At a time when the medical profession and other such bodies are finally attempting, at least in certain areas, to move away from this message, we of all people are stampeding towards it.

It is common of course for young members of any new movement to become more conservative with age; and if acknowledged, this can be a part of a natural and healthy human process. The first stage of the process being a stretching out and a time of questioning the rules, but not being defined by those rules. This then is followed by a movement of coming 'back to base' and of consolidating and making manifest the discoveries; discarding some, affirming others. And then the synthesis of these – not falling into the trap of the dominating principle of either/or but allowing the process to meander; a process inclusive of the need to stretch and break through existing boundaries, and the reflex response to that of pulling back and refusing to be carried off in a wave of innovation without having the grounded awareness to support it. And then a new generation or a fresh impetus of movement is born. But now those within the field want to halt this evolutionary process. They want to build a wall around the present status quo and legislate how the new unfolding should be allowed to proceed. And phrases such as 'consumer choice', 'protection of clients' and 'higher standards' are projected out so loudly that many of us get caught defending ourselves, protesting that we care just as much about these issues and thus let ourselves get lost in the wrong debate. A debate in which we are often relegated to being the ones less concerned about the standard of trainings or of the potential abuse that may occur within the client–therapist relationship. This is not actually what the debate is about at all, and we undermine what we are offering if we get caught up in it.

I am sure that the vast majority of both camps are genuine in their concern for these issues, but those of us against accreditation etc. are simply saying that we need to have a far broader understanding of how best we can grapple with these concerns. But now it seems to me important that we focus our energy not on what has gone wrong but on creating and living a new way. Not even to go on along as before, in spite of being blighted, but to use this as an opportunity to allow something wholly new to emerge. To own the accreditation etc. occurrence as part of our *own* process – not keep insisting that it is happening *to* us, but take responsibility for allowing all our buttons to be pressed and take responsibility for the fact that we still long for outside validation from those in authority (even if we do not act on it) – then we can allow truly creative growth to emerge. And *only* then will it be born of our collective adulthood rather than from our fearful and reactive child consciousness. And this is where the Independent Practitioners Network (IPN) comes in.

I feel really grateful to those who have dared not only to have the ideas but also to live the ideas, thereby making available for me, and others like me, a space and a helping hand into an alternate reality to the consensus one of fear that is so predominant. I came away from my first meeting with IPN in March 1997 with a renewed commitment to acknowledge and deal with my own fears about registration and accreditation – authority issues – giving my power away – my addiction to outside validation – wanting permission from 'out there' etc. I have a lot of fears – a lot! But I am learning that the best way of dealing with them is not always to stick with them and try to process them through but instead to retrieve some of my energy from the 'current picture' (my reality of fear and within it, of course there really are things to be fearful of!) and open to the possibility of a 'larger picture'. If I stubbornly continue to argue for my limitations and justify to myself and others why I really *should* be scared – then, with little or no effort at all, I will win. It is a lot more risky to see beyond my fear and acknowledge that however scary it gets I still have a choice – the choice of whether to feed my fears or the choice to have enough humility to accept that there just *might* be a different potential reality out there that I have hitherto been blinded to.

Rather than spending hours (and years in therapy!) trying to process through my fears around registration etc., *I could step beyond my present consciousness and enter into a different paradigm. One where I am no longer trying to deny or to justify my fears – but one where fear is no longer the foundation.*

I want to break away from the consensus reality and yet I keep turning back to get its approval of my breaking away. I want to be a part of evolving something new, and yet underlying that is a fear that at any moment I could be stopped or 'told off'. This fear is of course part of the hook to the consensus. I am rebelling yet surreptitiously peeking over my shoulder to check out what impact I am having. Which means of course that I am still in the same dynamic – still playing on the same 'game board'. Still wanting to prove 'them' wrong, thus never being free of 'them', their power and my fear. The only way is to create a new 'game board' – not a better one but a *different* one.

It seems to me that we have played and grown as much as we can on the present 'game board' – have reasoned, reacted, rebelled, denied, pleaded, etc. But we now need to keep on moving and allow a new paradigm to evolve. One where we give *ourselves* the permission and the authority to create, live and stand by alternative ways of assessing, challenging, supporting and supervising each other, and alternative ways of offering excellent, safe, supportive and healing space for clients. Until we really, deep down, believe this is possible, that it is us, on the micro level, that need to give *ourselves* permission and authority (not waiting for some outside source to tell us it is OK), until we really do, we will constantly draw obstacles, threats and potential clamp-downs.

However real the threats and potential clamp-downs are, I shall never know how much they need *really* affect me until I also own my projected fear – my faulty belief that I have no power unless someone 'out there' says I'm allowed to.

Are we still wanting *them* (other 'respectable' authorities) to acknowledge us and to acknowledge IPN, rather than fully acknowledging it ourselves and then getting on with the business of living it? It feels that now is the time to step off the verge into the kind of world that we protest so much that we want. Instead of blaming these 'organising bodies' for getting in our way, acknowledge that it's *our fear* that is getting in the way, have compassion for ourselves and each other and then, consciously, just decide to keep on walking.

I am not talking about an 'airy-fairy' denial of the reality. I am talking about taking responsibility for the present reality that we have all co-created and then taking responsibility for creating a different, more growthful and expanded reality.

Learning by Mistake: Client–Practitioner Conflict in a Self-Regulated Network V.6

Nick Totton

A spectre is haunting psychotherapy

Try again. Fail again. Fail *better*.
(Samuel Beckett)

Undoubtedly the most difficult and frightening aspect of a self-regulated network for practitioners is the idea of *complaint*. Complaint has a double face. On the one hand, there is the looming shadow of condemnation – all our chickens coming home to roost at once, the final exposure of our dreadful inadequacy to the role of psychotherapist or counsellor – the guilt, the failure, the shunning – all more or less well defended against with a front of toughness and counter-attack. On the other hand, there is, perhaps, our genuine empathy with how hard it is to be a *client* – our sincere wish to *do no harm*, and our hope that we can stay undefensive enough to make some sort of useful dialogue possible when things have broken down.

The legalistic approach of the Complaints Procedure can only support the first version – what I will call the 'shame and defence' model. I have so far been involved in two formal complaints – once supporting the practitioner being complained against, and once supporting the person complaining. What was identical in these two very different situations was that *no one got what they needed* – no one involved felt satisfied or helped by these incredibly laborious and long-drawn-out processes. Everything I hear convinces me that this is the usual result of the 'shame and defence' approach. I have also supported someone who felt injured by their ex-therapist through an ad hoc process which we all improvised stage by stage. After a lot of pain and difficulty, *both* parties now feel satisfied with the outcome. (I should emphasise that the client still feels clear that they were badly abused.)

This chapter was originally written as a discussion document for the IPN.

The Complaints Procedure has as its top priority to show that something is being done – properly, thoroughly, exhaustively, formally. Its intended outcome is either punishment or exoneration. In this it mimics a system of criminal justice. There is very little emphasis on learning; on reconciliation; on healing; or even on understanding. Quite frequently someone with a problem is eventually told that the system cannot process their problem *at all*: it doesn't fall within the terms of the procedure. Rather than the problem determining the procedure, the procedure determines whether it is allowed to count as a problem!

So is there an alternative to the complaints procedure? I think so, and I want to lay out some of its key elements.

A model for problem-solving between practitioner and client

1. ***We don't use the word* 'complaint'.** Shingles is a complaint. Or else a complaint is some sort of feeble, whiney, whingey moan. Or else it's what we do at some bureaucratic, Monty Python-type office – I wish to register a complaint .... None of these have much to do with problem-solving between client and practitioner. Another useful term which would often be applicable is *conflict resolution*, which allows us to move into a whole different register – one in which a good deal of wisdom has been accumulated in recent years. Conflict is scary too, but I suggest it's a much fresher, more expansive sort of scariness than the contracted, defensive scariness that complaints bring up. Complaints assume some arbitrating authority which can decide for or against. Conflict doesn't.

2. ***The practitioner immediately* apologises.** This is the hard one! – or so I find from sharing these ideas with colleagues. My thinking here is that, if the therapeutic relationship has broken down to the point that other people have to get involved, we must have failed in *some* way. This is OK, we don't have to feel guilty about it; it happens all the time. Undoubtedly the client has failed in some way as well. But saying 'Yes, you're right, I'm sorry', about at least some *tiny* part of what we are being attacked for – or simply saying 'I can hear that you're hurt/angry and I'm sorry for anything I've done to help create that' – is (a) liberating for us and (b) liberating for the client. Surprisingly often, it is the central thing that the client wants. Surprisingly, seldom do they get it.

I'll come back to this below; but I just want to emphasise that I am not trying to create a *rule* that we *have* to say 'sorry'. Such a response, as several people have pointed out to me, has to come from the heart if it is to have any meaning or value. What I am suggesting is more that in this situation, we sit with the question: *Is* there something here that I want to apologise for? If not, why not? Am I being fully honest about this? Am I being defensive? Do I *really* think that my behaviour has been *faultless*?

3. ***Everyone gets supported.*** This is a high priority for any peer group involved in a conflict. When an ex-client[1] writes or phones to say that they have an unresolved conflict with a member of the group (they may well initially phrase this as 'I want to make a complaint'), the first response must be to suggest that they talk things over with one of you – or, if they feel unable to trust one of the practitioner's peer group, with someone in a linked group. When you do talk, an early question should be, 'Do you have support? Would you like us to help you find some support?'[2] Equally, the *practitioner* will no doubt need support; and so will those doing the facilitation work. Everyone needs to be able to draw on people less centrally involved, and so on outwards as far as necessary. *Conflict is a collective problem that needs a collective response.* (What I mean by support is – unconditional uncritical attention for as long as necessary, followed by problem-solving work *if* requested.)

4. ***The focus is on* outcome *and* process.** Another early question of the ex-client needs to be: 'What would you like to have happen about this?' The range of possible answers includes 'I want them to listen to me'; 'I want them to acknowledge their mistake and apologise'; 'I want them never to do this to anyone else' – which might mean 'I want them to learn to be better practitioners' or 'I want them to stop practising'; 'I want them to pay me back all my fees'; 'I want them to go to prison'; and many others .... What happens next should be very different depending on the answer to this question (which may be a combination of answers). In most complaints procedures, it seems to make little or no difference.

   The practitioner involved also needs to express their sense of desired outcome, and this will also affect what happens next; but of course neither person is guaranteed that they will get what they want

– this is, after all, a *conflict*. Through negotiation and exchange one would hope that divergent desired outcomes could come together, either through compromise or through shifting on to another level.

One area of difficulty here is that the ex-client may want an outcome which the person listening to them feels is inappropriate, impossible, and/or actually bad for the ex-client. (The equivalent may be true for the practitioner's desired outcome.) What do we do? I suggest that we examine our feelings to see whether we can quietly leave our own views on one side and continue to support the client in seeking what they want – trusting that, if our assessment is right, time will lead them to the same understanding. If we simply can't support them, even on this provisional basis, then we need to explain this and help them find someone who can.[3]

It's important that an emphasis on *outcome* doesn't take our attention away from process. It's through the fine detail of process – what happens, what happens without anyone intending it to, what we feel and dream about it all – that our sense of desired outcome can change and grow; that other levels of experience and feeling can express themselves. Through attending to process we learn about the next thing.

5. ***We make it up as we go along.*** I can't help thinking that the main effect of having a fixed procedure is to deny anxiety. In most concrete situations I know about, the procedure has turned out not to fit the reality (and to deny process). It doesn't matter how long people have spent *imagining* things, what happens is almost always something else. Maybe we can acknowledge our extreme anxiety, get support for it, and work out what the best move seems to be on the spot rather than by consulting a book of rules. Problem solving is a creative process. (This obviously doesn't prevent us from learning by experience, including other people's experience. That is in fact how I have come up with these ideas.[4])

Therapy is never having to say you're sorry, but saying it anyway

I've been putting forward the idea that saying sorry is a good practitioner response to criticism for some while now, and very few people like it. This seems to be because it sounds like 'giving in,' 'taking the blame', 'making ourselves too vulnerable'. If someone tells us their mother has died, though, we usually say how sorry we are – not in the sense of taking the blame, but as an expression of sympathy and empathy. This is a very basic way in which 'I'm sorry' will always be an appropriate response.

However, I want to go further than that and argue for a shading of 'I'm sorry' which *does* include the sense 'I apologise for the shortcomings of the role I have taken in this situation'.

I am starting out here from Arnold Mindell's idea that the only way *not* to be vulnerable to criticism is 'to be shot so full of holes that there's nothing left to hit'. Arny's whole stance represents a personal ideal for me: he models a humility which is completely dignified and respectful of both self and other. When asked in a group of two hundred people why he did something that worked out badly, he'll say 'Because I'm incredibly stupid – but I'm trying to learn.'

Mistakes and failures are integral to the practice of psychotherapy and counselling, because they are integral to life. In both life and therapy, mistakes are invaluable because they *bring us up against reality* – force us to recognise what is real, rather than what we imagine, fear or hope for. In therapy, in particular, mistakes by the practitioner which are hurtful for the client tend to be *created by the field between the two*, often so as to allow a here-and-now re-experiencing of earlier traumatic interactions.

So we don't need to be afraid of mistakes: they are both inevitable, and potentially invaluable.[5] Our responsibility is to try to allow them to unfold their value, by *keeping them within the therapeutic space*: which we do through keeping them *symbolic* – I go over your boundaries not by having sex with you, but by sitting a bit too close to you, say, or by not hearing something you are telling me – and through *bringing awareness to them* – noticing that something has happened which is disturbing for the client (and/or ourselves), saying so, discussing and studying what has happened and what it means both in the here and now and in the there and then.

And not being afraid of mistakes, seeing them as potentially creative and enlightening, also liberates us to be *free to apologise*. That's the way I want to think about it: can I be free enough to apologise? Not as a penance, but as a *gift*.

This work demands of us, I believe, not that we are perfect, but that we fail *impeccably* – honestly, openly, over and over again. The really dreadful acts of oppression and exploitation of clients tend to take place in secret, in the closet, in denial. Being part of a peer group at all militates against such acts, though it doesn't prevent them. It is a move in the opposite direction from client abuse to join such a peer group, to expose oneself to the gaze of colleagues.

One very noticeable feature of thinking about 'complaints' is that it pulls us into the 'What if …?' syndrome. What if someone in the group turned out to abuse clients? What if we all colluded around it? What if I can't trust my face-to-face judgement of other people's integrity? My first level answer is – then I'm in the wrong job, since I have to rely constantly on my face-to-face judgement and reactions. My deeper answer is: then I will have learnt something new, something complex and humbling about human fallibility and capacity for illusion and collusion. Then I will have to share the responsibility for what has happened. Then I will have to come together with other hurt people to try to build some healing. Then I may reach a better understanding of the reality of the situation: that there is no absolute safety, and no absolute unsafety, anywhere.

• • •

These notes on problem-solving/conflict resolution in a self-regulated therapeutic network are provisional and incomplete. They await correction by experience. The biggest problem I can see with them is that the approach they suggest will probably not be what aggrieved ex-clients *expect*. This approach may *appear* evasive and elusive; the rationale behind it may not be easy to grasp. We need to find ways of developing a transparency which still gives people something solid to get hold of; but without compromising our own understanding of what needs to happen. This sort of approach *is* radical; but it is also, I believe, common sense. Following on from that, I have a strong preference for finding a common-sense *language* in which to communicate about them – talking to people in an ordinary, unalienating way.

Endnotes

1. They have to be an ex-client; otherwise the best response is highly likely to be one of supporting them in taking the conflict to their next session. Conflicts will also occasionally arise with those close to clients and ex-clients, who feel disturbed by something that (they think, rightly or wrongly) has happened.

2. The *first* question, of course, is 'What's the problem?'

3. Discussing this issue with other practitioners, an interesting question came up about revenge. Is it possible or desirable to support someone in seeking revenge (that is, seeking to harm the person they feel has harmed them)? Personally, at this point in my development, I can imagine circumstances in which I would be willing to do so – even though I know that revenge, if we actually get it, is unlikely to be as satisfying as we expect. If nothing else, people who have been hurt often need support in completing their experiencing of that hurt. Looking for revenge can be a part of doing that (and can also be a way of avoiding doing that).

4. This is an appropriate point to acknowledge the very helpful feedback I've had from a number of people about this piece, in particular John Talbut, Marion Abernethy, Denis Postle, Richard House and Arny Mindell. Of course none of them are responsible for anything I say here.

5. Richard House has put it neatly as: 'the therapeutic experience MUST at some important level be a failure, a disappointment'.

Participatory Ethics in a Self-Generating Practitioner Community V.7

Richard House

> To encourage and maintain diversity is a part of the ethical imperative of participating in the riches of creation. In the very idea of participation are contained ethical signposts concerning how we should treat all other forms of life. They are part of the family, part of ourselves.
> (Skolimowski, 1994: 373)

Introduction

The conventional didactic approach to ethical standards within the therapy field is well summarised by the radical behaviourist Glynn Owens (1987: 107, 112):

> professional bodies should be … in a position to control the actions of their members … those in such positions should be required to subscribe to an explicit and public code of conduct. Therapists should be subject to strict external control of their activities …. Simply appealing to the personal characteristics of the therapist is not enough ….

It is now almost two decades since John Heron (1978) wrote a key paper in which he developed the notion of a 'self-generating culture'. More recently he has defined a self-generating culture as:

> a society whose members are in a continuous process of co-operative learning and development, and whose forms are consciously adopted, periodically reviewed and altered in the light of experience, reflection and deeper vision. Its participants continually recreate it through cycles of collaborative inquiry in living.
> (Heron, 1996: 4; see also his Chapter IV.4, this volume)

Clearly, the question of ethics must loom large in any full articulation of a mature and responsible practitioner community, and in this chapter I address head on the difficult question of how a responsible ethics might organically emerge in a healthy and flourishing practitioner community.

A central theme of this book has been that the fields of activity called 'psychotherapy' and 'counselling' simply do not, and cannot in principle, cohere into anything remotely approaching a 'profession', as that term is conventionally understood. If we accept Mearns's recently expressed linkage of Ethics and Professionalisation ('Developing a Code of Ethics is a *necessary* part of establishing a profession' – 1997: 10, emphasis added), then to question the very idea of a sustainable profession may well in turn lead us to question the view that a centralised, universal code of ethics is appropriate for our field of activity.

Another recurring theme of this book has been that of challenging repeatedly the didacticism that is so endemic in the institutional professionalisation process. If a central goal of the therapeutic endeavour is that of client self-empowerment and autonomy (Holmes and Lindley, 1989), then in organising our own vocational practices it surely behoves us to embrace an approach to ethical practice which models the core values of our work. Nowhere, perhaps, is this such an important issue as in the realms of accountability and ethics. It is a telling indictment of the field of therapy in general that the *epistemology* of ethics tends to receive so little coverage, and that questions of ethics tend to be hived off into institutional top-down code-building procedures. As Holmes and Lindley (1989: 115) have it, 'Practitioners would on the whole rather think about technique than ethics'.

In the United States there is an increasingly influential movement of progressive and critical psychologists who are questioning the foundational assumptions of conventional institutional ethics (Lerman and Porter, 1990; Payton, 1994; Vasquez and Eldridge, 1994; Rave and Larsen, 1995; Brown, 1997), and this final chapter is very much aligned with these critical perspectives.

Code-of-ethics-mindedness

The philosopher Dale Beyerstein has tellingly written that:

> [The question] 'What ought I to do?' is not equivalent to the question, 'What is the consensus of my colleagues about what to do?'.... What makes [a given action] right has nothing to do with the numbers of

> people who take it to be so. Therefore, the fact that your professional colleagues have agreed to put a rule in your code does not *make* this the right action.
>
> (1993: 422, emphasis added)

It is far easier, and less personally demanding, of course, to follow an externally derived code of ethics than it is to take full responsibility for creating, owning and embodying one's own. In Chapter I.4 of this volume. Robin Shohet addresses a difficult ethical dilemma with honesty and openness, and in the very process of writing the chapter he makes his own authentic and congruent decision based on the spirit of the work as he himself sees it, rather than following to the letter an externally derived, didactically imposed code of ethics. Shohet is open about the deep fears his dilemma triggered, and the almost knee-jerk, infantile pull towards grabbing an external rule-book to tell him what to do, and so absolve him of taking the responsibility for fully addressing and making his own decision about a complex and sensitive ethical issue. This experience echoes the statement made by Blackham over 20 years ago, that '[The counsellor] is personally responsible, and there is no substitute for his considered judgement. This irreducibility of personal responsibility is why the simplicity of an ethical code is liable to be a snare and a delusion' (1974: 8).

What, then, seem to be the implicit assumptions lying behind the shibboleth that a practitioner community necessarily requires a centralised, universal code of ethical practice? Here are some that immediately come to mind:

- that practitioners can't be trusted to be, or are incapable of being, responsible for their own authentic ethical decision-making;
- that the therapeutic process is sufficiently programmatic and articulatable that it is in principle possible to devise universal statements about what does and what does not constitute ethical practice, regardless of the living uniqueness of the context;
- that we should be preoccupied with things not going wrong in therapeutic work – a kind of 'Thou Shalt Not …' mentality (a fear-driven and limiting way of being), rather than working openly and congruently with whatever emerges in the work (a creative and open way of being).

I'm sure there are many other important assumptions behind code-of-ethics-mindedness, but this short list will do for current purposes.

If there is anything at all in the increasingly fashionable constructivist view that we actively, even self-fulfillingly, create our own realities through the belief systems that we have about those realities, then it follows that the holding of the foregoing assumptions could well actively render practitioners less trustworthy, and less capable of making their own embodied and appropriate ethical decisions based on their own intrinsic authority. Not only does such an ideology reveal a deeply pessimistic view about human nature – one which is highly contestable (Fromm, 1949/1971) – but far worse than this, *it actively and self-fulfillingly creates that which it assumes ….*

Enhancing the quality of therapeutic practice? …

Now if it could be demonstrated logically and/or empirically that the existence of universal codes of ethics enhances the quality of therapeutic work and prevents client abuse, then there would exist a strong prima facie case for adopting such a code. But the logical and evidential basis for such a view is entirely lacking. First, what effect is it likely to have on my therapeutic work if I implicitly embrace the view that I am not intrinsically trustworthy, that I'm not capable of drawing on my own intrinsic authenticity to make decisions about my ongoing work – and, for that matter, that my clients necessarily need to be protected from me, or from anyone else, in this way? Not only does everyone – practitioner and client alike – become infantilised by such an assumptive base (cf. House, 1996a, b), but the result may be the cultivation of a climate of untrustworthiness and inadequacy. As Joyce McDougall has recently argued, the way we think about our clients cannot but have a significant influence on how they can be (McDougall, 1995: 171); and in the same way, how we *think about* ourselves as practitioners cannot but have a similarly profound impact upon how we are in our work with clients.

Of course, there is always the danger of self-delusion; but delusion is just as likely to occur in the case of practitioners who embrace didactic and institutional ethical codes as it is with practitioners who struggle to take personal responsibility for their own ethical standards. Indeed, it could plausibly be argued that self-delusion is actually more likely to occur when practitioners tacitly leave it to external institutional authority to decide for them what is and is not ethical practice, rather than take full personal responsibility for their own ethical practice. Mowbray (1995: Chapter 17; see also Chapter I.3, this volume) argues that clients might well relax their normal and quite healthy discriminatory instincts if they rely upon a practitioner's credentials in choosing a therapist, rather than trusting their own perceptions and feelings about a practitioner. In the same way, practitioners who rely upon on externally imposed code of ethics can easily eschew their natural and intrinsic capacity to determine their own authentic and 'being-centred' ethical standards that emerge organically from their own personhood.

Far from enhancing the quality of therapeutic work, then, the mind-set and the 'energy' that will tend to accompany code-of-ethics-mindedness can easily and surreptitiously detract from those qualities of being and responsibility-taking which are surely central to effective practitionership.

Preventing client abuse? ...

Another important point concerns whether the existence of institutional codes of ethics actually prevents client abuse (or put more fully, whether institutional ethical codes lead to less client abuse than would occur in a plausible counterfactual situation in which the question of ethical practice were left to the integrity of peer-supported or 'supervised' individual practitioners and practitioner groups). Of course, it is very difficult to see how it might be possible to conduct 'objective' empirical research on such a question; but again, the strictly logical case for such a view is at best flimsy. The naive, behaviourally informed view that it is the existence of didactic rules that prevents people behaving badly or abusively, for fear of punishment, simply doesn't stand up to scrutiny. Brown (1997: 57) also describes coming across the attitude that 'as long as the letter of the law is strictly followed and no one gets caught, the spirit of the law can be violated'.

And even if it were true that the existence of institutional ethical codes led practitioners to behave less abusively according to the codes' criteria, the idea that such a purely behavioural outcome somehow deals with the problem of client abuse is, again, simplistically naive – as is the view that it is somehow possible to 'ban' abuse! (Holmes and Lindley, 1989: 196). And of course this has central implications for the quality of therapeutic work; for the potentially abusive practitioner's propensity to abuse will simply tend to be 'redistributed' to another part of the work not explicitly covered by the code's criteria, rather than somehow organically eliminated or transcended. So again, we can see that *didactic codes of ethics can have the effect of simply redistributing abusive behaviour to less visible parts of the work rather than removing it*; that the ideology of didactic codes of ethics can actually collude with abuse by giving the erroneous impression that their existence somehow magically expunges abusive behaviour from therapeutic work.

Overall, then, those who favour didactic ethical codes as a means of securing ethical practice need to demonstrate that the net effect of such a code is to enhance the quality of therapeutic work compared with a no-code environment in which practitioners and practitioner groups themselves are trusted to draw upon their own intrinsic integrity to define 'good practice'. Given the lack of any empirical evidence on this question, we can only really rely upon a rational-logical assessment of the dynamic impact upon the whole field of alternative approaches to ethics. Certainly, the view that the embracing of an institutional ethical code necessarily improves the overall quality of therapeutic work, or 'protects the clients or patients from bad practice' (Holmes and Lindley, 1989: 194), are nothing more than unsubstantiated assertions. And there is abundant evidence that institutional ethical codes often have more to do with public relations and *practitioner* protection than they do with protection of the public (e.g. Collins, 1979: 136–7; Brown, 1997: 51).

The dynamics of power, and the didactic form

So far I have not mentioned power, which must surely be central to any discussion of abuse and any institutional attempt to prevent it. Yet it seems clear that the unproblematised adoption of institutional codes of ethics entails major (and unarticulated) assumptions about power. I agree with Steiner (quoted in Embleton Tudor and Tudor, 1994: 400) when he writes that 'the greatest antidote to the authoritarian use of power ... is for people to develop individual power in its multidimensional forms and to dedicate themselves to passing on that power to as many others as can be found in a lifetime'. Surely, we have hardly begun to understand in anything like a thoroughgoing way just how the deep dynamics of power and powerlessness impact upon the human psyche (both in interpersonal and group contexts), and in turn feed through into our political behaviour, structures – and posturings (see House, 1995a).

Again, therefore, we are faced with the uncomfortable reality that Codes-of-Ethics mindedness can easily draw attention *away from* the intrinsically complex, paradoxical and ineffable dynamics of power, powerlessness and abuse, by effectively peddling the comforting but highly complacent message that 'The code of ethics will take care of it so you needn't grapple with these issues any further. We, the authority on the matter, have invented the wheel for you, and you needn't bother to invent it again.'

There is a wider question, too, concerning the function that a didactic code of ethics is purported to perform, and whether the very didactic form itself is appropriate to the unique field of counselling and psychotherapy. A useful starting point is that of Gaie Houston's statement that 'A code of ethics is an abstraction into generality of what was once personal and passionate. At best, ethical codes are a useful shortcut to save us emoting and thinking the same questions over and over' (Houston, 1993: 6). I profoundly disagree that in the therapy field, ethical injunctions should be obeyed as a short cut in order to render unnecessary the emotional work that should organically underpin the ethical values upon which therapeutic practitionership is based. Rather, from a humanistic standpoint I believe that we must *re-invent the wheel every time* – for surely what competent and flexible therapists should aspire to is an authentically embodied and lived ethics that is experientially based, rather than one which is handed down as a solemn commandment from on high.

Dangerousness, chaos and 'defensive therapy'

I turn now to what I see as the *intrinsic dangerousness of therapeutic work* – dangerous not least because of the essential unknowability and mystery of human relationship, and of life itself (Groddeck, 1951: 40; cf. Spinelli, 1996). There is a danger of a bland kind of 'defensive psychotherapy' (Clarkson, 1995; Mowbray, 1995: 151–4) taking hold in an environment where practitioners take the energy-dynamics of fear, punishment and rule-following into their client work. When one works at depth with clients, such work is often risky and dangerous, and goes close to the edge of tolerance, holding and rational understanding – and for these reasons requires a great deal of trust and courage on the part of the therapist (House, 1995b). It follows, then, that how we respond as practitioners to the intrinsic dangerousness of the work will be crucial regarding the quality and depth of healing experience that one can offer. We can either act out from our fear of danger by fleeing into a safe, defensive therapy, buttressed on all sides by didactic ethical codes, external moral injunctions and insurance policies – thereby sacrificing the creativity of the work on the altar of our own scarcely containable anxieties; or we can furnish new approaches to ethics or 'principled practice' that enhance our capacities to embrace the intrinsic difficulties and *impossibilities* (Malcolm, 1982; Totton's Chapter II.5, this volume) inherent in therapeutic work.

A recent paper by Ernesto Spinelli (1996), provocatively titled 'Do therapists know what they're doing?', boldly maintains that 'there exists precious little about therapy that we can say with any certainty .... One is driven to the simple conclusion that psychotherapists do not know what they are doing and cannot train others to do it, whatever it is' (pp. 56, 57; cf. Lomas's Chapter IV.2, and my Chapter II.2, this volume). From this challenging deconstructive perspective (which is very consistent with New Paradigm thinking – cf. House's Chapter IV.3, this volume), perhaps the tendency to embrace programmatic ethical standards and guidelines is an unconscious acting-out – an unacknowledged fleeing from the existential anxiety that at some crucial level, the therapeutic process is *intrinsically* unknowable. And if this view is anything like right, then perhaps the adoption of relatively comforting didactic codes of ethics can easily become a self-deluding distraction from, rather than a facilitator of, effective and creative practitionership.

Recent developments in Chaos Theory and Complexity Theory contain important learnings in this regard. Here is biologist Brian Goodwin: 'Chaos combines order and irregularity in a subtle way .... Too much order is bad for you! ... Living on the edge of chaos is the best place to be if you want to live a creative life' (1997). So-called New Paradigm perspectives (see my Chapter IV.3, this volume) are telling us that the physical world (let alone the social world!) is so intrinsically complex that it is *in principle* beyond human rational understanding, predictability and control, and a concomitant of this realisation is that we have no choice but to be full participants in nature, and in relationship (cf. Goethe's view of science – Bortoft, 1996), rather than detached manipulators, deluding ourselves that we can control the process in which we are so indissolubly and irreducibly embedded. To quote Goodwin again, 'it is the intrinsic dynamics of creation and transformation that we now need to grapple with'; and it seems to me that the energy that accompanies didactic ethical codes is quite antithetical to these imperatives, and is defensively fixed within, and limited by, old-paradigm ways of apprehending the world.

Participatory ethics in a pluralistic practitioner culture

The writings of Fromm (1949/1971), Skolimowski (1994) and Heron (1996, and in this volume) provide a more than adequate philosophical foundation for the participative ethical practices which I will now outline. Fromm's inspiring vision of a humanistic ethics repays particularly close study. For him:

> Humanistic ethics takes the position that if man [*sic*] is alive he knows what is allowed .... As long as anyone believes that his ideal and purpose is outside him ..., he will look for solutions and answers at every point except the one where they can be found – within himself.
> (1949/1971: 248–9, emphasis added)

I have argued that the most sustainable ethical standards are those founded upon a full engagement with the existential complexities, paradoxes and ineffabilities of living and loving in the context of our developmental histories; the question remains as to the most creative form that a decentralised, non-didactic ethical practitioner environment might take.

Participatory ethics in the IPN

Gartrell (1994) writes of 'bringing ethics alive'; and Brown's statement that 'ethical behavior is a process, not a static outcome' (1997: 65) captures well the spirit informing ethical practice within the Independent Practitioners Network, which addresses the question of ethics by each practitioner-group taking full responsibility for devising its own ethical code or 'principles of good practice' (Chapter V.3, this volume). Such a process typically involves a *real living dialogue* between group members, who together struggle with and organically devise embodied and lived principles of practice that directly emerge from their own life and work-related experience, and which reflect the richness of diversity that each practitioner-group represents.

Lindsay (now Grace) Cooke, a member of the IPN practitioner-group 'Six of One', once said to me that, for her, what matters about the principle of confidentiality is its *spirit of respect* rather than the *letter* of its procedural detail; and I want to argue that this notion of *the spirit of principled practice* is appropriate for the ethics field in general. As quoted earlier, Brown (1997: 57) also makes the telling point that under an institutional code, she has sometimes found the attitude that 'as long as the letter of the law is strictly followed and no one gets caught, the spirit of the law can be violated'.

I will refer briefly to the Code of Ethics devised by the 'Six of One' practitioner-group, a full member group of the IPN (Six of One, 1994). One feature that stands out is that the code consists almost entirely of *positive* statements about principled practice rather than endless lists of negative statements about what the practitioner *shouldn't* do. The code is divided into ten 'Principles', and the care and attention to detail that the devisors brought to their task shines through every word. The only negative, 'Thou Shalt Not ...' principle is their 'Non-exploitation principle', which simply states that: 'We will not exploit people financially, sexually, emotionally or practically. We will not use our role for personal aggrandisement. We will not endeavour to keep people in therapy contrary to their own interests or wishes.' The 'Honesty Principle' also really catches the eye: 'We are open and honest with the people we work with about our experience and training. We are willing to discuss with people the personal beliefs and values which underpin our work as therapists.' Note the first-person ('we ...') usage: this is a group of practitioners who are publicly declaring to the world their principles of practice, and taking full ownership of, and responsibility for, those principles. On reading the code, then, I am left with a real sense of freshness, richness and vitality, which I'm sure directly reflects the quality and energy which the practitioners in question bring to their work. From a New Paradigm perspective (see Heron's Chapter IV.4 and my Chapter IV.3, this volume), this approach to principled ethical 'praxis' is a vibrant, living, creative example of what Skolimowski (1994: 371–82) calls 'participatory ethics'.

The contrast between this experience and that of reading one of the institutional codes, could hardly be more stark, and I would challenge anyone drawn to the didactic form of ethical regulation of the field to read a rich, alive and embodied code of ethical practice derived by those who use and personally stand by it, and a didactic code drawn up by one of the professional institutions in the field. Thus, in the UKCP Ethical Guidelines (Clarkson and Pokorny, 1994: 521–6), in the space of just three pages we find the phrase 'Psychotherapists are required to …' no less than 13 times; and Holmes and Lindley list five 'injunctions, which could plausibly find their way into … a code' (1989: 197) – all of which begin 'A psychotherapist must not …'. In such an atmosphere it comes as no surprise, therefore, to find Holmes and Lindley writing that 'In the next two chapters we shall consider proposals for tackling the problem of practitioner compliance ….'(p. 187).

Participatory ethics in the Feminist Therapy Institute (FTI)

Another highly relevant example of the participative ethical process is described by Laura Brown (1997: 62–5) – viz. the FTI's devising of its own ethical guidelines due to their disillusionment with existing institutional codes. Importantly, it is intentionally 'a work in progress' (p. 62), and privileges values which are anti-hierarchical, liberatory and aspirational rather than legalistic (p. 63). There are close echoes with the IPN's participative ethical process, for: 'The process of writing the code was itself an exercise in the ethics it attempted to codify. No one person was set up as the ethics expert; everyone was assumed to have valuable input' (ibid.). Clients were also actively involved in the code's creation, and 'it was written by and for the community' (ibid.). Furthermore, the FTI practitioner is assumed to be continuously involved in the process of ethical decision-making, both in her work and in her life more generally (p. 65).

Perhaps the greatest difference between these two very different approaches to ethics lies in the pessimism and fear-driven nature of the didactic institutional model, and the optimistic, positive and aspirational orientation of the IPN/FTI approach. Skolimowski's vivid description of *non*-participatory ethics serves as an excellent commentary on the kinds of institutional codes of ethics I have been challenging in this chapter:

> non-participatory ethics … appears appealing on the surface. Yet ultimately it makes the individual estranged from the larger context of participation and, in the end, deeply unfulfilled within his/her inner core. Non-participatory ethics satisfies the ego, but leaves the soul and the inner person deeply unsatisfied.
>
> (1994: 372)

By contrast, 'to participate is to be responsible. The larger the reach of our participation the larger the scope of our responsibility' (ibid.: 382).

Conclusion

A self-generating community of therapeutic practitioners will tend to gravitate towards some kind of commonality of values – not least in terms of some focal or unifying account of the broad principles by which its participants stand (I am grateful to John Heron for this insight). In other words, what I have written about here is a *unifying metacode of ethical decentralisation* (in the same way that in his Chapter IV.4, Heron commends a central metavalue to the effect that it is inherently healthy and mature for practitioners to generate their own values in local groups). Heron (personal communication, 1997) describes the shift from a centralised institutional code to a plurality of self-generated ethical standards, thus:

> A mature profession or body of practice shifts centralisation from the overcontrolling idea of one code for all, to the releasing idea of a metacode which affirms a situational pluralism of codes .... The central secretariat shifts from controlling hierarchy, seeking to contain local autonomy ... within a uniform mass, to empowering hierarchy, which seeks to affirm local autonomy and co-operation in a pluralism of codes and practices.

There are increasing signs within our culture that the trend towards ever more centralised, large-scale organisational forms, and institutionalisation more generally, is gradually being challenged and replaced by 'power-with', responsibility-taking forms of organisation and ways of being, and it would surely be a tragedy if the field of counselling and psychotherapy were one of the last to get the message.

In closing, I would like to quote the Buddha, who said,

> Be ye lamps unto yourselves.
> Be your own reliance.
> Hold to the truth within yourselves as to the only lamp.
> (Quoted in Fromm, 1949/1971: v)

Acknowledgements

My thanks and gratitude to Cal Cannon, John Heron, Richard Mowbray, Denis Postle and Nick Totton for helpful comments.

References

Beyerstein, O. (1993) 'The functions and limitations of professional codes of ethics', in E. R. Winkler and J. R. Coombs (eds), *Applied Ethics: A Reader*, Oxford: Blackwell, pp. 416–25.

Blackham, H. J. (ed.) (1974) *Ethical Standards in Counselling*, London: Bedford Square Press.

Bortoft, H. (1996) *The Wholeness of Nature: Goethe's Way of Science*, Edinburgh: Floris Books.

Brown, L. S. (1997) 'Ethics in psychology: *Cui Bono?*', in D. Fox and I. Prilleltensky (eds), *Critical Psychology: An Introduction*, London: Sage, pp. 51–67.

Clarkson, P. (1995) *The Therapeutic Relationship*, London: Whurr.

Clarkson, P. and Pokorny, M. (eds) (1994) *The Handbook of Psychotherapy*, London: Routledge.

Collins, R. (1979) *The Credential Society: An Historical Sociology of Education and Stratification*, New York: Academic Press.

Embleton Tudor, L. and Tudor, K. (1994) 'The personal and the political: power, authority and influence in psychotherapy', in P. Clarkson and M. Pokorny (eds), *The Handbook of Psychotherapy*, London: Routledge, pp. 384–402.

Fromm, E. (1971) *Man for Himself: An Inquiry into the Psychology of Ethics*, London: Routledge & Kegan Paul. (Original work published 1949)

Gartrell, N. K. (ed.) (1994) *Bringing Ethics Alive: Feminist Ethics in Psychotherapy Practice*, New York: Haworth.

Goodwin, B. (1997) 'Challenges to Darwinian orthodoxy', paper presented to the Scientific and Medical Network conference on 'Science, Heresy and the Challenge of Revolutionary Ideas', London, May.

Groddeck, G. (1951) *The World of Man*, London: Vision.

Heron, J. (1978) *Project for a Self-Generating Culture*, Guildford: University of Surrey.

Heron, J. (1996) *Co-operative Inquiry: Research into the Human Condition*, London: Sage.

Holmes, J. and Lindley, R. (1989) *The Values of Psychotherapy*, Oxford: Oxford University Press.

House, R. (1995a) 'The dynamics of power', *Counselling News*, 20 (December): 24–5.

House, R. (1995b) 'Legislating against the abuse of clients in therapy: a cautionary view', *Self and Society*, 23 (2): 34–9.

House, R. (1996a) 'In the wake of "Watchdog"', *Counselling*, 7 (2): 115–16.

House, R. (1996b) 'The professionalisation of counselling: a coherent "case against"?', *Counselling Psychology Quarterly,* 9 (4): 343–58.

Houston, G. (1993) 'The meanings of power', *Self and Society,* 21 (4): 4–9.

Lerman, H. and Porter, N. (eds) (1990) *Feminist Ethics in Psychotherapy*, New York: Springer.

McDougall, J. (1995) *The Many Faces of Eros: A Psychoanalytic Exploration of Human Sexuality*, London: Free Association Books.

Malcolm, J. (1982) *Psychoanalysis: The Impossible Profession,* New York: Vintage Books.

Mearns, D. (1997) 'The future of individual counselling' (The Ben Hartop Memorial Lecture), Durham University, 7 May (mimeo).

Mowbray, R. (1995) *The Case Against Psychotherapy Registration: A Conservation Issue for the Human Potential Movement*, London: Trans Marginal Press.

Owens, G. (1987) 'Radical behaviourism and the ethics of clinical psychology', in G. and S. Fairbairn (eds), *Psychology, Ethics and Change*, London: Routledge and Kegan Paul, pp. 91–114.

Payton, C.R. (1994) 'Implications of the 1992 Ethics Code for diverse groups', *Professional Psychology: Research and Practice*, 25: 317–20.

Rave, E. J. and Larsen, C. L. (eds) (1995) *Ethical Decision-Making in Therapy: Feminist Perspectives*, New York: Guilford Press.

Samuels, A. (1992) 'Foreword', in W. Dryden and C. Feltham (eds), *Psychotherapy and Its Discontents,* Buckingham: Open University Press, pp. xi–xv.

Six of One Practitioner-Group (1994) 'Code of Ethics', Norwich, November (mimeo).

Skolimowski, H. (1994) *The Participatory Mind: A New Theory of Knowledge and of the Universe*, London: Arkana/Penguin.

Spinelli, E. (1996) 'Do therapists know what they're doing?', in I. James and S. Palmer (eds), *Professional Therapeutic Titles: Myths and Realities*, Leicester: British Psychological Society, Division of Counselling Psychology, Occasional Papers Vol. 2, pp. 55–61.

Vasquez, M. J. T. and Eldridge, N. S. (1994) 'Bringing ethics alive: training practitioners about gender, ethnicity and sexual orientation issues', in N. K. Gartrell (ed.), *Bringing Ethics Alive: Feminist Ethics in Psychotherapy Practice*, New York: Haworth.

Conclusion to the First Edition

> The discontented are the therapists of psychotherapy ... allowing these discontented writers to be the therapists of psychotherapy will be no fun at all.
>
> (Andrew Samuels)

Implausible Professions was – quite literally – conceived in a dream; was an inordinate time in the gestation; and has finally burst into the world through a birth process free of external intervention and full of the richness, creativity and vitality which are in the best tradition of the pluralism and autonomy for which it argues. The book will now, of course, have its own life, its own momentum; and what impact it will make on the field of psychotherapy and counselling will depend on what chord it strikes with the thousands of practitioners, trainers and trainees who make up what is still, if diminishingly, a plurally diverse ecosystem of therapeutic practice in the UK.

Radical ideas that challenge established orthodoxies are typically met with defensiveness; all the more so when they also challenge entrenched interests and power structures. However, our strong sense, based on much personal experience, is of a sizeable disquiet and disillusionment with the process of professionalisation, institutionalisation, didactic control and commodification: disquiet which is even expressed by some of those deeply involved in the process itself. (This usually happens privately – but see the papers in James and Palmer, 1996, and Emmy van Deurzen's Foreword to Howard, 1996.) Such disquiet can be mobilised by the realisation that there *is* a viable alternative – just what has been so volubly denied by the UKCP and others.

If there is an alternative, then we believe that many people will want to explore it; because it is becoming more and more clear that therapy and counselling stand in danger of losing their soul. Many people are looking with alarm across the Atlantic, and wondering if an equivalent blight might be striking here. Last autumn one of us wrote to Arthur C.

Bohart and Karen Tallman to congratulate them on their paper 'The active client' (Bohart and Tallman, 1996). Professor Bohart wrote back from California to say 'I'm sorry to hear about the fight over licensure in Great Britain ... The battle, of course, is over here, and we are busy becoming more and more medical-like, rapidly losing our human souls. But we are a "Profession". I wish you luck in your fight.'

> There is something inherently schismatic in the field of psychotherapy ... psychotherapy has never been and holds little prospect of becoming a unified field.
>
> (Feltham and Dryden, 1992: 254–5; cf. Hinshelwood, 1985)

It seems clear that psychotherapy and counselling will remain incorrigibly diverse and indefinable, no matter how much 'therapy' the field receives – either from its discontented radicals, or from the proponents of establishment and professionalisation. The fear is not so much that the latter will succeed in changing a delicate ecosystem of organic interdependence – and competition! – into a centrally controlled hierarchy of 'expert' knowledge; more, that it will have the typical effect of human intervention on natural complexity – turning a rich rainforest into a desert (see Postle, Chapter III.2). Trying to control 'what psychotherapy *is*' may end up preventing it from being anything worth having.

However, the activity of therapy and counselling seems to have considerable resilience; as we said in the Introduction, there are grounds for quiet optimism. The State seems highly unlikely to intervene; and more and more practitioners are becoming alienated by the new institutions. (Many of the worst horror stories here unfortunately cannot be shared, for reasons of either confidentiality or legal restriction; but by now perhaps most practitioners have heard at least one.)

When one of us took the initiative in 1993–4 of floating the idea of an alternative framework for accountability, we half-expected a deafening silence. Instead, there is the thriving and constantly growing Independent Practitioners Network – whose events are often described to us as 'the only meetings that are actually *fun* to go to'. The contributions to Part V of this book show quite conclusively that practical pluralistic alternatives to institutional and didactic professionalisation not only exist, but are viable, sustainable and effective in securing accountability and supporting good practice. The only remaining question is whether we paralyse ourselves through fear of our intrinsic personal power, and through our transference onto the institutions of professionalisation; or, instead, embrace those alternatives, responsibly shape them according to our needs and preferences – and make them work. We invite our readers to dare to join us – either in an existing network, or by forming your own.

> The Post-Professional Ethos will hopefully result in a social panorama more colourful and diverse than all the cultures of past and present taken together.
>
> (Illich, 1977: 39)

References

Bohart, A. C. and Tallman, K. (1996) 'The active client: therapy as self-help', *Journal of Humanistic Psychology*, 36 (3): 7–30.

Feltham, C. and Dryden, W. (1992) 'Concluding comments' in W. Dryden and C. Feltham (eds), *Psychotherapy and its Discontents*, Buckingham: Open University Press.

Hinshelwood, R. (1985) 'Questions of training', *Free Associations*, 2: 7–13.

Howard, A. (1996) *Challenges to Counselling and Psychotherapy*, London: Macmillan.

Illich, I. et al. (1977) *Disabling Professions*, London: Marion Boyars.

James, I. and Palmer, S. (eds) (1996) *Professional Therapeutic Titles: Myths and Realities*, British Psychological Society Division of Counselling Psychology Occasional Paper, Vol 2, Leicester: BPS.

Conclusion to the Second Edition

Richard House

Bob Mullan: What are your thoughts about the 'registration' process?

Peter Lomas: I am appalled by it .... I am not sure whether we wouldn't be better without it altogether .... I do not think that people realise how dangerous [a register] is and how careful one should be with it ... [O]ne should be very careful about what is considered irresponsible ... [T]he control, the monitoring of the training of therapists is very destructive of creativity .... [T]he greatest threat to our creativity is the register.
(Quoted in Mullan, 1996: 87–8)

When approached by our publisher about the possibility of a second edition of *Implausible Professions*, one question that immediately came to mind was whether it will have stood the test of time, and will have as much relevance today as it had when originally published in 1997 (as a whole raft of very favourable reviews indeed attested at the time). We assume that most of us will, at times, have had the rather chastening experience of reading things we've written in the past, and positively cringing at some of the content! – and so it was with some uncertainty that I took on the task of closely re-reading the 1997 text in its entirety. Happily for us, we quickly found that the themes repeatedly addressed in this book are perennial ones that speak to the very heart and soul of working with the human condition in psy contexts – themes which are at least as fresh and prescient today as they were in the 1990s; indeed, perhaps even more so, given the current state of the drive to statutorily regulate the psy field (to which my co-editor Nick Totton also refers in our new Introduction).

In the first, 1997 edition, our cover blurb referred to a number of the core issues raised in the book – viz. can therapy be reduced to a set of 'expert' skills? is a 'core theoretical model' necessary or even possible? how can we develop accountability structures that are true, rather than antithetical, to the values of our unique kind of work? can effective practitionership be 'trained in'? are there viable practical alternatives to current models of professionalisation?... We could add a host of other equally pertinent, even urgent themes to this indicative list, at a time when the psy professionalisation process is up for such schismatic contestation, and all of which are also squarely addressed in the book: for example, what is the appropriate balance between art and science in the practice of therapy? what are the implications for the activity of therapy of viewing it as *spiritual* activity, or from spiritual or political perspectives? what are the effects of the many observable tensions that exist between vested professionalised interests and the nurturing of creative, pluralistic practice? how might ecological metaphors throw light on the nature of therapy work? and, how do we understand therapy in the context of the modernity/postmodernity (so-called) 'paradigm war', and the associated critiques of the medicalising, psychopathologising and audit-driven tendencies in psy work? – and so on ....

There will inevitably be lacks and omissions in any book such as this – and two that come to mind immediately are that *power* (whilst it is addressed tangentially in the first edition in a myriad of ways) is not directly addressed (see, for example, Totton, 2006); and that more consideration might have been given to the phenomenon of rivalries and competition within and between the organisations and practitioners in the field (e.g. Young, 1997; Clark, 2002). It is perhaps rather foolhardy to single out anything from the book to highlight in this editorial Conclusion; but with that caveat in mind, I have chosen one aspect of the first edition that, for me, speaks to the relevance of the book's message to the present day. Specifically, I wish to highlight the contributions of the 'elder statesman' of the human potential movement, John Heron, whose impeccably systematic articulation of what he terms a 'self-generating practitioner community' makes a perfect complement to his brilliant 1990 paper that begins the book. Heron's 'self-generating practitioner community' notion (see Chapter IV.4) also gives a wonderfully coherent and substantial 'New Paradigm' rationale for the Independent Practitioners Network (see Chapter V.3), of which the co-editors were both founding members in 1994, and which continues to thrive nearly two decades on, notwithstanding the predictions of many sceptics at the time that such a Network could not succeed in the current profession-centred era. The Network has been at the forefront of showing the psy world that there *is* another (and better) way to facilitate accountability in our work, and Heron's statement, reproduced below, sums up beautifully the *raison d'être* for self-regulation in psy work, and why this book, and the IPN, are so necessary in the field:

> Counsellors and psychotherapists need to find a model for institutional forms and processes which are free of centralised over-control and compulsive factionalism, and which have the sort of empowering hierarchy which serves the flourishing of autonomy and co-operation among its members. It seems fairly clear that if professional helpers are incapable of practising these values in their own working lives, they are in no place to empower their clients to do so.
>
> (p. 245, this volume)

Some 14 years on from the first edition of the book, we think that it is a fitting epigraph to this editorial Conclusion (see above) to quote one of our contributors, the late and much respected Peter Lomas (to whom this second edition is dedicated), who made such an important contribution to humanising and introducing critical self-reflexive thinking into the field of psychoanalytic theory and training. Whilst Lomas is speaking in this quotation about the specific case of 'the register', it seems clear that his sentiments can also be read as a commentary upon the wider issue of the *over-professionalisation* of the psy field, with the attendant harm that it does to the core values and practices of our work (see *European Journal of Psychotherapy and Counselling*, 2011; House, 2011a).

Peter Lomas would very likely have been a strong supporter of what is a relatively new, politically engaged movement within the psy field, the Alliance for Counselling and Psychotherapy Against State Regulation, of which both this book's co-editors and a number of the book's contributors were founder-members. The Alliance – a pluralistic organisation, if ever there was one – has been raising many of the issues that are squarely addressed in this book – not least, whether there is any conceivable case for statutorily regulating therapy work. The message that goes out from this book is a resounding 'no' – and perhaps the most telling commentary on the advisability or otherwise of statutory involvement in the psy field is that since the mid-1990s, there have been a significant number of books dedicated to the theme of professionalisation, all of which have argued strongly against the state or statutory regulation of the field (namely, Bates and House, 2003; House, 2003, 2010; King and Moutsou, 2010; Mowbray, 1995; Parker and Revelli, 2008; Postle, 2007; Postle and House, 2009 – and with more to come, too – e.g. Postle, 2011; Totton, 2011; Tudor, 2011) – and without a single published text to date making a systematic case *for* such regulation, despite repeated calls by regulation's critics to do so. Even accounting for the fact that it is commonly seen as being easier to challenge and criticise than it is to write in support of the conventional wisdom, this dramatic lack of balance in the literature is surely symptomatic of something very important; namely, that when looked at in any conceivable way, the extant literature on the professionalisation of the psychological therapies comes out unambiguously and resoundingly against the beneficence of the kinds of professionalising developments and political manoeuvrings (often driven by economic interests) that are still, alas, striving to dominate the field.

Returning for a moment to the internal 'politics' of the psy field, it was surely a key moment in the unfolding psychodrama which is the professionalisation of the field when one of our contributors, Professor Andrew Samuels, was elected as Chair of the United Kingdom Council for Psychotherapy (UKCP) in 2010, which had previously been one of the most aggressive and single-minded organisational proponents of the state register. The fact that a substantial majority of the UKCP membership could vote in a secret ballot for someone whose critical views on centralised state regulation were widely known, when added to the several thousands of therapists who have publicly supported the Alliance's position, surely means that no longer will the psy organisations be able to drag their sleepy memberships into the state or statutory regulation of the field without, at the very least, substantial discussion and widespread consultation – and with, as I write, viable and principled alternatives to didactic accountability structures now being actively developed. The new edition of this book can also hopefully contribute to these deliberations by helping to open up a creative space for critical and courageous thinking about the future of the field, and according to the poignant precept advocated by Juliana Brown and Richard Mowbray many years ago, when they so incisively wrote: 'Where there is a genuine need for [accountability] structures, we should develop structures that foster our values rather than betray them' (quoted in Mowbray, 1995: 225).

More generally, with a major new book having just been published (Cooper and Mcleod, 2010) that claims to be proposing a 'new pluralistic paradigm' for therapy, we are left somewhat perplexed as to how such a claim for a '*new* paradigm' in therapy could be made in 2010, some 14 years after the publication of the first edition of the present volume, in which the subtitle refers to '*Arguments for Pluralism* and Autonomy in Psychotherapy and Counselling'. Without in any way wishing to assert a churlish claim to have 'got there first' with our own book, I are reminded of the way in which Martin Seligman found a way to launch his 'new' school of 'positive psychology around a decade ago (e.g. Seligman and Csikszentmihalyi, 2000) with virtually no acknowledgement of the substantial work done on well-being and human potential in the Humanistic Psychology field over the preceding decades (e.g. Taylor, 2001; Slife and Richardson, 2008). Quasi-schoolist power-moves are perhaps alive and kicking in our own field, too; and we would certainly wish to distance ourselves from the quasi-modernist approach to 'pluralism' that Mick Cooper and John Mcleod are proposing in their new book (see House, 2011b).

In conclusion, we commend this new edition of what, we believe, continues to be a leading-edge text in the fields of counselling and psychotherapy, and one which has a freshness and a vested-interest-free orientation that is arguably increasingly difficult to find in the highly competitive and power-infused publishing industry, in which 'schoolist' approaches and orientations continue to jostle for position in a resources-scarce environment that arguably generates all manner of 'dysfunctional' institutional dynamics (cf. Wasdell's Chapter I.2, this volume). Following Andrew Samuels' approach to pluralism as described in this volume, one might say that there remains plenty that divides us; and that those divisions and differences should be positively welcomed and celebrated rather than fudged or denied – for as the great and eminently non-registerable poet and mystic William Blake wrote in *The Marriage of Heaven and Hell*, 'Without contraries is no progression'.

Yet we might also say that in terms of preserving the 'soul' of this precious work in a recognisable and values-congruent form (cf. Edwards, 1992), what unites the editors and the contributors to this book is far, far more important than what divides us; and we hope that our diverse strugglings to stay true to the heart and soul of our work will find resonances with readers, whatever their orientation or level of experience in the fields (still, thankfully, statutorily unregulated) of psychotherapy and counselling.

References

Bates, Y. and House, R. (eds) (2003) *Ethically Challenged Professions: Enabling Diversity and Innovation in Psychotherapy and Counselling.* Ross-on-Wye: PCCS Books.

Clark, J. (ed.) (2002) *Freelance Counselling and Psychotherapy: Competition and Collaboration*, London: Routledge.

Cooper, M.and Mcleod, J. (2010) *Pluralistic Counselling and Psychotherapy*, London: Sage.

Edwards, G. (1992) 'Does psychotherapy need a soul?', in W. Dryden and C. Feltham (eds), *Psychotherapy and Its Discontents*, Buckingham: Open University Press, pp. 194–224.

European Journal of Psychotherapy and Counselling (2011) Special issue on the work of Peter Lomas, volume 13 (1) (in press).

House, R. (2003) *Therapy Beyond Modernity: Deconstructing and Transcending Profession-Centred Therapy*, London: Karnac Books.

House, R. (2010) *In, Against and Beyond Therapy: Critical Essays towards a 'Post-Professional' Era*, Ross-on-Wye: PCCs Books.

House, R. (2011a) 'Conference Report: The legacy of Peter Lomas, 1923–2010; Cambridge Society for Psychotherapy, Cambridge, Saturday 6 November 2010', *Self and Society*, 38 (3) (in press).

House, R. (2011b) Commentary on Cooper and Mcleod's new pluralistic paradigm, *Therapy Today*, 22 (1) (in press).

King, L. and Moutsou, C. (eds) (2010) *Rethinking Audit Cultures: A Critical Look at Evidence-Based Practice in Psychotherapy and Beyond*, Ross-on-Wye: PCCS Books.

Mowbray, R. (1995) *The Case Against Psychotherapy Registration: A Conservation Issue for the Human Potential Movement*, London: Trans Marginal Press; downloadable as a pdf file free of charge at: www.transmarginalpress.co.uk

Mullan, B (ed.) (1996) *Therapists on Therapy*. London: Free Association Books.

Parker, I. and Revelli, S. (eds) (2008) *Psychoanalytic Practice and State Regulation*, London: Karnac Books.

Postle, D. (2007) *Regulating the Psychological Therapies – From Taxonomy to Taxidermy*, Ross-on-Wye: PCCS Books.

Postle, D. (2011) *Regulating the Psychological Therapies, eIpnosis Vol. 2,* title to be confirmed, Ross-on-Wye: PCCS Books.

Postle, D. and House, R. (eds) (2009) *Compliance? Ambivalence? Rejection? – Nine Papers Challenging Health Professions Council Regulation*. London: Wentworth Learning Resources.

Seligman, M. E. P. and Csikszentmihalyi, M. (2000) 'Positive psychology: an introduction', *American Psychologist*, 55: 5–14.

Slife, B. D. and Richardson, F. C. (2008) 'Problematic ontological underpinnings of positive psychology: a strong relational alternative', *Theory and Psychology*, 18 (5): 699–723.

Taylor, E. (2001) 'Positive psychology and humanistic psychology: A reply to Seligman', *Journal of Humanistic Psychology*, 41 (1): 13–29.

Totton, N. (2011) *Wild Therapy: Undomesticating Inner and Outer Worlds*, Ross-on-Wye: PCCS Books.

Totton, N. (ed.) (2006) *The Politics of Psychotherapy: New Perspectives*, Maidenhead: Open University Press.

Tudor, K. (ed.) (2011) *The Turning Tide: Pluralism and Partnership in Psychotherapy in Aotearoa New Zealand*, Auckland, Aotearoa New Zealand: LC Publications.

Young, R. M. (1997) 'The psychodynamics of psychoanalytic organisations', mimeo, http://www.human-nature.com/culture/ppo1.html (retrieved January 2011).

Contributors

Marion Abernethy: I started out as an actress and worked in the theatre until I completed my training as a psychotherapist in 1996. I then worked for seven years at Newmarket House Clinic (in-patient treatment centre for people with severe eating disorders) providing the one-to-one intensive therapy. I also taught monthly workshops and ran retreats for over ten years. I now live a much quieter, contemplative life with my husband in the Norfolk countryside, and work with individuals in private practice.

Val Blomfield left grammar school at 15 and discovered the joys of a more compassionate education at her commercial college. She went on to train as a teacher, then studied counselling on the SW London College Counselling Course. She then taught on this course for ten eventful years. She later trained in Psychosynthesis. Her work as a school counsellor in an Inner London boys' school informed her in helping, alongside Jane Weinberg, to set up the radical school counselling service at Thomas Tallis School. She has a private therapy and supervision practice in Greenwich, London, an MA in Creative Writing from Sussex University and is a published poet and dramatist. She is shortly to be ordained into the Triratna Buddhist Community.

Jill Brooks works as an Advisory Support Teacher in Early Years and Behaviour in Norfolk. My recent secondment with a colleague making accessible our Solution-Focused Learning and Development Programme to multi-disciplinary and multi-agency practitioners and teams brought me up against the same tensions as 15 years ago: How do I work to the good within large systems such as Children's Services without losing my integrity? I still don't know, yet I still have a passion for the efficacy of 'alongside', of 'power with', of belief in the capability, competence and courage of 'clients', be they three-year-olds, their parents or those who work to engage and empower them.

Cal Cannon is still working in East Anglia as a freelance therapist and supervisor (2011), and still fascinated by the endeavour even as the wider context changes, ebbs and flows, presents challenges, and elicits a myriad of feelings and responses. To sit alongside so many people, and to witness their stories over so many years, is a humbling and mysterious adventure.

Michael Eales has worked as a group facilitator for 27 years. He initially trained with John Heron, and was part of the staff team of the Human Potential Research Project at Surrey University. In 1984 he co-founded, with Anouk Graav, one of the first management consultancies drawing on Humanistic Psychology, with major projects in both the public and private sectors (see www.globalresonance.com). He facilitated five Postgraduate Diplomas in Humanistic Psychology and has trained many practitioners in the field. Michael has written for film and television, most notably in the 1990s 'Exceptional Leave to Remain' (Channel 4) about asylum seekers refused refugee status. More recently he co-wrote (with Anna Campion) and acted in the film 'Inertia', which opened at the London Raindance Film Festival, and 'Bipolar' which premiered in 2006 at the Edinburgh Film Festival. He is co-author of *The Personal Management Handbook* (ed. John Mulligan) and *The Coaching Cube*. He is currently developing a web-based leadership tool with Steve Radcliffe Associates.

Colin Feltham is Emeritus Professor of Critical Counselling Studies, Sheffield Hallam University.

Guy Gladstone is a humanistic psychology practitioner. He has been a member of the Open Centre in London since 1984, where he offers a full programme of groupwork – long-term ongoing groups, weekend groups, and occasional themed workshops. He also works one to one and supervises practitioners in a variety of settings. He is in a full member group of IPN and is an active founder member of The Alliance for Counselling and Psychotherapy Against State Regulation. He completed training with the IDHP in 1982, with the IPSS in 1985, with BAABP in 1995, and is accredited by UKAHPP for groupwork and bodywork.

Sue Hatfield: I live in a small village in West Norfolk, where I spend my time tending my garden, growing vegetables and walking in the forest near my home. Tending to my personal spiritual journey is an important part of my life. I am involved locally with the Transition Towns movement.

Catherine Hayes: I studied Fine Art at Brighton Polytechnic (1977–80) and was a founder member of the Brixton Artists Collective. I trained as a person-centred counsellor at the University of East Anglia in 1995–96 and as a trainee trainer in 1996–97. Since then I have been fortunate to be employed as a counsellor working for local charities in and around East Anglia. I had a few years as an editor and briefly as managing editor for *PCQ* (the membership magazine of BAPCA) and am also a tutor and lecturer on a Person-Centred Counselling degree course at University College Suffolk, based in Great Yarmouth.

John Heron is currently a Co-director the South Pacific Centre for Human Inquiry in New Zealand. He was Founder and Director of the Human Potential Research Project, University of Surrey, UK; Assistant Director, British Postgraduate Medical Federation,

University of London; Director, International Centre for Co-operative Inquiry, Tuscany, Italy. He is a researcher, author, facilitator and trainer in peer self-help psychotherapy, co-operative inquiry, educational development, group facilitation, management development, personal and transpersonal development, professional development in the helping professions. His books include *Feeling and Personhood*, Sage, 1992; *Co-operative Inquiry*, Sage, 1996; *Sacred Science*, PCCS Books, 1998; *The Complete Facilitator's Handbook*, Kogan Page, 1999; *Helping the Client*, Sage, 2001; *Participatory Spirituality*, Lulu Press, 2006.

Richard House, Ph.D., is Senior Lecturer in Psychotherapy and Counselling, Department of Psychology and the Research Centre for Therapeutic Education, Roehampton University. A trained counsellor and psychotherapist and a therapy practitioner since 1990, his books include *In, Against and Beyond Therapy* (PCCS Books, 2010), *Therapy Beyond Modernity* (Karnac, 2003), *Against and For CBT* (co-editor Del Loewenthal, PCCS Books, 2008) and *Childhood, Well-being and a Therapeutic Ethos* (co-editor Del Loewenthal, Karnac, 2009). Richard is a co-founder of the Independent Practitioners Network, in which he has participated since 1995, and of the Alliance for Counselling and Psychotherapy Against State Regulation. Richard is also a trained Steiner Kindergarten and class teacher, co-founding the Open EYE early childhood campaign in 2007, and, with author Sue Palmer, co-orchestrating the two press Open Letters on 'toxic childhood' and 'play, in 2006 and 2007, helping to precipitate a global media debate about the state of childhood in modern technological culture.

Juliet Lamont: I practised as a psychotherapist from 1988 until 2008. I joined the Independent Practitioners' Network in 1994 and remained an active and enthusiastic member until my retirement. I was partially trained with Gestalt South West, a nonhierarchical training organisation and later gave up on the accreditation process when psychotherapy started to be defined as a 'postgraduate profession'. I ran a therapy centre in Bristol for several years alongside my own practice. I now let space to psychotherapists in my home and I've recently taken up drawing and other creative endeavours, where I am back at the stage of conscious incompetence.

Peter Lomas trained at the Institute of Psychoanalysis and worked in the NHS for several years. He practised independently as a psychotherapist in Cambridge and was a founder member of the Cambridge Society for Psychotherapy. He was married and had three children. He was the author of *True and False Experience*, *The Limits of Interpretation*, *The Psychotherapy of Everyday Life*, *Cultivating Intuition* and *Personal Disorder and the Family*. Peter died in 2010.

Michael McMillan wrote this chapter after completing a postgraduate Diploma in Counselling from the University of East Anglia (1995–96).

Katharine Mair was a consultant forensic psychologist at Royal Cornhill Hospital, Aberdeen until she retired. She has previously worked as a clinical psychologist in both England and Scotland. She is co-author of *Voices from the Middle Class* (Hutchinson, 1975) and has published papers on a variety of clinical and forensic topics in professional journals. She has a special interest in the problems of eliciting reliable testimony in both clinical and forensic settings, and is on the Scientific and Professional Advisory Board of The British False Memory Society.

Richard Mowbray is a practitioner of Primal Integration, a form of human potential work, and has been in group and individual practice for over 30 years. He is co-director, with Juliana Brown, of the Primal Integration Programme in London, and has been a member of the Open Centre, one of the UK's longest established growth centres, since 1979. He is co-author with Juliana Brown of a chapter on Primal Integration in *Innovative Therapy: A Handbook* (Open University Press, 1994) and author of *The Case Against Psychotherapy Registration: A Conservation Issue for the Human Potential Movement* (Trans Marginal Press, 1995); www.transmarginal.co.uk

Denis Postle: Over the past 25 years my work has developed from transpersonal, co-counselling and primal beginnings into a core practice of personal and professional development, supervision, training and consultancy. Much of the last 15 years has been devoted to participation in the Independent Practitioners Network, and parallel with this, of finding ways of resisting state regulation of the psychological therapies, principally through writing for, and maintaining, the eIpnosis website. Early books on high energy physics and *Catastrophe Theory* were followed by *Letting the Heart Sing: The Mind Gymnasium*, a compendium of humanistic psychology translated into six languages, later republished in a much expanded CD-ROM version and recently, a free eBook library of selected chapters. These books were followed by a collection of the first five years of eIpnosis web texts '*Regulating the Psychological Therapies*', which will shortly be joined by another volume of the eIpnosis chronology of events in the regulation debate (PCCS Books, in press).

Andrew Samuels is well known internationally for his contributions to the politics of the professions of psychotherapy and counselling with particular reference to inclusivity and equal opportunities and, in recent years, to the problem of state regulation. He has also contributed to visions of how these professions might contribute to politics in the wider sense. He is Professor of Analytical Psychology at Essex and holds visiting chairs at New York, Goldsmiths and Roehampton; Training Analyst of the Society of Analytical Psychology and Chair of the United Kingdom Council for Psychotherapy; Board Member, International Assocation for Relational Psychoanalysis and Psychotherapy; co-founder Psychotherapists and Counsellors for Social Responsibility; Consultant Editor, *Psychotherapy and Politics International*. His books have been translated into 19 languages and include *The Plural Psyche*, *The Political Psyche*, and *Politics on the Couch*. www.andrewsamuels.com

Robin Shohet is a psychotherapist, supervisor, trainer and consultant and he combines his work as a trainer with team coaching and culture change in organisations, using Appreciative Inquiry. He lives with his family in Findhorn, Scotland. His interests include the interface between psychotherapy and spirituality, particularly as expressed in *The Course in Miracles*. He is co-author with Peter Hawkins of *Supervision in the Helping Professions* (Open University Press, 3rd edn, 2006), and editor of *Passionate Supervision* (Jessica Kingsley, 2008). His next book, *Supervision as Transformation*, will be published by Jessica Kingsley in 2011.

David Smail is a retired NHS clinical psychologist and former Special Professor in Clinical Psychology at the University of Nottingham. He is the author of several books on psychotherapy and society; the most recent, *Power, Interest and Psychology,* was published by PCCS Books in 2005.

Annie Spencer, with an Oxford MA and postgraduate diplomas in humanistic psychology (IDHP) and education (PGCE), started her professional work as a humanistic psychotherapist and group facilitator nearly 30 years ago. Introduced to Native American Medicine Wheel teachings in 1982, Annie found these to be a natural next step from her psychology work: 'earth-based ceremony can provide a strong gateway to healing'. Annie has always been an innovator. In the 1980s she co-founded Openings, a centre of psychotherapy and groupwork that today is an integral part of the Bath psychotherapy landscape. In the 1990s she was a founder member of the Independent Practitioners Network (IPN); and, moving in a different direction, established the groundbreaking Women's Mysteries programme. Recently Annie broadened her work further and now develops and co-leads grant-aided courses for teenagers. In all her work, Annie finds ways to include the principles of self and peer assessment that she writes about. Annie can be contacted through her website: www.Hartwell.eu.com.

Brian Thorne is Emeritus Professor of Counselling at the University of East Anglia, Norwich. He is also a Founder Member of the Norwich Centre, Britain's first counselling agency committed to the person-centred approach. He is a leading person-centred scholar and has contributed substantially to the professional literature. Among his books are *Carl Rogers* (2nd edn, Sage, 2003) and the best-selling *Person-Centred Counselling in Action* (3rd edn, Sage, 2007) which he co-authored with Dave Mearns. Brian has a particular concern for the spiritual dimension in counselling and in 2005 was made a Lay Canon of Norwich Cathedral in recognition of his contribution to pastoral theology.

Nick Totton: I am a therapist and trainer with over 25 years' experience. Originally a Reichian body therapist, my approach has become broad based and open to the spontaneous and unexpected. I have an MA in Psychoanalytic Studies, and have worked with Process Oriented Psychology and trained as a craniosacral therapist. I have a 24-year-old daughter. I have written or edited 12 books, including *Body Psychotherapy:*

An Introduction; *Psychotherapy and Politics*; *Press When Illuminated: New and Selected Poems*; and *Wild Therapy* and am editor of the journal *Psychotherapy and Politics International*. There is an extensive website at www.erthworks.co.uk. I live in Calderdale with my partner and grow vegetables.

David Wasdell is in psychotherapeutic practice (analytic/integrative) with individuals presenting in life-crisis. He also offers supervision, mentoring and training with organisational consultants, managers and psychotherapists. David also does consultancy research with a range of organisations and institutions undergoing rapid change in a context of low resource and high stress. Since 1981 he has been Founder and Director of the Unit for Research into Changing Institutions, London; since 1987, International Coordinator of the Meridian Programme (formerly the Manhattan Project of the Behavioural Sciences); and since 2007, Director of the Apollo-Gaia Project.

Name Index

Subject Index

Index compiled by Richard House

In, Against and Beyond Therapy

critical essays towards a post-professional era

RICHARD HOUSE

ISBN 978 1 906254 32 2

Richard House assembles 15 years of updated critical writings and provocative commentaries on the professionalisation process, the client voice, therapeutic education and training, and research. He discusses the deadening effect of institutional professionalisation, 'audit-culture' obsessions with 'evidence-based practice', and the psychopathologising of clients.

In this panoramic view of the state of therapy today that, unusually, has a view of the world outside therapy, Richard House writes with energy and purpose, providing us with arguments and reflections that are a delight to read.

Professor Ian Parker, Discourse Unit, Manchester Metropolitan University

No one personally located within a mainstream professional organisation, whether an umbrella body like UKCP or a smaller training body, should ignore this book.

Andrew Samuels, Professor of Analytical Psychology, University of Essex

---

Wild Therapy

undomesticating inner and outer worlds

NICK TOTTON

ISBN 978 1 906254 36 0

In our 'civilised' society, wild has come to mean dangerous, savage, crazy or being out of control. This highly original book restores the balance to the meaning of wild, suggesting that wildness – both of the human psyche and of the land – is vital for our sanity. Drawing together insights from psychotherapy, geography, ecology and anthropology, Nick Totton suggests that wild mind, like wild nature, has an order of its own. Furthermore, that 'wild therapy' can support the restoration of this balance inherent in our psyche.

Wild therapy is a welcome contribution to new paradigm thinking. These ideas are sorely needed at a time when the domestication of our planet is out of control, threatening the health and sanity of the human animal, our communities and the lives of other species.

www.ingramcontent.com/pod-product-compliance
Ingram Content Group UK Ltd.
Pitfield, Milton Keynes, MK11 3LW, UK
UKHW021240300926
15471UKWH00014B/861

9 781906 254339